Role of Nutrition in Allergic Diseases

Role of Nutrition in Allergic Diseases

Editor: Hilary Dawsey

AMERICAN
MEDICAL PUBLISHERS
www.americanmedicalpublishers.com

AMERICAN
MEDICAL PUBLISHERS
www.americanmedicalpublishers.com

Cataloging-in-Publication Data

Role of nutrition in allergic diseases / edited by Hilary Dawsey.
p. cm.
Includes bibliographical references and index.
ISBN 978-1-63927-800-8
1. Allergy. 2. Allergy--Nutritional aspects. 3. Allergy--Diet therapy. 4. Nutrition.
5. Diet therapy. I. Dawsey, Hilary.
RA645.A44 R65 2023
618.929 7--dc23

American Medical Publishers,
41 Flatbush Avenue,
1st Floor, New York,
NY 11217, USA

ISBN 978-1-63927-800-8 (Hardback)

Contents

Preface

Allergic diseases refer to several conditions which are primarily caused through hypersensitivity of the immune system to commonly found harmless substances in the atmosphere. There are various types of allergic diseases such as atopic dermatitis, hay fever, anaphylaxis, food allergies and allergic asthma. The symptoms involve sneezing, shortness of breath, red eyes, swelling, an itchy rash and a runny nose. The usual allergens involve certain foods and pollen. Metals and other substances can also lead to such difficulties. Severe reactions can be caused through medications, food and insect stings. Diagnosis is usually dependent on a person's medical history. Some cases may include testing of the blood or skin. There are several foods that cause allergic reactions, such as tree nuts, cow's milk, shellfish, wheat, soy, fish, eggs and peanuts. Allergies can be managed by avoiding the triggers and taking medication for improving the symptoms. This book unravels the recent studies focused on the role of nutrition in allergic diseases. It presents researches and studies performed by experts across the globe. This book is appropriate for students seeking detailed information in this area as well as for experts.

All of the data presented henceforth, was collaborated in the wake of recent advancements in the field. The aim of this book is to present the diversified developments from across the globe in a comprehensible manner. The opinions expressed in each chapter belong solely to the contributing authors. Their interpretations of the topics are the integral part of this book, which I have carefully compiled for a better understanding of the readers.

At the end, I would like to thank all those who dedicated their time and efforts for the successful completion of this book. I also wish to convey my gratitude towards my friends and family who supported me at every step.

Editor

1

Nutritional Interventions to Improve Asthma-Related Outcomes through Immunomodulation

Lieve van Brakel [1], Ronald P. Mensink [1], Geertjan Wesseling [2] and Jogchum Plat [1,*]

[1] Department of Nutrition and Movement Sciences, NUTRIM (School of Translational Research in Metabolism), Maastricht University Medical Center, 6200 MD Maastricht, The Netherlands; lieve.vanbrakel@maastrichtuniversity.nl (L.v.B.); r.mensink@maastrichtuniversity.nl (R.P.M.)

[2] Department of Respiratory Medicine, Maastricht University Medical Center, 6200 MD Maastricht, The Netherlands; g.wesseling@mumc.nl

* Correspondence: j.plat@maastrichtuniversity.nl

Abstract: Asthma is a chronic inflammatory disease of the airways, characterized by T-helper (Th) 2 inflammation. Current lifestyle recommendations for asthma patients are to consume a diet high in fruits and vegetables and to maintain a healthy weight. This raises the question of whether other nutritional interventions may also improve asthma-related outcomes and whether these changes occur via immunomodulation. Therefore, we systematically reviewed studies that reported both asthma-related outcomes as well as immunological parameters and searched for relations between these two domains. A systematic search identified 808 studies, of which 28 studies met the inclusion criteria. These studies were divided over six nutritional clusters: herbs, herbal mixtures and extracts ($N = 6$); supplements ($N = 4$); weight loss ($N = 3$); vitamin D3 ($N = 5$); omega-3 long-chain polyunsaturated fatty acids (LCPUFAs) ($N = 5$); and whole-food approaches ($N = 5$). Fifteen studies reported improvements in either asthma-related outcomes or immunological parameters, of which eight studies reported simultaneous improvements in both domains. Two studies reported worsening in either asthma-related outcomes or immunological parameters, of which one study reported a worsening in both domains. Promising interventions used herbs, herbal mixtures or extracts, and omega-3 LCPUFAs, although limited interventions resulted in clinically relevant results. Future studies should focus on further optimizing the beneficial effects of nutritional interventions in asthma patients, e.g., by considering the phenotypes and endotypes of asthma.

Keywords: asthma; nutrition; immune system; inflammation; lifestyle

1. Introduction

Asthma is a chronic inflammatory disease of the respiratory system, which affects over 300 million people worldwide [1]. The inflammation is characterized by infiltration of immune cells into the airways, among others the T-helper (Th) cells. In asthma patients, these cells predominantly secrete the Th2 cytokines interleukin (IL) 4, IL-5 and IL-13 [2]. The release of these cytokines activates a cascade of reactions, including mast cell activation and immunoglobulin E (IgE) production. Ultimately, airway inflammation leads to symptoms such as wheezing, cough and shortness of breath [2]. The Global Initiative for Asthma (GINA) provides treatment steps to determine the type of treatment [3]. Frequently, asthma patients have prescribed a combination of short-acting β2-agonists for short-term relief and inhaled corticosteroids in order to suppress the airway inflammation, thereby preventing exacerbations. Compliance to inhaled corticosteroids is generally low and was previously estimated to be between

22% and 63%, whereas short-acting β2-agonists are often used too frequently [4,5]. Noncompliance to inhaled corticosteroids could lead to a gradual worsening of the airway and even systemic inflammation in asthma patients over time [4,6]. This does not only worsen asthma severity, but long-term continuous low-grade systemic inflammation may also contribute to the simultaneous development of disorders related to low-grade inflammation, such as cardiovascular diseases [7]. Therefore, asthma patients could benefit from acceptable and easily applicable strategies in conjunction with pharmacological treatment to decrease airway inflammation and asthma symptoms.

In recent years, there has been a growing interest in the effects of lifestyle and, more particularly, nutrition in the prevention of noncommunicable diseases [8–10]. For example, the importance of nutrition in the prevention of common lifestyle-related diseases such as diabetes and cardiovascular diseases is well known and has been described in various reviews and meta-analyses [10–13]. The role of nutrition in relation to asthma has also been studied extensively. Over the past decades, numerous nutrients, foods, diets or even dietary patterns have been suggested to lower exacerbation rates, improve lung function and asthma control, or even decrease inflammatory markers [14,15]. According to several reviews and meta-analyses, vitamin D [16], omega-3 long-chain polyunsaturated fatty acids (LCPUFAs) [17], and increased fruit and vegetable intake [18] are promising interventions for asthma patients. In line with these observations, the current GINA guidelines state that the use of non-pharmacological strategies on top of asthma medication could contribute to the improvement of asthma control [3]. These guidelines advise clinicians to recommend their asthma patients to follow a healthy lifestyle. More specifically, they recommend to quit smoking [19,20], lose weight in case of obesity (with [21,22] or without [23] bariatric surgery), and consume a diet high in fruit and vegetables. Furthermore, regular physical activity is recommended to reduce cardiovascular disease risk [24] and improve quality of life [25]. However, as mentioned above, asthma severity may be reduced by many more dietary approaches than just by increasing the intake of fruit and vegetables. Moreover, it is relevant to emphasize that most of these interventions potentially affect the immune system, which could explain the decrease in inflammation of the respiratory system and the consequent reduction in asthma complaints. An example is a suggestion made in a review that vitamin D could have a direct effect on the immune system, since a variety of immune cells involved in asthma pathology express the vitamin D receptor [26]. However, despite promising results of vitamin D interventions [16], data are inconsistent. This may at least partly be related to the different doses of vitamin D supplemented in the various studies [26,27]. Therefore, a better understanding of mechanisms underlying the immunomodulatory effects of nutritional components is needed to support dietary approaches to improve asthma control. However, a systematic evaluation of randomized controlled trials studying these effects is missing. Therefore, the aim of this review is to provide an overview of nutritional interventions in asthma patients and reported asthma-related outcomes as well as immunological parameters and to search for possible relations.

2. Materials and Methods

2.1. Search Strategy

The preferred reporting items for systematic review and meta-analyses (PRISMA) checklist was used to structure this systematic review [28]. The aim of the search was to find controlled intervention studies in which the effects of a dietary intervention on asthma-related outcomes as well as on immunological parameters in asthma patients were reported. Three databases (Medline, Embase and the Cochrane Controlled Register of Trials) were used to conduct the search strategy. The abstracts of papers present in these databases were searched in August 2019 without any restriction on publication date. The following search string was used: asthma and immune system or immune function or immunology or inflammation or inflammatory or immunity and trial or clinical study or intervention or RCT and nutrition* or food or diet* or supplement* or micronutrient* or antioxidant*.

2.2. Selection of Studies

After the removal of duplicates, two researchers (LvB and JP) screened the articles that were retrieved from the databases. The screening consisted of two rounds. First, titles and abstracts were screened to determine potential eligible papers. Second, all these papers were read and included in the systematic review if they met all inclusion criteria. Relevant papers present in the reference lists of selected articles were screened as well. The following inclusion criteria were used: (1) randomized-controlled trials, (2) written in English, (3) scientific papers, (4) publication in a peer-reviewed journal, (5) used a nutritional intervention, (6) the subjects used medication for allergic asthma, (7) at least one immunological parameter was reported, (8) at least one asthma-related outcome was reported. Studies were excluded if they did not have a control group or were not randomized. Additionally, conference abstracts or posters were excluded. Differences in selection by the two researchers were solved by discussion. If two articles referred to the same study, both were included in the review, provided that both articles presented either different asthma-related outcomes or immunological parameters. Data of articles describing the same study were merged and presented as one study in tables. In this systematic review, this occurred twice and has been mentioned as a footnote of the corresponding table.

2.3. Data Extraction

After the second screening, data were extracted from the eligible papers and transferred to Excel. The following characteristics were extracted: (1) study information (first author, year of publication, study design, duration, subgroups, intervention, type of asthma, participants' health status, medication use, dietary requirements during the study) (2) baseline characteristics (number of subjects, gender, age, body mass index (BMI)), (3) immunological parameters measured, and (4) asthma-related outcomes measured. For each paper, data were extracted for the experimental and control groups separately. If outcome parameters were only presented in a figure, corresponding means or medians were estimated using a pixel ruler [29]. If not presented in the paper, within-group changes were calculated by subtracting the mean or median outcome of the baseline measurement from the mean or median of the final measurement in that group for both parallel and crossover studies [30–32].

For asthma-related outcomes, a wide variety of parameters was reported. Therefore, we decided that the three most reported questionnaires (asthma control test (ACT), asthma control questionnaire (ACQ) and asthma quality of life questionnaire (AQLQ)) and the three most reported lung function parameters (forced expiratory volume in one second (FEV_1), forced vital capacity (FVC) and peak expiratory flow (PEF)) were the focus of this review. Moreover, a study was classified to result in improved asthma-related outcomes if at least one of these parameters was significantly improved as compared to control treatment. For immunological outcomes, there was an even wider variation in outcome parameters. Therefore, we decided to focus on markers that were reported by at least five different studies. A study was classified to result in improved immunological outcomes if at least one of these five parameters was significantly improved as compared to control treatment. If a study did not report one of the three most used asthma questionnaires or lung function parameters, results were still included in the systematic review and listed under the heading "other" in the corresponding tables. The same applies to studies that only used immune markers that were not measured in five or more studies. Interventions that observed statistically significant changes in both asthma-related outcomes and immunological parameters were used to search for possible relations between these two outcome domains.

FEV_1 and FVC were reported as the percentage of the predicted value unless the original paper only reported these outcomes in liters. If FEV_1 or FVC were reported in milliliters, the unit was transformed into liters. PEF was also reported as the percentage of the predicted value unless the original paper reported PEF in L/min. The total score of the AQLQ was calculated from domain scores if the total score was not presented in the original paper. Units for the immunological parameters IgE, IL-10 and C-reactive protein (CRP) were transformed into IU/mL, pg/mL and mg/L, respectively.

Units for eosinophils in blood were transformed into 10^9 cells/L unless the original paper reported eosinophils as a percentage of total leukocytes.

2.4. Methodological Quality Assessment

The methodological quality of the trials was assessed by calculating the Jadad score [33]. Studies received a total score ranging from 0 to 5 based on methodological aspects, including randomization, blinding and description of withdrawals. Outcomes are described in Supplemental Table S1.

3. Results

The search resulted in 808 records, and six other papers were identified through other sources. In the end, 30 articles were included in this review after removal of duplicates, the title and abstract screening (first screening round) and the full-text screening (second screening round) (Figure 1). These articles described 28 individual studies.

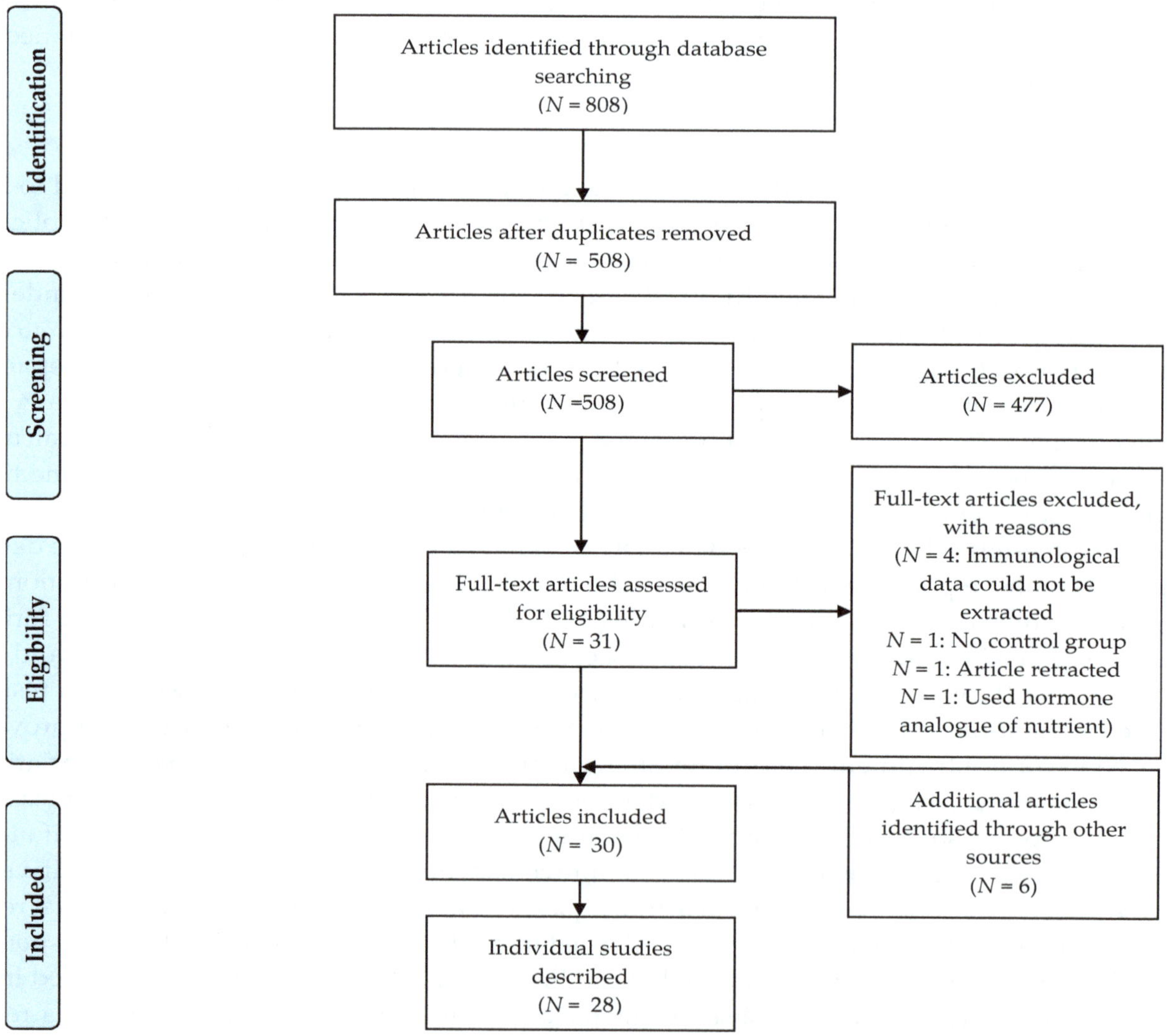

Figure 1. PRISMA flow diagram of study selection. In total, 30 articles describing 28 studies were included in the review.

These 28 studies were clustered based on the nutritional interventions used. The following six clusters (with their respective number of articles) were formed: herbs, herbal mixtures and extracts ($N = 6$); supplements ($N = 4$); weight loss ($N = 3$); vitamin D3 ($N = 5$); omega-3 LCPUFAs ($N = 5$); and whole-food approaches ($N = 5$). An overview of the clusters and selected studies with their characteristics is presented in Table 1.

Table 1. Study characteristics.

Cluster	First Author (Year)	Study Design	Population	Asthma Diagnosis	Intervention and Dose ##	Study Duration	*n*	Age (Years)	Male (%)
Herbs, herbal mixtures and extracts	Barlianto (2017) * Barlianto (2018) * [34,35]	Parallel	Children with asthma	GINA guidelines	*Nigella sativa* oil 15–30 mg/kg/day	8 weeks	28	9 #	39 #
	Hosseini (2018) ** Zilaee (2019) ** [36,37]	Parallel	Adults with mild-to-moderate asthma	GINA guidelines	Saffron 100 mg/day	8 weeks	76	41 #	63 #
	Khayyal (2003) [38]	Parallel	Adults with mild-to-moderate asthma	National Institutes of Health and GINA guidelines	Aqueous extract of propolis 13% solution, equivalent to active constituents in 2 mL of aqueous extract of propolis per day	2 months	46	Range: 19–52	78 #
	Koshak (2017) [39]	Parallel	Adults with asthma	GINA guidelines and ACT score	*Nigella sativa* oil 1 g/day	4 weeks	80	41 #	41 #
	Salem (2017) [40]	Parallel, 3 arms	Adults with asthma	Previous physician's diagnosis and National Institutes of Health criteria	*Nigella sativa* (low dose) 1 g/day *Nigella sativa* (high dose) 2 g/day	12 weeks	76	38 #	34 #
	Yugandhar (2017) [41]	Parallel	Adults with bronchial asthma	Previous physician's diagnosis	Extract of *B. serrata gum* resin and *A. marmelos* fruit 200 mg/day	56 days	29	39 #	41 #
Supplements	Ghaffari (2014) [42]	Parallel	Children with moderate asthma	Previous physician's diagnosis	Vitamin E 50 mg/day	8 weeks	240	9 #	54 #
	Pearson (2004) [43]	Parallel	Adults with asthma	Previous physician's diagnosis and medication use	Vitamin E 500 mg/day	6 weeks	72	48	46
	Smith (2015) [44]	Parallel	Children and adults with asthma	Previous physician's diagnosis, symptoms and medication use	Soy isoflavone 100 mg/day	6 months	386	36	34
	Wood (2008) [45]	Crossover, 3 arms	Adults with stable asthma	Previous physician's diagnosis, symptoms and airway hyper-responsiveness	Tomato extract 45 mg lycopene/day Tomato juice 45 mg lycopene/day	7 days	22	52	36
Weight loss	Dias-Junior (2014) [46]	Parallel	Obese adults with severe asthma	Previous physician's diagnosis and treatment according to GINA guidelines	Low-calorie intake, use of sibutramine (10 mg/day) and use of orlistat (max. 120 mg/day)	6 months	33	43 #	6 #
	Jensen (2013) [47]	Parallel	Obese children with asthma	Previous physician's diagnosis	Energy reduction (−500 kcal/day) and counseling sessions	10 weeks	28	12 #	61 #
	Toennesen (2018) [1] [48]	Parallel, 4 arms	Adults with asthma	ACQ score and positive diagnostic test	High protein and low glycemic index diet Combination of diet and exercise	8 weeks	125	40 #	31 #
Vitamin D3	Bar Yoseph (2015) [49]	Parallel	Children with mild asthma	Previous physician's diagnosis, positive methacholine challenge test	Vitamin D3 14.000 IU/week	6 weeks	39	13 #	64 #
	Castro (2014) [50]	Parallel	Adults with symptomatic asthma	Previous physician's diagnosis, evidence of bronchodilator reversibility or airway hyper-responsiveness	Vitamin D3 100.000 IU once, followed by 4000 IU/day	28 weeks	408	40 #	32 #

Table 1. *Cont.*

Cluster	First Author (Year)	Study Design	Population	Asthma Diagnosis	Intervention and Dose ##	Study Duration	*n*	Age (Years)	Male (%)
	de Groot (2015) [51]	Parallel	Adults with nonatopic asthma	Evidence of bronchodilator reversibility or airway hyper-responsiveness	Vitamin D3 (cholecalciferol) 400.000 IU single dose	9 weeks	44	56 #	59 #
	Kerley (2016) [52]	Parallel	Children with uncontrolled asthma	Previous physician's diagnosis and medication use according to GINA guidelines	Vitamin D3 2000 IU/day	15 weeks	39	8 #	62 #
	Martineau (2015) [53]	Parallel	Adults with asthma	Previous physician's diagnosis, evidence of bronchodilator reversibility	Vitamin D3 (Vigantol oil) 120.000 IU/2 months	1 year	250	48 #	44 #
Omega-3 LCPUFA	Emelyanov (2002) [54]	Parallel	Adults with mild-to-moderate atopic asthma	American Thoracic Society asthma definition	Lipid extract of the New Zealand green-lipped mussel 200 mg/day EPA + DHA	8 weeks	46	39 #	26 #
	Hodge (1998) [55]	Parallel	Children with asthma and a history of episodic wheeze in the last 12 months and airway hyperresponsiveness to histamine	Symptoms and airway hyper-responsiveness	Omega-3 fatty acid-rich diet and omega-3 fatty acid supplementation 1200 mg/day EPA + DHA	6 months	39	10 #	41 #
	Mickleborough (2013) [56]	Crossover	Adults with mild-to-moderate persistent asthma	Previous physician's diagnosis	Marine lipid fraction PCSO-524™ 400 mg/day omega-3 LCPUFA, of which 120 mg/day EPA + DHA	3 weeks	20	23	60
	Moreira (2007) [57]	Parallel	Adults with stable, persistent asthma	Previous physician's diagnosis and use of inhaled corticosteroids	N-3 PUFA 780 mg/day EPA+DHA 10 mg/day vitamin E	2 weeks	20	38 #	0
	Schubert (2009) 2 [58]	Parallel	Adults with asthma and house dust mite allergy	Unknown	N-3 PUFA-enriched fat blend 750 mg/day (of which 630 mg/day EPA + DHA)	3 weeks	23	24 #	43 #
Whole food approaches	Bseikri (2018) [59]	Parallel	Obese adolescents with asthma	Previous physician's diagnosis and ACQ score	Nutrient-dense bar (CHORI-bar) 2 bars/day	2 months	56	15 #	55 #
	Papamichael (2019) [60]	Parallel	Children with mild asthma	Previous physician's diagnosis and GINA guidelines	Two meals with fatty fish per week as part of the Greek Mediterranean diet	6 months	64	8 #	52 #
	Sexton (2013) [61]	Parallel, 3 arms	Adults with symptomatic asthma	Previous physician's diagnosis, bronchodilator reversibility or PEFR variability during run-in	High-intervention: encouraged to adopt a Mediterranean diet and received intensive initial advice and 41 h of consultation sessions with a dietitian Low intervention: received less intensive advice and spent 2 h with a dietitian	12 weeks	35	38 #	29 #
	Sudini (2016) [62]	Parallel	Adults with asthma and a positive skin test to an indoor allergen	Previous physician's diagnosis	Broccoli sprouts 100 g/day	3 days	40	34 #	40 #
	Wood (2012) 2 [63]	Parallel	Adults with stable asthma	Previous physician's diagnosis, symptoms and airway hyper-responsiveness	High antioxidant diet	14 days	137	57 #	42 #

Abbreviations: ACT = asthma control test; ACQ = asthma control questionnaire; DHA = docosahexaenoic acid; EPA = eicosapentaenoic acid; GINA = Global Initiative for Asthma; IU = international unit; (LC)PUFA = long-chain polyunsaturated fatty acid; PEFR = peak expiratory flow rate; 1 = exercise arm not included in this review; 2 = not all data of this article could be extracted; */** = articles were based on the same study; # = calculated; ## = habitual intake and reference data for nutritional interventions is presented in Supplemental Table S2.

3.1. Herbs, Herbal Mixtures and Extracts

Asthma-related outcomes: The results for the cluster "Herbs, Herbal Mixtures and Extracts" are shown in Table 2. Lung function parameters were reported in five studies in the "herbs, herbal mixtures or extracts" cluster. Saffron, *Nigella sativa* or an extract *of B. serrata* gum resin and *A. marmelos* fruit caused an increase in these parameters as compared to the control group [36,40,41]. In contrast, no effect of *Nigella sativa* was found on airway function in another study [39]. Only within-group changes were reported in a study using an extract of propolis. Therefore, no statement could be made if the change of the intervention group differed significantly from the change in the control group [38]. Improvements in asthma control as measured via the ACT were reported in three studies using *Nigella sativa* [35,39,40]. Furthermore, an extract of *B. serrata* gum resin and *A. marmelos* fruit improved asthma-related quality of life [41].

Immunological parameters: *Nigella sativa* oil did not change fractional exhaled nitric oxide (FeNO) [40] but caused a decrease in the number of eosinophils in blood [39].Th1 cytokines were reported in four studies. *Nigella sativa* and an extract of *B. serrata* gum resin and *A. marmelos* fruit increased interferon-γ (IFN-γ) [34,40,41]. Th1 cytokines were reported in a study using an extract of propolis, but between-group changes were not presented. Therefore, no statement could be made if the change of the intervention group differed significantly from the change in the control group [38]. Th2 cytokines or IgE were reported in four studies. *Nigella sativa* and an extract of *B. serrata* gum resin and *A. marmelos* fruit caused decreases in these parameters [34,41]. In contrast to the *Nigella sativa* intervention by Barlianto et al. (2017) [34], two other *Nigella sativa* interventions did cause a significant effect on Th2 cytokines or IgE [39,40]. Treg cytokines were analyzed in two studies. *Nigella sativa* had no effect on these parameters [40]. Only within-group changes were reported in a study using an extract of propolis [38]. Proinflammatory markers were reported in three studies and only decreased after saffron supplementation [36]. *Nigella sativa* did not change these markers [40]. Only within-group changes were reported in a study using an extract of propolis [38].

Overlap between both domains: Five out of six studies from this herb, herbal mixture, or extract cluster showed significant improvements in both asthma-related as well as immunological parameters, compared to the control group [34–37,39–41]. *Nigella sativa* ($N = 3$) increased ACT score in children with 1.9 points [34,35], and in adults with 1.3, 1.4 [40] or 2.1 points [39]. It also increased PEF variability with 8.2 and 5.8 L/min in adults, depending on the dose used [40]. *Nigella sativa* also increased IFN-γ with 7.8 pg/mL in children [34,35] and with 0.5 or 0.9 pg/mL in adults [40]. It decreased IL-4 with 0.3 pg/mL in children [34,35] and eosinophils in blood with 65 cells/μL in adults. Saffron ($N = 1$) increased FEV_1 with 5% and FVC with 1% and decreased CRP with 37.5 ng/mL in adults [36,37]. A mixture of *B. serrata* gum resin and *A. marmelos* fruit ($N = 1$) improved PEF with 46.2 L/min, the AQLQ score with 0.5 points, increased IFN-γ with 7.6 pg/mL and decreased IL-4 with 0.4 pg/mL in adults [41].

3.2. Supplements

Asthma-related outcomes: The results for the cluster "Supplements" are shown in Table 3. All six studies that used supplements as intervention reported lung function parameters. Soy isoflavone supplementation decreased FVC [44]. Using vitamin E, tomato juice, or a tomato extract did not cause changes in lung function [43,45]. Another study with vitamin E supplements only reported within-group changes. Therefore, no statement could be made if the change of the intervention group differed significantly from the change in the control group [42]. No effects were found of soy isoflavones on ACT score [44] or a tomato extract or juice on ACQ score [45].

Table 2. Changes in asthma-related outcomes and immunological parameters as compared to the control group for the herbs, herbal mixtures and extracts cluster.

First Author (Year)	Jadad Score ***	Intervention and Dose	Asthma-Related Outcomes					Immunological Parameters					
			Lung Function			Asthma Control	QoL						
			FEV_1	FVC	PEF	ACT	(P)AQLQ	FeNO	Cells (Sputum, Blood)	Th1	Th2, IgE	Treg	Pro-Inflammatory Markers
Barlianto (2017) * Barlianto (2018) * [34,35]	2	*Nigella sativa* oil 15–30 mg/kg/day				↑ [1]				↑	↓		
Hosseini (2018) ** Zilaee (2019) ** [36,37]	5	Saffron 100 mg/day	↑	↑					=				↓
Khayyal (2003) [38]	2	Aqueous extract of propolis 13% solution, equivalent to active constituents in 2 mL of aqueous extract of propolis per day	N/A	N/A	N/A					N/A		N/A	N/A
Koshak (2017) [39]	5	*Nigella sativa* oil 1 g/day	=		=	↑			↓		=		
Salem (2017) [40]	3	*Nigella sativa* (low dose) 1 g/day	=	=	↑	↑		=		↑	=	=	=
		Nigella sativa (high dose) 2 g/day	=	=	↑	↑		=		↑	=	=	=
Yugandhar (2017) [41]	4	Extract of *B. serrata gum* resin and *A. marmelos* fruit 200 mg/day	=		↑		↑			↑	↓		

Abbreviations: FEV_1 = forced expiratory flow in one second; FVC = forced vital capacity; PEF = peak expiratory flow; ACT = asthma control test; (P)AQLQ = (pediatric) asthma quality of life questionnaire; FeNO = fractional exhaled nitric oxide; Th = T helper cell; IgE = immunoglobulin E; Treg = regulatory T cell; QoL = quality of life; ↑ = significant increase as compared to the control group; ↓ = significant decrease as compared to the control group; = = no change as compared to the control group; N/A = between-group changes not reported; * = based on the same study; ** = based on the same study; *** = Jadad score was calculated to assess the methodological quality of the RCTs. The calculation of the Jadad score can be found in Supplemental Table S1; [1] = both articles presented ACT data; only between-group changes are shown here since comparing changes results in less bias than comparing scores at the final time point. Quantitative data showing the within-group changes is presented in Supplemental Tables S3–S7.

Table 3. Changes in asthma-related outcomes and immunological parameters as compared to the control group for the supplements cluster.

First Author (Year)	Jadad Score *	Intervention and Dose	Asthma-Related Outcomes						Immunological Parameters		
			Lung Function			Asthma Control					
			FEV_1	FVC	PEF	ACT	ACQ	FeNO	Cells (Sputum, Blood)	Th2, IgE	Pro-Inflammatory Markers
Ghaffari (2014) [42]	3	Vitamin E 50 mg/day	N/A	N/A						N/A	
Pearson (2004) [43]	5	Vitamin E 500 mg/day	=	=	=					=	
Smith (2015) [44]	5	Soy isoflavone 100 mg/day	=	↓	=	=		↑	=		=
Wood (2008) [45]	3	Tomato extract 45 mg lycopene/day	=	=			=	=	↓; =		
		Tomato juice 45 mg lycopene/day	=	=			=	=	↓; =		

Abbreviations: FEV_1 = forced expiratory flow in one second; FVC = forced vital capacity; PEF = peak expiratory flow; ACT = asthma control test; ACQ = asthma control questionnaire; FeNO = fractional exhaled nitric oxide; Th = T helper cell; IgE = immunoglobulin E; ↑ = significant increase as compared to the control group; ↓ = significant decrease as compared to the control group; = = no change as compared to the control group; N/A = between-group changes not reported; * = Jadad score was calculated to assess the methodological quality of the RCTs. The calculation of the Jadad score can be found in Supplemental Table S1. Quantitative data showing the within-group changes is presented in Supplemental Tables S3–S7.

Immunological parameters: Two studies reported the effect of their intervention on FeNO, but no effects were reported for a tomato extract or tomato juice [45]. Soy isoflavone supplementation even worsened FeNO concentrations [44]. The number of immune cells in sputum or blood was reported by two studies. Tomato extract and tomato juice decreased the number of immune cells in sputum [45]. Soy isoflavones had no effect [44]. Two studies reported Th2 cytokines or IgE, and one study reported proinflammatory markers. Vitamin E did not change IgE levels [43]. Another study using vitamin E supplements only reported within-group changes. It is unknown if the change of the intervention group differed significantly from the change in the control group [42]. Soy isoflavones did not change proinflammatory markers [44].

Overlap between both domains: None of the studies reported improvements in both asthma-related outcomes and immunological parameters. In adults, soy isoflavones worsened both asthma-related outcomes and immunological outcomes, as FVC was decreased by 0.1 L and FeNO increased with 4.9 ppb compared to the control group [44].

3.3. Weight Loss

Asthma-related outcomes: The results for the cluster "Weight Loss" are shown in Table 4. Lung function parameters were reported in all three studies of the weight loss cluster. Low caloric intake combined with weight loss medication (sibutramine and orlistat) caused a reduction in BMI of 5.3 kg/m^2 in the intervention group and improved FVC compared to the control group [46]. A high protein and low glycemic index diet, high-intensity interval training, or a combination of this diet and high-intensity interval training caused weight losses of 2.3 kg, 1.0 kg and 3.1 kg, respectively [48]. Combining energy restriction and counseling sessions resulted in a weight loss of 3.4 kg and a reduction in BMI z-score of 0.2 [47]. No changes were found in lung function parameters in these two studies [47,48]. Additionally, asthma control was evaluated in all studies. Low caloric intake combined with weight loss medication and energy restriction together with counseling sessions improved asthma control [46,47]. The study evaluating diet and high-intensity interval training reported an improvement in asthma control in the group that combined the diet with high-intensity interval training [48]. Asthma-related quality of life was increased after this same diet combined with high-intensity interval training [48], but not after energy reduction combined with counseling sessions [47].

Immunological parameters: FeNO was reported as an immunological outcome in all studies, but no significant improvements were found. The number of immune cells was also evaluated by all three studies. Energy reduction, combined with counseling sessions, decreased sputum lymphocyte numbers [47]. The other interventions did not change immune cell numbers [46,48]. Low caloric intake, combined with weight loss medication, did not change IgE levels [46]. Proinflammatory markers were reported in all studies. Only energy reduction in combination with counseling sessions decreased CRP [47].

Overlap between both domains: Energy reduction in combination with counseling sessions in children significantly decreased ACQ score by 0.6 points, decreased sputum lymphocyte numbers with 0.1×10^6 cells/mL, and decreased CRP with 1.1 mg/L compared to the control group [47].

3.4. Vitamin D3

Asthma-related outcomes: The results for the cluster "Vitamin D3" are shown in Table 5. Lung function parameters were evaluated in four out of five studies from the vitamin D3 cluster, but no significant improvements were found [50–53]. The effect of vitamin D3 on asthma control was also evaluated in four studies, but none found significant improvements [50–53]. The effect of vitamin D3 on asthma-related quality of life was reported in two studies, although no changes were reported [51,52]. Finally, Bar Yoseph et al. (2015) did not find an effect of vitamin D3 on the provocative dose causing a 20% fall in FEV_1.

Table 4. Changes in asthma-related outcomes and immunological parameters as compared to the control group for the weight loss cluster.

First Author (Year)	Jadad Score *	Intervention and Dose	Asthma-Related Outcomes						Immunological Parameters		
			Lung Function		Asthma Control		QoL				
			FEV_1	FVC	ACT	ACQ	(P)AQLQ	FeNO	Cells (Sputum, Blood)	Th2, IgE	Pro-Inflammatory Markers
Dias-Junior (2014) [46]	3	Low-calorie intake, use of sibutramine (10 mg/day) and use of orlistat (max. 120 mg/day)	=	↑	↑	↓		=	=	=	=
Jensen (2013) [47]	3	Energy reduction (−500 kcal/day) and counseling sessions	=	=		↓	=	=	↓; =		↓; =
Toennesen (2018) [48]	3	High protein and low glycemic index diet	=	=		=	=	=	=		=
		Combination of diet and exercise	=	=		↓	↑	=	=		=

Abbreviations: FEV_1 = forced expiratory flow in one second; FVC = forced vital capacity; ACT = asthma control test; ACQ = asthma control questionnaire; (P)AQLQ = (pediatric) asthma quality of life questionnaire; FeNO = fractional exhaled nitric oxide; Th = T helper cell; IgE = immunoglobulin E; QoL = quality of life; ↑ = significant increase as compared to the control group; ↓ = significant decrease as compared to the control group; = = no change as compared to the control group; * = Jadad score was calculated to assess the methodological quality of the RCTs. The calculation of the Jadad score can be found in Supplemental Table S1. Quantitative data showing the within-group changes is presented in Supplemental Tables S3–S7.

Table 5. Changes in asthma-related outcomes and immunological parameters as compared to the control group for the vitamin D3 cluster.

First Author (Year)	Jadad Score *	Intervention and Dose	Asthma-Related Outcomes							Immunological Parameters				
			Lung Function			Asthma Control		QoL						
			FEV_1	FVC	PEF	ACT	ACQ	(P)AQLQ	Other	FeNO	Cells (Sputum, Blood)	Th2, IgE	Treg	Pro-Inflammatory Markers
Bar Yoseph (2015) [49]	4	Vitamin D3 14.000 IU/week							= [1]	=	=	=		=
Castro (2014) [50]	5	Vitamin D3 100.000 IU once, followed by 4000 IU/day	=			=					=			
de Groot (2015) [51]	4	Vitamin D3 (Cholecalciferol) 400.000 IU single dose	=				=	=		=	↓ [2]	=		
Kerley (2016) [52]	3	Vitamin D3 2000 IU/day	=	=		=		=					=	↑
Martineau (2015) [53]	5	Vitamin D3 (Vigantol oil) 120.000 IU/2 months	=		=	=				=				

Abbreviations: FEV_1 = forced expiratory flow in one second; FVC = forced vital capacity; PEF = peak expiratory flow; ACT = asthma control test; ACQ = asthma control questionnaire; (P)AQLQ = (pediatric) asthma quality of life questionnaire; FeNO = fractional exhaled nitric oxide; Th = T helper cell; IgE = immunoglobulin E; Treg = regulatory T cell; QoL = quality of life; ↑ = significant increase as compared to the control group; ↓ = significant decrease as compared to the control group; = = no change as compared to the control group; * = Jadad score was calculated to assess the methodological quality of the RCTs. The calculation of the Jadad score can be found in Supplemental Table S1; [1] = provocative dose causing a 20% fall in FEV_1; [2] = significant difference after correction for baseline. Quantitative data showing the within-group changes is presented in Supplemental Tables S3–S7.

Immunological parameters: FeNO was reported in three studies, but no changes were found [49,51,53]. Only a single dose of 400.000 IU vitamin D3 decreased sputum eosinophilia after adjustment for baseline values [51]. Other interventions did not change the number of eosinophils in sputum [50] or blood [49]. Th2 cytokines and IgE were reported twice [49,51], as well as Treg cytokines [49,52]. No changes in these parameters were reported. Two studies reported proinflammatory markers. One study using a daily dose of 2.000 IU vitamin D3 reported an increase in CRP [52], whereas no effect on CRP was found in another study using the same dose of vitamin D3 [49].

Overlap between both domains: None of the vitamin D3 interventions resulted in improvements in both asthma-related outcomes and immunological parameters.

3.5. Omega-3 LCPUFAs

Asthma-related outcomes: The results for the cluster "Omega-3 LCPUFAs" are shown in Table 6. Lung function parameters were evaluated in all five studies of the omega-3 LCPUFA cluster [54–58]. PEF increased after using a lipid extract of the New Zealand green-lipped mussel [54,56]. Omega-3 LCPUFA supplementation, an omega-3 LCPUFA rich diet or an omega-3 LCPUFA enriched fat blend did not improve lung function parameters [55,57,58]. ACQ score did not change after omega-3 LCPUFA supplementation [57].

Immunological parameters: FeNO was reported by three studies and decreased after using an extract of the New Zealand green-lipped mussel and a fat blend enriched with omega-3 fatty acids [56,58]. Another study did not find any changes [57]. Furthermore, the number of sputum eosinophils was not changed after increasing omega-3 LCPUFA intake [55,58]. Finally, Emelyanov et al. showed that an extract of the New Zealand green-lipped mussel decreased exhaled H_2O_2 [54].

Overlap between both domains: Two studies that used lipid extracts of the New Zealand green-lipped mussel as intervention found significant improvements in asthma-related outcomes as well as immunological parameters in adults, compared to the control group [54,56]. Combined morning and evening PEF increased with 21.8 L/min and FeNO decreased with 9.9 ppb in one study [56], whereas morning PEF increased with 80.4 L/min and exhaled H_2O_2 decreased with 0.1 uM in the other study [54].

3.6. Whole Food Approaches

Asthma-related outcomes: The results for the cluster "Whole Food Approaches" are shown in Table 7. Lung function parameters were reported in all five studies using a whole-food approach intervention [59–63]. Consuming a high antioxidant diet increased FEV_1 and FVC [63]. The other interventions did not change lung function parameters. Additionally, asthma control was evaluated in all studies. However, no changes in ACT or ACQ score were found. The Mediterranean diet did not improve asthma-related quality of life [60,61].

Immunological parameters: FeNO was reported in four studies [59,60,62,63]. Consuming two meals with fatty fish per week as part of the Mediterranean diet decreased FeNO [60]. A nutrient-dense bar [59], broccoli sprouts [62] and a high antioxidant diet [63] did not have an effect on FeNO concentrations. The Mediterranean diet and a high antioxidant diet did not change Th1 cytokines [61,63]. In the same study on the Mediterranean diet, no changes in Treg cytokines and immune cell count were found [61]. Using a nutrient-dense bar or broccoli sprouts did not change Th2 cytokines or IgE [59,62]. Proinflammatory markers were not changed after using a nutrient-dense bar, the Mediterranean diet, a high antioxidant diet or broccoli sprouts as an intervention [59,61–63].

Table 6. Changes in asthma-related outcomes and immunological parameters as compared to the control group for the omega-3 long-chain polyunsaturated fatty acids (LCPUFA) cluster.

First Author (Year)	Jadad Score *	Intervention and Dose	Asthma-Related Outcomes			Immunological Parameters		
			Lung Function		Asthma Control			
			FEV_1	PEF	ACQ	FeNO	Cells (Sputum, Blood)	Other
Emelyanov (2002) [54]	5	Lipid extract of the New Zealand green-lipped mussel 200 mg/day EPA+DHA	=	↑; =				↓[1]
Hodge (1998) [55]	4	Omega-3 fatty acid-rich diet and omega-3 fatty acid supplementation 1200 mg/day EPA+DHA	=				=	
Mickleborough (2013) [56]	5	Marine lipid fraction PCSO-524™ 400 mg/day omega-3 LCPUFA, of which 120 mg/day EPA+DHA		↑		↓		
Moreira (2007) [57]	5	N-3 PUFA 780 mg/day EPA+DHA 10 mg/day vitamin E	=		=	=		
Schubert (2009) [58]	4	N-3 PUFA-enriched fat blend 750 mg/day (of which 630 mg/day EPA+DHA)	=			↓	=	

Abbreviations: FEV_1 = forced expiratory flow in one second; PEF = peak expiratory flow; ACQ = asthma control questionnaire; FeNO = fractional exhaled nitric oxide; ↑ = significant increase as compared to the control group; ↓ = significant decrease as compared to the control group; = = no change as compared to the control group; * = Jadad score was calculated to assess the methodological quality of the RCTs. The calculation of the Jadad score can be found in Supplemental Table S1; [1] = exhaled H_2O_2. Quantitative data showing the within-group changes is presented in Supplemental Tables S3–S7.

Table 7. Changes in asthma-related outcomes and immunological parameters as compared to the control group for the whole-food approach cluster.

First Author (Year)	Jadad Score *	Intervention and Dose	Asthma-Related Outcomes						Immunological Parameters					
			Lung Function			Asthma Control		QoL						
			FEV_1	FVC	PEF	ACT	ACQ	(P)AQLQ	FeNO	Cells (Sputum, Blood)	Th1	Th2, IgE	Treg	Pro-Inflammatory Markers
Bseikri (2018) [59]	2	Nutrient-dense bar (CHORI-bar) 2 bars/day	=	=		=			=			=		=
Papamichael (2019) [60]	3	Mediterranean diet	=	=	=		=	=	↓ [1]					
Sexton (2013) [61]	2	Mediterranean diet (high intervention) [2]	=	=			=	=		=	=		=	=
		Mediterranean diet (low intervention) [2]	=	=			=	=		=	=		=	=
Sudini (2016) [62]	4	Broccoli sprouts 100 g/day	=	=		=			=			=		=
Wood (2012) [63]	3	High antioxidant diet	↑	↑			=		=	=	=			=

Abbreviations: FEV_1 = forced expiratory flow in one second; FVC = forced vital capacity; PEF = peak expiratory flow; ACT = asthma control test; ACQ = asthma control questionnaire; (P)AQLQ = (pediatric) asthma quality of life questionnaire; FeNO = fractional exhaled nitric oxide; Th = T helper cell; IgE = immunoglobulin E; Treg = regulatory T cell; QoL = quality of life; ↑ = significant increase as compared to the control group; ↓ = significant decrease as compared to the control group; = = no change as compared to the control group; * = Jadad score was calculated to assess the methodological quality of the RCTs. The calculation of the Jadad score can be found in Supplemental Table S1; [1] = significant difference after correction for baseline; [2] = High-intervention: encouraged to adopt a Mediterranean diet and received intensive initial advice and 41 h of consultation sessions with a dietitian. Low intervention: received less intensive advice and spent 2 h with a dietitian. Quantitative data showing the within-group changes is presented in Supplemental Tables S3–S7.

Overlap between both domains: None of the studies from this whole-food approach cluster found improvements in asthma-related outcomes and immunological outcomes simultaneously.

3.7. Effect Sizes in the Context of Minimal Clinically Important Difference

Eight studies found changes in asthma-related outcomes as well as in immunological parameters, which may indicate a link between immunological parameters with asthma-related outcomes. The magnitude of changes in asthma-related outcomes in comparison to the minimal clinically important difference is shown in Figure 2. In three of these eight studies, the changes as compared to those of the control group had an effect size that exceeded the minimal clinically important difference. These three interventions were part of the following clusters: herbs, herbal mixtures and extracts ($N = 1$), weight loss ($N = 1$) and omega-3 LCPUFAs ($N = 1$) and showed effects on PEF (extract of *B. serrata* gum resin and *A. marmelos* fruit; lipid extract of the New Zealand green-lipped mussel), ACQ (energy reduction combined with counseling) and AQLQ (extract of *B. serrata* gum resin and *A. marmelos* fruit). A minimal clinically important difference of FVC could not be found in the literature.

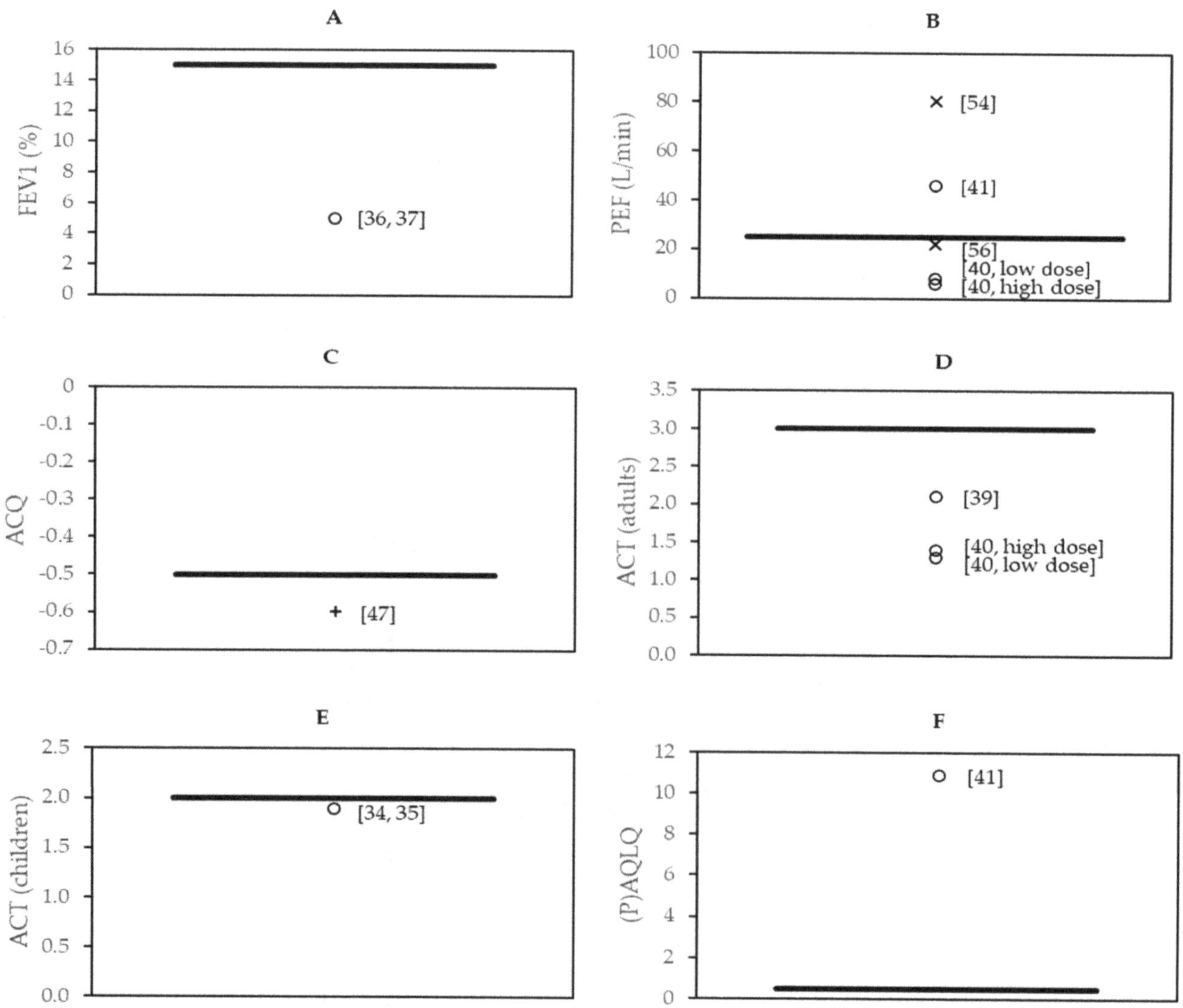

Figure 2. The magnitude of changes in asthma-related outcomes compared to the minimal clinically important difference for (**A**) FEV1; (**B**) PEF; (**C**) ACQ; (**D**) ACT for adults; (**E**) ACT for children; and (**F**) (P)AQLQ. The symbols (○ = herbs, herbal mixtures and extracts; x = omega-3 LCPUFA; + = weight loss) represent individual studies, and the line (−) indicates the minimal clinically important difference. Reference numbers for individual studies are noted next to the corresponding symbol.

4. Discussion

The aim of this systematic review was to provide an overview of studies that examined the effects of nutritional interventions in asthma patients on both changes in asthma-related outcomes as well as immunological parameters and search for possible relations. The reason for this approach was that we hypothesized that nutritional interventions might affect asthma severity via modulation of the immune system. Therefore, interventions that improved asthma-related outcomes, as well as immunological parameters, were considered as indications of a link between these two outcome domains, without claiming causality. Current guidelines for asthma patients do contain lifestyle recommendations, but only to a limited extent. It is only advised to increase fruit and vegetable intake and to maintain a healthy weight in order to improve asthma-related outcomes. Based on the results of our systematic review, it may be interesting to consider whether these lifestyle recommendations could be extended in the future. As shown in Tables 2–7, fifteen out of 28 controlled dietary intervention studies reported an improvement in at least one asthma-related outcome or immunological parameter. However, also two studies reported a worsening in one of the domains, of which one study using soy isoflavones observed a worsening in both domains. With respect to our hypothesis that nutritional interventions likely affect asthma severity via modulation of the immune system, we identified eight studies that showed a simultaneous improvement in asthma-related outcomes and immunological parameters. These studies used *Nigella sativa* (n = 3), saffron (n = 1), an extract of *B. serrata* gum resin and *A. marmelos* fruit (n = 1), energy reduction in combination with counseling sessions (n = 1) or a lipid extract of the New Zealand green-lipped mussel (n = 2) as an intervention. Regarding the clinical relevance of these results, we showed in Figure 2 that three out of the eight studies were able to find clinically relevant changes in asthma-related outcomes. Clinically relevant changes were found in lung function parameters, asthma control and quality of life.

In the context of identifying nutritional interventions that improve asthma-related outcomes via immunomodulation, the "herbs, herbal mixtures and extracts" cluster showed the most consistent and promising results. When interpreting the effects of this cluster, however, it should be noted that exact concentrations of the active compounds of herbal extracts are not always known, and concentrations of extracts could be variable. The use of *Nigella sativa* resulted in an improvement in asthma control and PEF, which was accompanied by a reduction in eosinophils numbers in blood, an increase of IFN-γ and an increase in IL-4 [34,35,39,40]. An intervention with saffron increased FEV_1 and FVC and simultaneously decreased CRP levels [36,37]. An increase in PEF and asthma-related quality of life was observed after using an extract of *B. serrata* gum resin and *A. marmelos* fruit. These changes in asthma-related outcomes occurred simultaneously with an increase in the Th1 cytokine IFN-γ and a decrease in the Th2 cytokine IL-4 [41]. These results suggest that the improvement in asthma-related outcomes after using these herbal interventions is mediated by affecting the Th1/Th2 balance, thereby dampening the Th2 driven pathological process. Since the Th1/Th2 balance in asthma is disturbed as asthma is characterized by Th2 mediated inflammation, asthma patients could benefit from interventions that increase Th1 activity, thereby contributing to restoring the Th1/Th2 balance [64]. Based on mouse models, it has been suggested that increased production of Th1 cytokines, such as IFN-γ, could contribute to a decrease in immune cell infiltration in the lungs and eventually to a decrease in local inflammation [64–66]. This suggested mechanism is supported by the findings in this review and is in accordance with previous research. For example, the main constituent of *Nigella sativa* oil, thymoquinone, stimulates IFN-γ production and decreases IL-4 production in animal models of asthma [64,67,68]. Moreover, lowering Th2 cytokine concentrations is part of the suggested mechanism underlying the effects of crocin, which is the main active component of saffron [69]. However, there are additional pathways that can be modulated by thymoquinone [70] and crocin [71], which indicates that herbal interventions could reduce asthma-related complaints via several mechanisms.

The second cluster that showed promising results was the omega-3 LCPUFA cluster. Two studies using a lipid extract of the New Zealand green-lipped mussel both showed an increase in PEF, which occurred simultaneously with a decrease in FeNO concentrations in one study [56] and a decrease in exhaled H_2O_2 in the other study [54]. FeNO and exhaled H_2O_2 are both markers for airway inflammation and can be analyzed in exhaled breath, and correlate positively with eosinophils in induced sputum [72,73]. Furthermore, FeNO can provide information on the asthmatic state that is consistent with other biomarkers for inflammation in asthma [74] and also decreases after treatment with inhaled corticosteroids [75,76]. The results found in this cluster suggest that the effects of interventions with omega-3 LCPUFAs on asthma-related outcomes are mediated by a decrease in airway immune cell infiltration and local inflammation. These anti-inflammatory effects of omega-3 LCPUFAs and their mediators, such as resolvins and protectins, are generally acknowledged and are in line with earlier findings [77]. Several findings in mouse models confirm the results of the studies described in this review. For example, a study in mice suggested that administration of resolvin E1 to an experimental asthma model resulted in an increased IFN-γ production and a decrease in the proinflammatory lipid mediator leukotriene B4 [78]. Leukotriene B4, as well as other leukotrienes, may be involved in immune cell recruitment in lung tissue of asthma patients [79,80]. Also, leukotriene B4 production in neutrophils was previously found to be reduced after human subjects were supplemented with omega-3 LCPUFA and omega-6 short-chain fatty acids [81]. Another study in Fat-1 transgenic mice, which can endogenously produce omega-3 from omega-6 fatty acids, showed that Fat-1 mice had decreased concentrations of Th2 cytokines IL-5 and IL-13 in their lung tissue as compared to wildtype mice [82]. In short, these results suggest that mediators of eicosapentaenoic acid (EPA) and docosahexaenoic acid (DHA) stimulate IFN-γ production by Th1 cells and inhibit the production of Th2 cytokines and other proinflammatory markers such as leukotrienes, at least in asthma conditions. This could ultimately lead to an inhibition of immune cell recruitment into the airways and therefore contribute to an improvement in asthma-related outcomes. However, not all omega-3 LCPUFA intervention studies in this review showed improvements in asthma-related outcomes that were mediated by the immune system. Strikingly, the three studies with the lowest daily doses of EPA and DHA were the studies that showed beneficial effects on asthma-related outcomes as well as immunological parameters. These studies used intakes between 120 and 300 mg/day. Additionally, one study using a daily dose of EPA and DHA of 630 mg only reported a decrease in FeNO concentrations, but not in asthma-related outcomes [58]. Studies using higher daily intakes of 780 mg or even 1200 mg did not report changes in asthma-related outcomes or in immunological parameters [55,57]. The Food and Agriculture Organisation/World Health Organization set an acceptable macronutrient distribution range for omega-3 LCPUFA between 250 and 2.000 mg/day [83]. Based on the results of this systematic review, asthma patients may benefit from the immunomodulatory effects of omega-3 LCPUFAs when doses on the lower side of this range are consumed. Regarding the effects of higher doses, Yin et al. (2009) showed that supplementing the diet of mice with high doses of fish oil (2% *w/w* and 4% *w/w*) increased the levels of Th2 cytokines IL-5 and IL-13 in lung tissue [84]. It is possible that this mechanism explains why the studies using higher doses of EPA and DHA described in this review did not find the improvements in asthma-related outcomes as observed with the lower doses. The underlying mechanism of the dose-response effect of omega-3 LCPUFAs in asthma patients should be explored further.

The least promising clusters were the supplement cluster, the vitamin D3 cluster and whole-food approaches. Since many different interventions were part of the supplement and whole-food approach clusters, we cannot conclude that these types of interventions will never affect asthma-related outcomes. For vitamin D3, the evidence remains contradictory. We found no indications that vitamin D3 is beneficial for asthma patients. However, future studies should take into account the vitamin D status at the start of the study, dose, timing of the dose (single dose versus multiple doses) and parameters that could be affected by vitamin D3, e.g., immune cells that express the vitamin D receptor.

The current GINA guidelines for asthma state that a diet high in fruit and vegetable intake, as well as weight loss, could improve asthma-related outcomes. Indeed, all interventions of the weight loss cluster had a positive effect on asthma-related outcomes and, more specifically, asthma control. This agrees with the systematic review of Okoniewski and colleagues, who reported that weight loss improved a variety of asthma-related outcomes [85]. However, these beneficial effects hardly coincided with improvements in the response of the immune system in our current review. An explanation for this could be that obesity-related asthma has lower eosinophilic inflammation compared to other phenotypes, and therefore the asthma-related changes after weight-loss were mediated by other mechanisms [86]. It has been suggested that adipokines such as leptin and adiponectin could be involved, which can directly affect airway reactivity [87]. Furthermore, two of the whole-food approaches targeted fruit and vegetable intake of asthma patients [62,63]. Only one of these studies, which used a high antioxidant diet, reported changes in asthma-related outcomes. None of these studies, unfortunately, reported changes in immunological parameters. The effect of fruit and vegetable intake on asthma has been described previously and indeed improved asthma-related outcomes, which has been attributed to their high anti-oxidant and fiber contents [18]. The high antioxidant capacity of fruit and vegetables, as well as the short-chain fatty acids formed from fiber by the microbiota have been suggested to reduce airway inflammation [18]. These suggestions are, unfortunately, not in accordance with the results of this review. However, the number of studies included in this review evaluating fruit and vegetable intake was limited, and these studies mainly addressed the short-term intake of fruits and vegetables. It remains unclear if fruit and vegetables may influence asthma-related outcomes via other routes than the immune system.

Finally, as shown in this review, studies using the same nutritional intervention do not always find similar effects on asthma-related outcomes and immunological parameters. This could be explained by several factors that influence the success of nutritional interventions in asthma patients in general. These factors that were unintendedly part of the study populations may certainly have influenced the interpretation of the results described. An example of such a factor is asthma severity at baseline. Scott and co-workers found that a 10-week weight loss intervention was more successful in participants with more severe asthma at baseline. They suggested that asthma severity could have been a motivator for this group of patients since the burden of the severity of asthma was a motivation for weight loss [88]. Moreover, nutritional status at the start of the intervention may influence the success of the nutritional intervention in asthma patients. Poor diet quality, which may lead to deficiencies of several micronutrients, has been associated with severe asthma [89]. Therefore, dietary interventions might be more successful in asthma patients that have deficiencies at baseline [16]. In addition, study duration could have influenced study outcomes. The studies in this review had durations varying from three days to one year but were, in general, relatively short (3–6 months). Therefore, we cannot exclude that longer-term nutritional interventions could result in more beneficial effects for asthma patients. Furthermore, pathophysiologic mechanisms differ between asthma endotypes [90], suggesting that characteristics of the study population (e.g., age, obesity) influence the success of nutritional interventions. We here show the data for the studies presented in this review did not suggest that the success of nutritional interventions was depended on age. However, other characteristics of the study population could have been of influence. Other examples are indications that vitamin C may be relevant in the prevention of viral-induced exacerbations [91], whereas weight loss interventions may be most relevant for the obesity-induced asthma phenotype [86]. Information on asthma phenotypes or endotypes was missing in many of the trials included in this review. A recommendation for future research is to provide this information since it is crucial in order to interpret the effect of nutritional interventions in asthma patients.

In summary, this review provides an overview of studies that examined nutritional interventions in asthma patients and reported changes in asthma-related outcomes as well as immunological parameters. Certain components from the herbs, herbal mixtures, and extract cluster, as well as the omega-3 LCPUFAs, are promising interventions in the context of improving asthma-related outcomes via immunomodulation. Only three interventions showed clinically relevant improvements. Future studies should now focus on how to optimize the beneficial effects of nutritional interventions in asthma patients, e.g., by considering the phenotypes and endotypes of asthma in the study population.

The potential of these interventions and underlying pathways should be explored further before any of these interventions could be added to lifestyle guidelines for asthma patients.

Author Contributions: L.v.B., J.P. and R.P.M. interpreted the data and wrote the manuscript. L.v.B. and J.P. conducted the literature review. G.W. reviewed and edited the manuscript. All authors have read and approved the manuscript.

References

1. Global Asthma Network. *The Global Asthma Report 2018*; Global Asthma Network: Auckland, New Zealand, 2018.
2. Maslan, J.; Mims, J.W. What is asthma? Pathophysiology, demographics, and health care costs. *Otolaryngol. Clin. N. Am.* **2014**, *47*, 13–22. [CrossRef] [PubMed]
3. Global Initiative for Asthma. *Global Strategy for Asthma Management and Prevention, 2020*. 2020. Available online: www.ginasthma.org (accessed on 24 March 2020).
4. Amin, S.; Soliman, M.; McIvor, A.; Cave, A.; Cabrera, C. Understanding patient perspectives on medication adherence in asthma: A targeted review of qualitative studies. *Patient Prefer. Adherence* **2020**, *14*, 541–551. [CrossRef] [PubMed]
5. Bårnes, C.B.; Ulrik, C.S. Asthma and adherence to inhaled corticosteroids: Current status and future perspectives. *Respir. Care* **2015**, *60*, 455–468. [CrossRef] [PubMed]
6. Dahl, R. Systemic side effects of inhaled corticosteroids in patients with asthma. *Respir. Med.* **2006**, *100*, 1307–1317. [CrossRef]
7. Tattersall, M.C.; Guo, M.; Korcarz, C.E.; Gepner, A.D.; Kaufman, J.D.; Liu, K.J.; Barr, R.G.; Donohue, K.M.; McClelland, R.L.; Delaney, J.A. Asthma predicts cardiovascular disease events: The multi-ethnic study of atherosclerosis. *Arterioscler. Thromb. Vasc. Biol.* **2015**, *35*, 1520–1525. [CrossRef]
8. Schulze, M.B.; Martínez-González, M.A.; Fung, T.T.; Lichtenstein, A.H.; Forouhi, N.G. Food based dietary patterns and chronic disease prevention. *BMJ* **2018**, *361*, k2396. [CrossRef]
9. Minihane, A.M.; Vinoy, S.; Russell, W.R.; Baka, A.; Roche, H.M.; Tuohy, K.M.; Teeling, J.L.; Blaak, E.E.; Fenech, M.; Vauzour, D. Low-grade inflammation, diet composition and health: Current research evidence and its translation. *Br. J. Nutr.* **2015**, *114*, 999–1012. [CrossRef]
10. Mozaffarian, D. Dietary and policy priorities for cardiovascular disease, diabetes, and obesity: A comprehensive review. *Circulation* **2016**, *133*, 187–225. [CrossRef]
11. Rosato, V.; Temple, N.J.; La Vecchia, C.; Castellan, G.; Tavani, A.; Guercio, V. Mediterranean diet and cardiovascular disease: A systematic review and meta-analysis of observational studies. *Eur. J. Nutr.* **2019**, *58*, 173–191. [CrossRef]
12. Khan, S.U.; Khan, M.U.; Riaz, H.; Valavoor, S.; Zhao, D.; Vaughan, L.; Okunrintemi, V.; Riaz, I.B.; Khan, M.S.; Kaluski, E. Effects of nutritional supplements and dietary interventions on cardiovascular outcomes: An umbrella review and evidence map. *Ann. Intern. Med.* **2019**, *171*, 190–198. [CrossRef]
13. Aune, D.; Giovannucci, E.; Boffetta, P.; Fadnes, L.T.; Keum, N.; Norat, T.; Greenwood, D.C.; Riboli, E.; Vatten, L.J.; Tonstad, S. Fruit and vegetable intake and the risk of cardiovascular disease, total cancer and all-cause mortality—A systematic review and dose-response meta-analysis of prospective studies. *Int. J. Epidemiol.* **2017**, *46*, 1029–1056. [CrossRef] [PubMed]
14. Garcia-Larsen, V.; Del Giacco, S.R.; Moreira, A.; Bonini, M.; Charles, D.; Reeves, T.; Carlsen, K.H.; Haahtela, T.; Bonini, S.; Fonseca, J. Asthma and dietary intake: An overview of systematic reviews. *Allergy* **2016**, *71*, 433–442. [CrossRef]
15. Allan, K.; Devereux, G. Diet and asthma: Nutrition implications from prevention to treatment. *J. Am. Diet. Assoc.* **2011**, *111*, 258–268. [CrossRef] [PubMed]
16. Wang, M.; Liu, M.; Wang, C.; Xiao, Y.; An, T.; Zou, M.; Cheng, G. Association between vitamin D status and asthma control: A meta-analysis of randomized trials. *Respir. Med.* **2019**, *150*, 85–94. [CrossRef] [PubMed]
17. Miyata, J.; Arita, M. Role of omega-3 fatty acids and their metabolites in asthma and allergic diseases. *Allergol. Int.* **2015**, *64*, 27–34. [CrossRef] [PubMed]
18. Guilleminault, L.; Williams, E.J.; Scott, H.A.; Berthon, B.S.; Jensen, M.; Wood, L.G. Diet and asthma: Is it time to adapt our message? *Nutrients* **2017**, *9*, 1227. [CrossRef]

19. Chaudhuri, R.; Livingston, E.; McMahon, A.D.; Lafferty, J.; Fraser, I.; Spears, M.; McSharry, C.P.; Thomson, N.C. Effects of smoking cessation on lung function and airway inflammation in smokers with asthma. *Am. J. Respir. Crit. Care Med.* **2006**, *174*, 127–133. [CrossRef]
20. Jang, A.S.; Park, S.W.; Kim, D.J.; Uh, S.; Kim, Y.H.; Whang, H.G.; Lim, G.; Park, C.S. Effects of smoking cessation on airflow obstruction and quality of life in asthmatic smokers. *Allergy Asthma Immunol. Res.* **2010**, *2*, 254–259. [CrossRef]
21. Boulet, L.P.; Turcotte, H.; Martin, J.; Poirier, P. Effect of bariatric surgery on airway response and lung function in obese subjects with asthma. *Respir. Med.* **2012**, *106*, 651–660. [CrossRef]
22. Dixon, A.E.; Pratley, R.E.; Forgione, P.M.; Kaminsky, D.A.; Whittaker-Leclair, L.A.; Griffes, L.A.; Garudathri, J.; Raymond, D.; Poynter, M.E.; Bunn, J.Y. Effects of obesity and bariatric surgery on airway hyperresponsiveness, asthma control, and inflammation. *J. Allergy Clin. Immunol.* **2011**, *128*, 508–515.e502. [CrossRef]
23. Scott, H.A.; Gibson, P.G.; Garg, M.L.; Pretto, J.J.; Morgan, P.J.; Callister, R.; Wood, L.G. Dietary restriction and exercise improve airway inflammation and clinical outcomes in overweight and obese asthma: A randomized trial. *Clin. Exp. Allergy* **2013**, *43*, 36–49. [CrossRef] [PubMed]
24. Warburton, D.E.R.; Nicol, C.W.; Bredin, S.S.D. Health benefits of physical activity: The evidence. *CMAJ* **2006**, *174*, 801–809. [CrossRef] [PubMed]
25. Brown, D.R.; Carroll, D.D.; Workman, L.M.; Carlson, S.A.; Brown, D.W. Physical activity and health-related quality of life: US adults with and without limitations. *Qual. Life Res.* **2014**, *23*, 2673–2680. [CrossRef] [PubMed]
26. Lange, N.E.; Litonjua, A.; Hawrylowicz, C.M.; Weiss, S. Vitamin D, the immune system and asthma. *Expert Rev. Clin. Immunol.* **2009**, *5*, 693–702. [CrossRef]
27. Mann, E.H.; Chambers, E.S.; Pfeffer, P.E.; Hawrylowicz, C.M. Immunoregulatory mechanisms of vitamin D relevant to respiratory health and asthma. *Ann. N. Y. Acad. Sci.* **2014**, *1317*, 57–69. [CrossRef]
28. Moher, D.; Liberati, A.; Tetzlaff, J.; Altman, D.G. Preferred reporting items for systematic reviews and meta-analyses: The PRISMA statement. *Ann. Intern. Med.* **2009**, *151*, 264–269. [CrossRef]
29. Online Ruler on Screen Pixel Ruler. Available online: https://www.rapidtables.com/web/tools/pixel-ruler.html (accessed on 24 March 2020).
30. Ras, R.T.; Hiemstra, H.; Lin, Y.; Vermeer, M.A.; Duchateau, G.S.M.J.E.; Trautwein, E.A. Consumption of plant sterol-enriched foods and effects on plasma plant sterol concentrations—A meta-analysis of randomized controlled studies. *Atherosclerosis* **2013**, *230*, 336–346. [CrossRef]
31. Trabuco, E.C.; Moorman, P.G.; Algeciras-Schimnich, A.; Weaver, A.L.; Cliby, W.A. Association of ovary-sparing hysterectomy with ovarian reserve. *Obstet. Gynecol.* **2016**, *127*, 819–827. [CrossRef]
32. Meropol, S.B.; Metlay, J.P. Accuracy of pneumonia hospital admissions in a primary care electronic medical record database. *Pharmacoepidemiol. Drug Saf.* **2012**, *21*, 659–665. [CrossRef]
33. Jadad, A.R.; Moore, R.A.; Carroll, D.; Jenkinson, C.; Reynolds, D.J.M.; Gavaghan, D.J.; McQuay, H.J. Assessing the quality of reports of randomized clinical trials: Is blinding necessary? *Control. Clin. Trials* **1996**, *17*, 1–12. [CrossRef]
34. Barlianto, W.; Rachmawati, M.; Irawan, M.; Wulandari, D. Effects of Nigella sativa oil on Th1/Th2, cytokine balance, and improvement of asthma control in children. *Paediatr. Indones* **2017**, *57*, 223–228. [CrossRef]
35. Barlianto, W.; Wulandari, D.; Chusniyah, M.; Chandra Kusuma, H.M.S.; Prawiro, S.R. Improvement of Th17/Treg balance and asthma control test score by nigella sativa supplementation in asthmatic children: A new approach to managing asthma. *Turk. J. Immunol.* **2018**, *6*, 1–7. [CrossRef]
36. Hosseini, S.A.; Zilaee, M.; Shoushtari, M.H.; Ghasemi dehcheshmeh, M. An evaluation of the effect of saffron supplementation on the antibody titer to heat-shock protein (HSP) 70, hsCRP and spirometry test in patients with mild and moderate persistent allergic asthma: A triple-blind, randomized placebo-controlled trial. *Respir. Med.* **2018**, *145*, 28–34. [CrossRef] [PubMed]
37. Zilaee, M.; Hosseini, S.A.; Jafarirad, S.; Abolnezhadian, F.; Cheraghian, B.; Namjoyan, F.; Ghadiri, A. An evaluation of the effects of saffron supplementation on the asthma clinical symptoms and asthma severity in patients with mild and moderate persistent allergic asthma: A double-blind, randomized placebo-controlled trial. *Respir. Res.* **2019**, *20*, 39–49. [CrossRef] [PubMed]
38. Khayyal, M.T.; El-Ghazaly, M.A.; El-Khatib, A.S.; Hatem, A.M.; De Vries, P.J.F.; El-Shafei, S.; Khattab, M.M. A clinical pharmacological study of the potential beneficial effects of a propolis food product as an adjuvant in asthmatic patients. *Fundam. Clin. Pharmacol.* **2003**, *17*, 93–102. [CrossRef] [PubMed]

39. Koshak, A.; Wei, L.; Koshak, E.; Wali, S.; Alamoudi, O.; Demerdash, A.; Qutub, M.; Pushparaj, P.N.; Heinrich, M. Nigella Sativa supplementation improves asthma control and biomarkers: A randomized, double-blind, placebo-controlled trial. *Phytother. Res.* **2017**, *31*, 403–409. [CrossRef]
40. Salem, A.M.; Bamosa, A.O.; Qutub, H.O.; Gupta, R.K.; Badar, A.; Elnour, A.; Afzal, M.N. Effect of Nigella sativa supplementation on lung function and inflammatory mediatorsin partly controlled asthma: A randomized controlled trial. *Ann. Saudi Med.* **2017**, *37*, 64–71. [CrossRef]
41. Yugandhar, P.; Rao, K.M.; Sengupta, K. A novel herbal composition containing extracts of Boswellia serrata gum resin and Aegle marmelos fruit alleviates symptoms of asthma in a placebo controlled double-blind clinical study. *Phytother. Res.* **2017**, *32*, 140–150. [CrossRef]
42. Ghaffari, J.; Hossaini, R.F.; Khalilian, A.; Nahanmoghadam, N.; Salehifar, E.; Rafatpanah, H. Vitamin E supplementation, lung functions and clinical manifestations in children with moderate asthma: A randomized double blind placebo- Controlled trial. *Iran. J. Allergy Asthma Immunol.* **2014**, *13*, 98–103.
43. Pearson, P.J.; Lewis, S.A.; Britton, J.; Fogarty, A. Vitamin E supplements in asthma: A parallel group randomised placebo controlled trial. *Thorax* **2004**, *59*, 652–656. [CrossRef]
44. Smith, L.J.; Kalhan, R.; Wise, R.A.; Sugar, E.A.; Lima, J.J.; Irvin, C.G.; Dozor, A.J.; Holbrook, J.T.; Hanania, N.; Sockrider, M.; et al. Effect of a soy isoflavone supplement on lung function and clinical outcomes in patients with poorly controlled asthma: A randomized clinical trial. *JAMA* **2015**, *313*, 2033–2043. [CrossRef] [PubMed]
45. Wood, L.G.; Garg, M.L.; Powell, H.; Gibson, P.G. Lycopene-rich treatments modify noneosinophilic airway inflammation in asthma: Proof of concept. *Free Radic. Res.* **2008**, *42*, 94–102. [CrossRef] [PubMed]
46. Dias-Junior, S.A.; Reis, M.; de Carvalho-Pinto, R.M.; Stelmach, R.; Halpern, A.; Cukier, A. Effects of weight loss on asthma control in obese patients with severe asthma. *Eur. Respir. J.* **2014**, *43*, 1368–1377. [CrossRef] [PubMed]
47. Jensen, M.E.; Gibson, P.G.; Collins, C.E.; Hilton, J.M.; Wood, L.G. Diet-induced weight loss in obese children with asthma: A randomized controlled trial. *Clin. Exp. Allergy* **2013**, *43*, 775–784. [CrossRef]
48. Toennesen, L.L.; Meteran, H.; Hostrup, M.; Wium Geiker, N.R.; Jensen, C.B.; Porsbjerg, C.; Astrup, A.; Bangsbo, J.; Parker, D.; Backer, V. Effects of exercise and diet in nonobese asthma patients—A randomized controlled trial. *J. Allergy Clin. Immunol. Pract.* **2018**, *6*, 803–811. [CrossRef]
49. Bar Yoseph, R.; Livnat, G.; Schnapp, Z.; Hakim, F.; Dabbah, H.; Goldbart, A.; Bentur, L. The effect of vitamin D on airway reactivity and inflammation in asthmatic children: A double-blind placebo-controlled trial. *Pediatr. Pulmonol.* **2015**, *50*, 747–753. [CrossRef]
50. Castro, M.; King, T.S.; Kunselman, S.J.; Cabana, M.D.; Denlinger, L.; Holguin, F.; Kazani, S.D.; Moore, W.C.; Moy, J.; Sorkness, C.A. Effect of vitamin D3 on asthma treatment failures in adults with symptomatic asthma and lower vitamin D levels: The VIDA randomized clinical trial. *JAMA* **2014**, *311*, 2083–2091. [CrossRef]
51. De Groot, J.C.; Van Roon, E.N.H.; Storm, H.; Veeger, N.J.G.M.; Zwinderman, A.H.; Hiemstra, P.S.; Bel, E.H.D.; Ten Brinke, A. Vitamin D reduces eosinophilic airway inflammation in nonatopic asthma. *J. Allergy Clin. Immunol.* **2015**, *135*, 670–675.e673. [CrossRef]
52. Kerley, C.P.; Hutchinson, K.; Cormican, L.; Faul, J.; Greally, P.; Coghlan, D.; Elnazir, B. Vitamin D3 for uncontrolled childhood asthma: A pilot study. *Pediatr. Allergy Immunol.* **2016**, *27*, 404–412. [CrossRef]
53. Martineau, A.R.; MacLaughlin, B.D.; Hooper, R.L.; Barnes, N.C.; Jolliffe, D.A.; Greiller, C.L.; Kilpin, K.; McLaughlin, D.; Fletcher, G.; Mein, C.A.; et al. Double-blind randomised placebo-controlled trial of bolus-dose vitamin D3 supplementation in adults with asthma (ViDiAs). *Thorax* **2015**, *70*, 451–457. [CrossRef]
54. Emelyanov, A.; Fedoseev, G.; Krasnoschekova, O.; Abulimity, A.; Trendeleva, T.; Barnes, P.J. Treatment of asthma with lipid extract of New Zealand green-lipped mussel: A randomised clinical trial. *Eur. Respir. J.* **2002**, *20*, 596–600. [CrossRef] [PubMed]
55. Hodge, L.; Salome, C.M.; Hughes, J.M.; Liu-Brennan, D.; Rimmer, J.; Allman, M.; Pang, D.; Armour, C.; Woolcock, A.J. Effect of dietary intake of omega-3 and omega-6 fatty acids on severity of asthma in children. *Eur. Respir. J.* **1998**, *11*, 361–365. [CrossRef] [PubMed]
56. Mickleborough, T.D.; Vaughn, C.L.; Shei, R.J.; Davis, E.M.; Wilhite, D.P. Marine lipid fraction PCSO-524TM (lyprinol/omega XL) of the New Zealand green lipped mussel attenuates hyperpnea-induced bronchoconstriction in asthma. *Respir. Med.* **2013**, *107*, 1152–1163. [CrossRef] [PubMed]
57. Moreira, A.; Moreira, P.; Delgado, L.; Fonseca, J.; Teixeira, V.; Padrao, P.; Castel-Branco, G. Pilot study of the effects of n-3 polyunsaturated fatty acids on exhaled nitric oxide in patients with stable asthma. *J. Investig. Allergol. Clin. Immunol.* **2007**, *17*, 309–313. [PubMed]

58. Schubert, R.; Kitz, R.; Beermann, C.; Rose, M.A.; Lieb, A.; Sommerer, P.C.; Moskovits, J.; Alberternst, H.; Bohles, H.J.; Schulze, J.; et al. Effect of n-3 polyunsaturated fatty acids in asthma after low-dose allergen challenge. *Int. Arch. Allergy Immunol.* **2009**, *148*, 321–329. [CrossRef] [PubMed]
59. Bseikri, M.; McCann, J.C.; Lal, A.; Fong, E.; Graves, K.; Goldrich, A.; Block, D.; Gildengoren, G.L.; Mietus-Snyder, M.; Shigenaga, M.; et al. A novel nutritional intervention improves lung function in overweight/obese adolescents with poorly controlled asthma: The Supplemental Nutrition in Asthma Control (SNAC) pilot study. *FASEB J.* **2018**, *32*, 6643–6654. [CrossRef]
60. Papamichael, M.M.; Katsardis, C.; Lambert, K.; Tsoukalas, D.; Koutsilieris, M.; Erbas, B.; Itsiopoulos, C. Efficacy of a Mediterranean diet supplemented with fatty fish in ameliorating inflammation in paediatric asthma: A randomised controlled trial. *J. Hum. Nutr. Diet.* **2019**, *32*, 185–197. [CrossRef]
61. Sexton, P.; Black, P.; Metcalf, P.; Wall, C.R.; Ley, S.; Wu, L.; Sommerville, F.; Brodie, S.; Kolbe, J. Influence of mediterranean diet on asthma symptoms, lung function, and systemic inflammation: A randomized controlled trial. *J. Asthma* **2013**, *50*, 75–81. [CrossRef]
62. Sudini, K.; Diette, G.B.; Breysse, P.N.; McCormack, M.C.; Bull, D.; Biswal, S.; Zhai, S.; Brereton, N.; Peng, R.D.; Matsui, E.C. A randomized controlled trial of the effect of broccoli sprouts on antioxidant gene expression and airway inflammation in asthmatics. *J. Allergy Clin. Immunol. Pract.* **2016**, *4*, 932–940. [CrossRef]
63. Wood, L.G.; Garg, M.L.; Smart, J.M.; Scott, H.A.; Barker, D.; Gibson, P.G. Manipulating antioxidant intake in asthma: A randomized controlled trial. *Am. J. Clin. Nutr.* **2012**, *96*, 534–543. [CrossRef]
64. Balaha, M.F.; Tanaka, H.; Yamashita, H.; Rahman, M.N.A.; Inagaki, N. Oral Nigella sativa oil ameliorates ovalbumin-induced bronchial asthma in mice. *Int. Immunopharmacol.* **2012**, *14*, 224–231. [CrossRef] [PubMed]
65. Iwamoto, I.; Nakajima, H.; Endo, H.; Yoshida, S. Interferon gamma regulates antigen-induced eosinophil recruitment into the mouse airways by inhibiting the infiltration of CD4+ T cells. *J. Exp. Med.* **1993**, *177*, 573–576. [CrossRef] [PubMed]
66. Mehta, A.A.; Mahajan, S. Role of cytokines in pathophysiology of asthma. *Iran. J. Pharmacol. Ther.* **2006**, *5*, 1–14.
67. Keyhanmanesh, R.; Boskabady, M.H.; Khamneh, S.; Doostar, Y. Effect of thymoquinone on the lung pathology and cytokine levels of ovalbumin-sensitized guinea pigs. *Pharmacol. Rep.* **2010**, *62*, 910–916. [CrossRef]
68. Rana Keyhanmanesh, L.P.; Omrani, H.; Mirzamohammadi, Z.; Shahbazfar, A.A. The effect of single dose of thymoquinone, the main constituents of Nigella sativa, in guinea pig model of asthma. *BioImpacts* **2014**, *4*, 75–81.
69. Xiong, Y.; Wang, J.; Yu, H.; Zhang, X.; Miao, C. Anti-asthma potential of crocin and its effect on MAPK signaling pathway in a murine model of allergic airway disease. *Immunopharmacol. Immunotoxicol.* **2015**, *37*, 236–243. [CrossRef]
70. Noorbakhsh, M.F.; Shaterzadeh-Yazdi, H.; Hayati, F.; Samarghandian, S.; Farkhondeh, T. Protective effects of thymoquinon on pulmonary disorders in experimental studies. *Tanaffos* **2018**, *17*, 211–222.
71. Pashirzad, M.; Shafiee, M.; Avan, A.; Ryzhikov, M.; Fiuji, H.; Bahreyni, A.; Khazaei, M.; Soleimanpour, S.; Hassanian, S.M. Therapeutic potency of crocin in the treatment of inflammatory diseases: Current status and perspective. *J. Cell. Physiol.* **2019**, *234*, 14601–14611. [CrossRef]
72. Berry, M.A.; Shaw, D.E.; Green, R.H.; Brightling, C.E.; Wardlaw, A.J.; Pavord, I.D. The use of exhaled nitric oxide concentration to identify eosinophilic airway inflammation: An observational study in adults with asthma. *Clin. Exp. Allergy* **2005**, *35*, 1175–1179. [CrossRef]
73. Fireman, E.; Shtark, M.; Priel, I.E.; Shiner, R.; Mor, R.; Kivity, S.; Fireman, Z. Hydrogen peroxide in exhaled breath condensate (EBC) vs eosinophil count in induced sputum (IS) in parenchymal vs. airways lung diseases. *Inflammation* **2007**, *30*, 44–51. [CrossRef]
74. Strunk, R.C.; Szefler, S.J.; Phillips, B.R.; Zeiger, R.S.; Chinchilli, V.M.; Larsen, G.; Hodgdon, K.; Morgan, W.; Sorkness, C.A.; Lemanske, R.F., Jr. Relationship of exhaled nitric oxide to clinical and inflammatory markers of persistent asthma in children. *J. Allergy Clin. Immunol.* **2003**, *112*, 883–892. [CrossRef] [PubMed]
75. Kharitonov, S.A.; Yates, D.H.; Barnes, P.J. Inhaled glucocorticoids decrease nitric oxide in exhaled air of asthmatic patients. *Am. J. Respir. Crit. Care Med.* **1996**, *153*, 454–457. [CrossRef] [PubMed]
76. Silkoff, P.E.; McClean, P.; Spino, M.; Erlich, L.A.; Slutsky, A.S.; Zamel, N. Dose-response relationship and reproducibility of the fall in exhaled nitric oxide after inhaled beclomethasone dipropionate therapy in asthma patients. *Chest* **2001**, *119*, 1322–1328. [CrossRef]
77. Calder, P.C. Marine omega-3 fatty acids and inflammatory processes: Effects, mechanisms and clinical relevance. *Biochim. Biophys. Acta Mol. Cell. Biol. Lipids* **2015**, *1851*, 469–484. [CrossRef]

78. Haworth, O.; Cernadas, M.; Yang, R.; Serhan, C.N.; Levy, B.D. Resolvin E1 regulates interleukin 23, interferon-γ and lipoxin A 4 to promote the resolution of allergic airway inflammation. *Nat. Immunol.* **2008**, *9*, 873–879. [CrossRef] [PubMed]
79. Ohnishi, H.; Miyahara, N.; Gelfand, E.W. The role of leukotriene B4 in allergic diseases. *Allergol. Int.* **2008**, *57*, 291–298. [CrossRef]
80. Yates, C.M.; Calder, P.C.; Rainger, G.E. Pharmacology and therapeutics of omega-3 polyunsaturated fatty acids in chronic inflammatory disease. *Pharmacol. Ther.* **2014**, *141*, 272–282. [CrossRef]
81. Weaver, K.L.; Ivester, P.; Seeds, M.; Case, L.D.; Arm, J.P.; Chilton, F.H. Effect of dietary fatty acids on inflammatory gene expression in healthy humans. *J. Biol. Chem.* **2009**, *284*, 15400–15407. [CrossRef]
82. Bilal, S.; Haworth, O.; Wu, L.; Weylandt, K.H.; Levy, B.D.; Kang, J.X. Fat-1 transgenic mice with elevated omega-3 fatty acids are protected from allergic airway responses. *Biochim. Biophys. Acta Mol. Basis Dis.* **2011**, *1812*, 1164–1169. [CrossRef]
83. FAO/WHO. *Expert Consultation on Fats and Fatty Acids in Human Nutrition: Fats and Fatty Acids in Human Nutrition: Report of an Expert Consultation, 10–14 November 2008, Geneva*; Food and Agriculture Organization of the United Nations: Rome, Italy, 2010.
84. Yin, H.; Liu, W.; Goleniewska, K.; Porter, N.A.; Morrow, J.D.; Peebles, R.S., Jr. Dietary supplementation of ω-3 fatty acid-containing fish oil suppresses F2-isoprostanes but enhances inflammatory cytokine response in a mouse model of ovalbumin-induced allergic lung inflammation. *Free Radic. Biol. Med.* **2009**, *47*, 622–628. [CrossRef]
85. Okoniewski, W.; Lu, K.D.; Forno, E. Weight loss for children and adults with obesity and asthma. A systematic review of randomized controlled trials. *Ann. Am. Thorc. Soc.* **2019**, *16*, 613–625. [CrossRef] [PubMed]
86. Farzan, S. The asthma phenotype in the obese: Distinct or otherwise? *J. Allergy* **2013**, *2013*. [CrossRef]
87. Sideleva, O.; Suratt, B.T.; Black, K.E.; Tharp, W.G.; Pratley, R.E.; Forgione, P.; Dienz, O.; Irvin, C.G.; Dixon, A.E. Obesity and asthma: An inflammatory disease of adipose tissue not the airway. *Am. J. Respir. Crit. Care Med.* **2012**, *186*, 598–605. [CrossRef] [PubMed]
88. Scott, H.A.; Gibson, P.G.; Garg, M.L.; Pretto, J.J.; Morgan, P.J.; Callister, R.; Wood, L.G. Determinants of weight loss success utilizing a meal replacement plan and/or exercise, in overweight and obese adults with asthma. *Respirology* **2015**, *20*, 243–250. [CrossRef] [PubMed]
89. Berthon, B.S.; Macdonald-Wicks, L.K.; Gibson, P.G.; Wood, L.G. Investigation of the association between dietary intake, disease severity and airway inflammation in asthma. *Respirology* **2013**, *18*, 447–454. [CrossRef]
90. Kuruvilla, M.E.; Lee, F.E.H.; Lee, G.B. Understanding asthma phenotypes, endotypes, and mechanisms of disease. *Clin. Rev. Allergy Immunol.* **2019**, *56*, 219–233. [CrossRef]
91. Han, Y.Y.; Forno, E.; Holguin, F.; Celedón, J.C. Diet and asthma: An update. *Curr. Opin. Allergy Clin. Immunol.* **2015**, *15*, 369–374. [CrossRef]

2

Dietary Habits in Children with Respiratory Allergies: A Single-Center Polish Pilot Study

Eliza Wasilewska [1,*], Sylwia Małgorzewicz [2], Marta Gruchała-Niedoszytko [2], Magdalena Skotnicka [3] and Ewa Jassem [1]

1 Department of Pulmonology and Allergology, Medical University of Gdansk, Debinki str 7, 90-211 Gdańsk, Poland; ejassem@gumed.edu.pl
2 Department of Clinical Nutrition, Medical University of Gdansk, Debinki str 7, 90-211 Gdańsk, Poland; sylwia.malgorzewicz@gumed.edu.pl (S.M.); marta.gruchala@gumed.edu.pl (M.G.-N.)
3 Department of Food Commodity Science, Medical University of Gdansk, Debinki str 7, 90-211 Gdańsk, Poland; skotnicka@gumed.edu.pl
* Correspondence: ewasilewska@gumed.edu.pl

Abstract: Background: The rising trend in allergic diseases has developed in parallel with the increasing prevalence of obesity, suggesting a possible association. The links between eating habits and allergies have not been sufficiently clarified. Aim: To evaluate the nutritional status, eating habits, and risk factors of obesity and pulmonary function in children with allergic rhinitis. Materials and methods: We evaluated 106 children with allergic rhinitis (mean age 12.1 ± 3.4 years; M/F 60/46) from the Department of Allergology. Clinical data were collected regarding allergies, physical activity, nutritional status (Bodystat), dietary habits (Food Frequency Questionnaire validated for the Polish population), skin prick test with aeroallergens (Allergopharma), and spirometry (Jaeger). Results: All children suffered from allergic rhinitis; among them, 43 (40.6%) presented symptoms of asthma. There were differences between children with only allergic rhinitis (AR group) and children with both rhinitis and asthma (AA group) in pulmonary function (forced expiratory volume in one second (FEV_1) 100 ± 11 vs. 92.1 ± 15.0; $p < 0.05$). A total of 84 children (79%) presented a normal body mass index (BMI) (10–97 percentile), 8 (7.5%) were underweight, and 14 (13.5%) were overweight or obese. There were no differences in body composition between the AR and AA groups. Incorrect eating habits were demonstrated by most of the children, e.g., consumption of three or fewer meals in a day (38%), sweets every day (44%), snacking between meals every day (80%), and eating meals less than 1 h before bedtime (47%). Compared to the AR group, the AA group was more likely to eat more meals a day ($p = 0.04$), snack more often ($p = 0.04$), and eat before sleeping ($p = 0.005$). Multiple regression analysis showed a significant association between high BMI and snacking between meals and low physical activity (adjusted $R^2 = 0.97$; $p < 0.05$). Conclusions: The risk factors for obesity in children with allergies include snacking and low physical activity. Most children with respiratory allergies, especially those with asthma, reported incorrect eating habits such as snacking and eating before bedtime. A correlation between pulmonary function and body composition or dietary habits was not found.

Keywords: nutritional status; obesity; dietary habits; allergy; pulmonary function; allergic rhinitis; asthma

---

1. Introduction

The incidence of allergic diseases in Poland is increasing concomitantly with improvements in living standards and the adoption of a Western lifestyle. The most common clinical manifestation of hypersensitivity to inhalant allergens is allergic rhinitis (AR), which is one of the strongest factors affecting the quality of life and contributing to missed or unproductive time at work and school. In Europe and the United States, a significant increase in allergic diseases has been observed in recent decades [1,2]. In addition, the multicenter, standardized, randomized Epidemiology of Allergic Disorders in Poland (ECAP) study showed a prevalence of AR among the Polish population of 36% based on self-reported nasal symptoms, and 29% as diagnosed by physicians [3].

Among children with allergies, decreased involvement in outdoor activities and increased problems with concentration, sleep problems, and headaches are seen; moreover, children with AR often also suffer from asthma [4]. It is estimated that up to 40% of people with AR also have asthma, and almost 70% of asthmatics present coexisting AR [5,6]. In the Polish population, the asthma rate was 8% in children and adolescents according to the ECAP study, of which 70% of asthmatics presented with AR, while asthma occurred in 40% of patients with AR [7].

It is known that not only hygiene habits and exposure to allergens, tobacco smoke, and environmental pollution, but also a poor-quality diet, high caloric intake, overweight, and obesity in children and adolescents are important environmental factors that are conducive to the development of allergies [8,9]. Epidemiological and clinical studies suggest a relationship between obesity and allergic rhinitis as well as bronchial asthma [10,11].

In recent years, a significant increase has been noted in the incidence of obesity in children and adolescents in many European countries [12]. Excess body mass was diagnosed in 2% of Polish children in the 1990s, and in 15% of children 20 years later [13–15]. The authors of these studies indicated increased changes in lifestyle and nutritional habits as the causes of increased childhood obesity, i.e., consumption of sweets and unhealthy food; limited consumption of fruits, vegetables, and whole grains; and limited physical activity. In recent decades, fast foods have become a significant component of the diet in Westernized high-income countries, and now also for young people in Poland.

Children with allergic diseases present numerous risk factors for poor nutrition status. There are few studies describing dietary habits and their impact on the nutritional status of people with respiratory allergies. Although allergies are chronic and common diseases, these issues have not yet been clarified. Moreover, early diagnosis of excess body weight in children with allergic diseases, including asthma, seems to be important due to the course and treatment of the disease [16]. Therefore, the aim of this work was to evaluate the pulmonary function, nutritional status, eating habits, and risk factors of obesity in children and adolescents with AR.

2. Methods

2.1. Study Design

In this single-center, cross-sectional study, we evaluated, for the first time pediatric patients with symptoms of persistent rhinitis who visited the Department of Allergology of the Medical University in Gdańsk, Poland, between 2015 and 2017. The study was performed in compliance with the Code of Ethics of the World Medical Association (Declaration of Helsinki). The study protocol was approved by the Gdańsk Medical University Ethics Committee, and written informed consent was obtained from the parents of each patient. The study was supported by local research grant no. ST-554.

2.2. Patients

Inclusion criteria for the study were as follows: (1) age 7–18 years old, (2) persistent allergic rhinitis (duration at least 6 months in the last 12 months) never diagnosed and never treated with antihistamine drugs, (3) ability to perform spirometry, and (4) signed consent from parents to participate in the study.

Patients were evaluated according to the study protocol by a multidisciplinary team (allergologist, pediatrician, dietician). Children with persistent rhinitis symptoms in the last 12 months who had never been diagnosed and treated with anti-allergic or anti-asthmatic drugs were enrolled in the study (Visit 1, screening). During the next visit (Visit 2), allergy was confirmed by skin prick test,

AR was diagnosed according to Allergic Rhinitis and Its Impact on Asthma (ARIA) [6], and asthma according to Global Initiative for Asthma (GINA) guidelines [17]. The medical history and spirometry results indicated newly diagnosed asthma in 43 patients; therefore, patients were divided into two groups: allergic rhinitis (AR group), and allergic rhinitis and asthma (AA group). Anthropometry, bioimpedance assessment, and dietary habits based on Food Frequency Questionnaire (FFQ-6) were collected and compared between the two groups. The scheme of the study is presented in Figure 1.

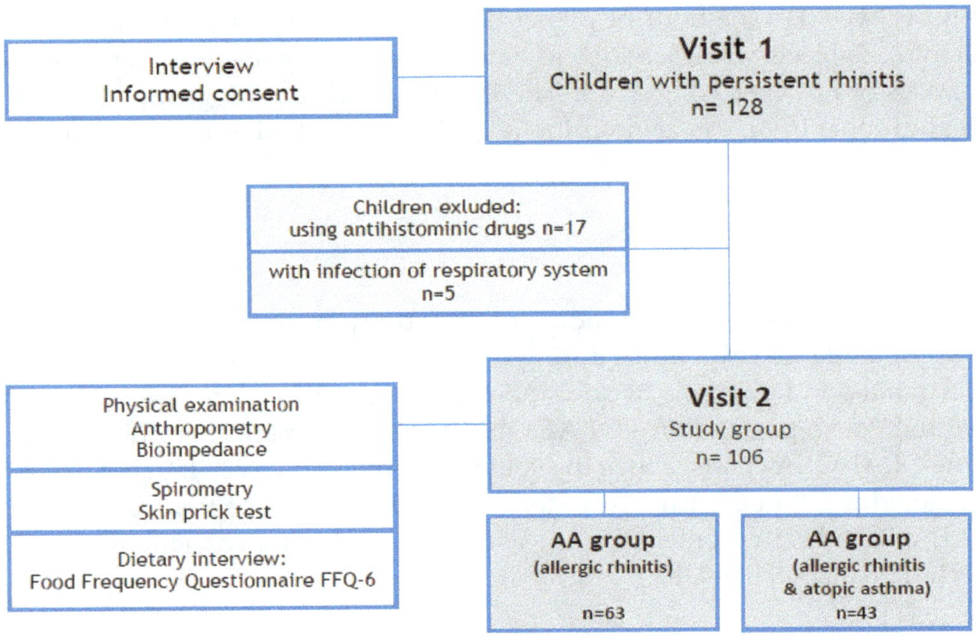

Figure 1. Study design.

Allergy background was confirmed with skin prick test to aeroallergens (*Dermatophagoides pteronyssinus*, *Dermatophagoides farinae*; cat, dog; *Alternaria alternata*, *Cladosporium herbarum*; pollens: grass mix, rye, birch pollen, alder, hazel; Allergopharma, Germany). Children with food allergies and atopic dermatitis were excluded from the study because of the frequent use of elimination diets.

Spirometry with a reversibility test (400 μg salbutamolum) was performed using a MasterScreen Pneumo spirometer, Jaeger Company, Germany. Forced expiratory volume in one second (FEV_1), forced vital capacity (FVC) and forced expiratory flow (FEF_{25-75}) were measured in accordance with the procedures recommended by the European Respiratory Society [18] and presented as percentage of predicted value (pv).

2.3. Nutritional Habits

Data were collected by face-to-face interviews using a researcher-designed standardized questionnaire based on the Food Frequency Questionnaire (FFQ-6) and validated for the Polish population [19]. The FFQ-6 is the most common dietary assessment tool used in large epidemiological studies of diet and health and is validated for the population. The self-administered FFQ-6 asks participants to report the frequency of consumption of approximately 62 line items over a defined period of time (last year). Each line item is defined by a series of foods or beverages. The FFQ-6 includes an assessment of eight food groups (sweets and snacks, dairy products and eggs, grain products, fats, fruits, vegetables and grains, meat products and fish, drinks). Respondents have a choice of six categories of food consumption frequency: (1) never or almost never, (2) once a month or less often, (3) several times a month, (4) several times a week, (5) daily, and (6) several times a day. The FFQ-6 also includes questions on eating habits, i.e., meal intake frequency and snacking between meals.

The following information was obtained: the number of meals in a day, amount of sweets consumed in a week, amount of fast-food eaten in a month, time of last meal before bedtime, and snacking between meals. Fast food was defined as mass-produced food prepared and served very quickly, with poor nutritional quality (hamburgers, takeaways, and carbonated soft drinks).

2.4. Physical Activity

The subjects were assigned to four categories depending on their level of physical activity: sedentary lifestyle (up to 2 h per week), low (3–5 h per week), moderate (6–7 h per week), and high (more than 8 h per week). One hour of physical activity corresponded to one hour of classroom attendance (45 min). Subjects were classified as having a sedentary lifestyle if only sometimes present during gym classes or not exercising at all. The low physical activity group attended gym class in school and an additional hour, e.g., swimming. Children identified as high activity trained in some kind of sport.

2.5. Nutritional Status

Body height was measured by stadiometer and body mass by electronic scale (Tanita Inc., Amsterdam, The Netherlands) by a nurse during the first visit. Body mass index (BMI) was calculated by dividing body mass in kilograms by the square of height in meters. Based on centile charts for sex and age for the Polish population—OLAF/OLA project—percentiles of BMI were specified [20]. According to the OLAF/OLA charts, above the 90th percentile is overweight, above the 97th percentile is obese, and below the 10th percentile is underweight. Body composition values of fat mass (FAT), fat-free mass (LEAN), and water content were measured via the bioimpedance method using a BodyStat 1500 (Bodystat Ltd., Ballafletcher, UK).

2.6. Statistical Analysis

Differences for somatic traits and between AR and AA groups were evaluated using Student's t-test or using the Mann-Whitney test for asymmetrical distributions. Distributions of values for somatic traits were evaluated using the Kołmogorov-Smirnov test. Differences between qualitative data were compared using the χ^2 test. The association between obesity risk factors and BMI percentile was determined using linear multivariate regression analysis. Differences were considered significant at $p < 0.05$. All analyses were carried out using the Statistica 10.0 software package.

3. Results

3.1. Patients

Allergic rhinitis was diagnosed in all 106 patients included in the study; among them, asthma was newly diagnosed in 43 (40.6%). Subjects with only allergic rhinitis were classified into the AR group and those with both allergic rhinitis and atopic asthma into the AA group (see Figure 1). All 106 children (100%) had a positive skin prick test to house dust mite (HDM; *D. farinae* and/or *D. pteronyssimus*), among which 40 (37.7%) were also positive to grass pollen (n = 29) and animals (n = 11).

Children in the AA group had a positive reversibility test and lower FEV_1 % predicted volume than children in the AR group. The basic characteristics of the study groups and the spirometry parameters are presented in Table 1.

3.2. Eating Habits and Physical Activity

The results of the eating habits and physical activity assessment are presented in Table 2.

Table 1. Clinical and lung function characteristics of patients.

Parameters	All Children * $n = 106$	AR Group $n = 63$	AA Group $n = 43$	p-Value AR vs. AA
M/F	60/46	38/25	22/21	0.34
Age (years) mean ± SD (range)	12.2 ± 3.5 (7–18)	13.3 ± 3.5 (7–18)	11.5 ± 3.2 (7–18)	0.01
Tobacco smoking exposure n (%)	21 (19.8%)	15 (24%)	6 (28%)	0.21
Animal at home n (%)	49 (50.7%)	32 (50.7%)	17 (39.5%)	0.25
Family allergies n (%)	65 (61%)	34 (53%)	31 (72%)	0.09
	Spirometry mean % pv ± SD			
FEV_1	95.4 ± 16.3	100.0 ± 11.1	92.1 ± 15.0	0.05
FVC	95.1 ± 10.0	97.1 ± 10.1	94.0 ± 10.9	0.13
FEV_1%FVC	108.8 ± 9.9	102.0 ± 4.4	99.0 ± 9.2	0.16
PEF	86.7 ± 16.0	90.2 ± 15.4	84.2 ± 15.9	0.06

AR: allergic rhinitis; AA: atopic asthma; FEV_1: forced expiratory volume in one second; FVC: forced vital capacity; PEF: peak expiratory flow; pv: predicted value; n: number of subjects. * All children ($n = 106$) had a positive skin prick test.

Table 2. Eating habits and physical activity assessment.

Parameters	All Patients $n = 106$	AR Group $n = 63$	AA Group $n = 43$
	Meals (number per day)		
2	4 (3.7%)	3 (4.7%)	1 (2.3%)
3	35 (33.0%)	19 (30.1%)	16 (37.2%)
4	31 (29.2%)	16 (25.6%)	15 (34.8%)
5 or more	36 (34.1%)	25 (39.6%)	11 (25.7%)
	Sweets (days per week)		
1	12 (11.5%)	7 (11.1%)	5 (11.6%)
2–3	29 (27.3%)	19 (30.1%)	10 (23.2%)
4–6	18 (16.9%)	10 (15.8%)	8 (18.6%)
every day	47 (44.3%)	27 (43.0%)	20 (46.6%)
	Fast food (days per month)		
never	17 (16.0%)	12 (19.0%)	5 (11.6%)
1	52 (49.0%)	32 (50.7%)	20 (46.6%)
2–3	27 (25.4%)	13 (20.6%)	14 (32.5%)
4–6	9 (8.7%)	6 (9.7%)	3 (7.0%)
every day	1 (0.9%)	0 (0.0%)	1 (2.3%)
	Last meal before sleep (hours to bedtime)		
<1	52 (49.0%)	30 (47.6%)	22 (51.1%)
1	20 (18.8%)	7 (11.1%)	13 (30.2%)
2	13 (12.4%)	11 (17.4%)	2 (4.6%)
>2	21 (19.8%)	15 (23.9%)	6 (14.1%)
	Snacking between meals		
yes	85 (80%)	50 (79.3%)	35 (81.4%)
no	21 (20%)	13 (20.7%)	8 (18.6%)
	Physical activity		
sedentary lifestyle	9 (8.4%)	4 (6.3%)	5 (11.6%)
low	58 (54.7%)	40 (63.4%)	18 (42.0%)
moderate	27 (25.4%)	12 (19.2%)	15 (34.8%)
high	12 (11.5%)	7 (11.1%)	5 (11.6%)

AR: allergic rhinitis; AA: atopic asthma; n: number of subjects.

3.2.1. Number of Meals

The majority of children reported eating three (33.4%), four (29.2%), or five (34.1%) meals per day. Children with AA ate more frequently than children with AR ($\chi^2 = 12.9$; $p = 0.04$).

Thirty-five children (34%) did not eat regularly; their meals were at different hours each day. There was no difference in meal regularity between AR and AA groups ($\chi^2 = 0.26$; $p = 0.60$).

3.2.2. Sweets

Almost half of the patients (47; 44.3%) ate sweets every day, in comparison to 12 (11.5%) who consumed sweets only one day per week. There was no difference in the consumption of sweets between AR and AA groups ($\chi^2 = 2.5$; $p = 0.88$).

3.2.3. Snacks

Eight-seven children (80%) snacked (sweet and salty snacks) between meals, 81.4% in the AA group and 79.3% in the AR group. There was no difference in snack consumption, but deeper analysis showed the AA group consumed more salty snacks than AR group ($\chi^2 = 0.59$; $p = 0.04$).

All overweight and obese children (AR and AA) snacked significantly more often between meals ($\chi^2 = 9.46$, $p = 0.01$) than children with normal BMI.

3.2.4. Fast Food

Seventeen patients (16.0%) had never eaten fast food. Most of the children (84%) ate fast food; half of them ($n = 52$) ate it very rarely (once a month) and 8.7% ate it 4–6 times per month. There was no difference in fast food consumption between AR and AA groups ($\chi^2 = 6.3$; $p = 0.50$).

3.2.5. Meals before Bedtime

It was found that children most often consumed their last meal of the day 0.5–2 h before bedtime; a total 12.4% ($n = 13$) did so 2 h before falling asleep, 19.8% ($n = 21$) did so much earlier (from 2.5 to 3 h before bedtime), and 49% ($n = 52$) ate the last meal <1 h before sleeping. Children with AA ate the last meal 1 h before sleep more frequently than those in the AR group ($\chi^2 = 19.4$; $p = 0.005$).

3.3. *Physical Activity*

The mean physical activity was 5 h per week. Most children (55%) reported 3–5 h/week physical activity. These children had only physical education (PE) at school and 1 h of additional activities after school (swimming or games). Children with AR reported low (63.4%; $n = 40$) and moderate (19.2%; $n = 12$) physical activity; similarly, children with AA reported low (42.0%; $n = 8$) and moderate (34.8%; $n = 15$) activity. There was no difference in physical activity between the AR and AA groups ($\chi^2 = 13.1$; $p = 0.15$). There was a negative correlation between physical activity level and BMI centile in the whole study population (Spearman's R = –0.19; $p < 0.05$).

3.4. *Nutritional Status and Body Composition*

Obesity was diagnosed in six children (6.0%) and eight were overweight (7.5%). In the AA group, obesity was present in 4.7% compared to 6.9% in the AR group ($\chi^2 = 3.58$; $p = 0.30$). The results of body composition measurement are presented in Table 3. There was no difference between the AR and AA groups.

3.5. *The Multifactorial Linear Regression Analysis*

Multifactorial linear regression analysis showed an association (independent of age) between BMI percentile and both snacking and physical activity level (see Figure 2 and Table 4).

Table 3. Nutritional status and body composition in studied groups.

Parameters	All Patients	AR Group $n = 63$	AA Group $n = 43$	p-Value AR vs. AA
Anthropometric data, mean ± SD (range)				
Weight (kg)	47.1 ± 17.9 (18–98.2)	51.3 ± 17.9 (21–95)	44.5 ± 17 (18–92)	0.06
Height (cm)	154.6 ± 19.1 (110–185)	160.3 ± 17.1 (116–182)	151.4 ± 19.2 (110–185)	0.03
BMI (percentile)	45.5 ± 32.1 (1–99)	41.6 ± 31.1 (5–99)	47.9 ± 33.1 (1–99)	0.63
BMI, n (%)				
Underweight BMI <10th percentile	8 (7.5%)	5 (7.9%)	3 (6.9%)	0.81
Normal BMI, 10th–90th percentile	84 (79.0%)	52 (82.5%)	32 (74.4%)	0.43
Overweight BMI, 90th–97th percentile	8 (7.5%)	3 (6.9%)	5 (11.0%)	0.57
Obesity BMI, >97th percentile	6 (6.0%)	3 (4.7%)	3 (6.9%)	0.89
Body composition; mean ± SD (range)				
Body fat (%)	29.6 ± 20.6 (1–90)	20 ± 15.4 (3–70)	21.5 ± 17 (1–90)	0.14
Body fat (kg)	9.2 ± 4.8 (1–30)	8.2 ± 4.7 (2–31)	7.9 ± 3.9 (1–17)	0.94
LEAN (%)	70.3 ± 20.6 (8.9–89)	79 ± 16.5 (21–89)	78.1 ± 17.1 (8.9–56)	0.42
LEAN (kg)	27.9 ± 17.3 (2–24)	39.5 ± 17.6 (6–24)	36.8 ± 17.4 (2–24)	0.23

AR: allergic rhinitis; AA: atopic asthma; BMI: body mass index; LEAN: lean body mass.

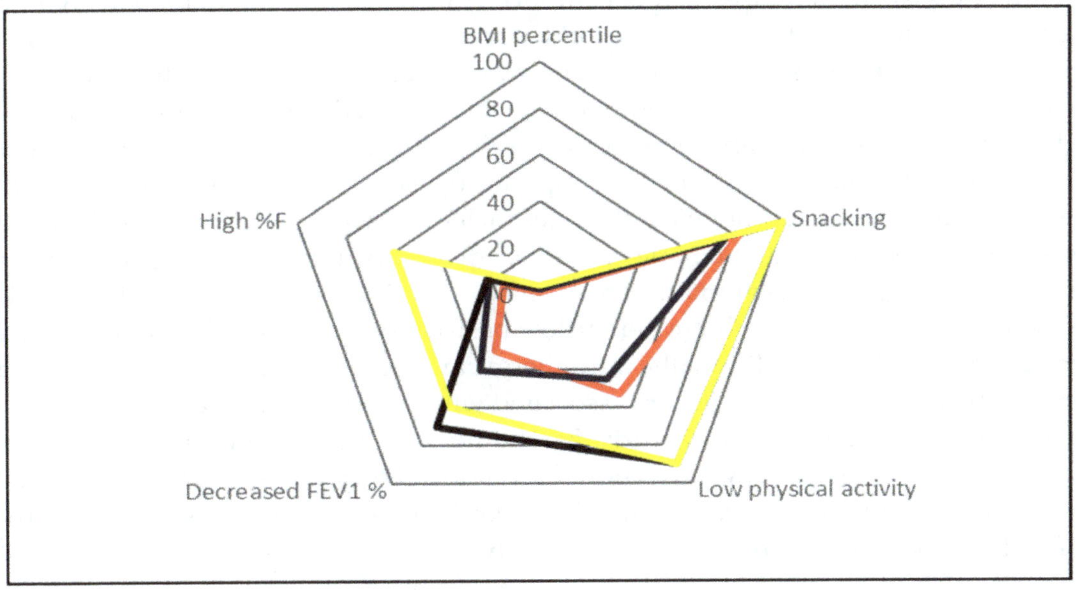

Figure 2. Association between body mass index (BMI) percentile and risk factors for obesity in all studied groups (adjusted $R^2 = 0.97$; $p < 0.05$). %F: percentage of body fat; FEV_1: forced expiratory volume in one second. Legend: red line means < 25th percentile, black line 25th–89th percentile, grey line 90th–97th percentile and yellow line >97th percentile.

Table 4. Multivariate regression model predicting BMI value (adjusted R^2 of the model was 0.97, $p < 0.05$).

Regression Model	B	Standard Error	Beta	p-Value
Constant	16.7	2.84		<0.001
Snacking	2.07	0.94	0.21	0.03
Fat%pv	−0.05	0.02	−0.21	0.058
FEV_1%pv	0.03	0.02	0.11	0.23
Physical activity	−1.02	0.46	−0.21	0.028

FEV_1: forced expiratory volume in one second; B: Regression coefficient B; Beta: beta standardized regression coefficient.

4. Discussion

In the present study, we evaluated the nutritional status and dietary habits of Caucasian children with allergic rhinitis alone or with co-existing asthma. Although all of the children presented respiratory allergy symptoms at least 12 months before the study, they were never diagnosed with allergies and had not previously been treated with an antihistamine or anti-asthmatic drugs before.

The most important finding of the study is that the majority of children with respiratory allergies reported incorrect eating habits and low physical activity, with 7.5% being overweight and 6.0% being obese. In the study population, excess body weight was significantly associated with snacking between meals and low physical activity.

4.1. Nutritional Status

Unexpectedly, the prevalence of overweight and obesity among allergic children was similar to the population of healthy children in Poland [13,14,21,22]. This aligned with data from the International Obesity Task Force (IOTF) showing that approximately 10% of children worldwide are overweight [12].

Although AR is a common disease, most authors focus on children with food allergies or asthma. These studies have suggested that adiposity indicators are associated with asthma, asthma severity, and atopy [23,24]. It is obvious that a positive energy balance is associated with changes in immune system functioning, including chronic inflammation, which is clearly an unfavorable phenomenon [22]. Overweight and obese children with allergic diseases have metabolic derangements, and obesity may have an impact on inflammation and clinical symptoms in asthma. The cause of impact of the obesity on asthma risk is still unknown. Potential etiologies include airway smooth muscle dysfunction from thoracic restriction, obesity-related circulating inflammation priming the lung, and obesity-related comorbidities mediating asthma symptom development. Studies suggest that obesity in children with asthma appears to be associated with greater airflow obstruction and a mildly diminished response to inhaled corticosteroids [25]. Additionally, anti-allergic and anti-asthmatic medications may be risk factors for obesity and physiological factors associated with puberty, also intensifying the tendency to gain weight in adolescents [23]. In our study, we did not take into account the effects of medicines because all of the children were newly diagnosed with respiratory allergies and had not been treated with an antihistamine or anti-asthmatic drugs. This may be one of the reasons for the relatively small number of children with obesity observed in our study.

Recent prospective evidence supports the notion that increased body weight precedes asthma development, but there is an ongoing debate as to whether obesity directly increases this risk or whether patients first experience asthma and then become overweight or obese, possibly because of respiratory constraints and reduced physical activity [26].

There are only a few studies on nutritional status and allergic rhinitis. A cross-sectional study of obesity indicators and AR in 8165 participants from the 2005–2006 National Health and Nutrition Examination Survey (NHANES) showed that overweight and obesity were associated with increased risk of AR in adults, but no such evidence was found among children [27].

Interestingly, in our study, although children with co-existing asthma were younger than and not as tall as the children with only AR, they had similar weight. However, there were no statistical differences between the number of overweight and obese children and body composition (FAT, LEAN) in the two groups. This is interesting because other authors have reported more than 50% of children with excessive body weight among children with asthma [28]. Spirometry parameters also did not correlate to BMI, body fat, and lean body mass content in the whole study group, although pulmonary function tests were lower in asthmatics. There were no differences in terms of family burden between allergy, asthma, obesity, exposure to tobacco smoke, and pet allergens.

4.2. Dietary Habits

Our study showed that incorrect eating habits were reported by most of the children with allergies, such as frequent consumption of fast foods and sweets, snacking between meals, and eating meals less than 1 h before bedtime.

Many studies have confirmed that fast-food consumption is linked to childhood obesity [29,30]. The multicenter International Study of Asthma and Allergies in Children (ISAAC) showed that fast food consumption is high in childhood (6–7 years), increases in adolescence (13–14 years), and is associated with higher BMI [31]. In our study, 35% of the children reported fast food consumption at least several times a month. This result is similar to the ISAAC results, showing that 27% of children and 52% of adolescents reported more than weekly fast food consumption [31]. We did not find an association between dietary habits and pulmonary function. There were also no differences in fast food consumption between children with asthma and those with only rhinitis. These results are different from those reported by other authors, suggesting that fast food consumption may contribute to the increasing prevalence of asthma, rhinoconjunctivitis, and eczema in adolescents and children [31]. Other results from case-control [32–34] and cross-sectional [35–40] studies indicate that consumption of fast foods is significantly related to current asthma and allergic rhinitis (pollen fever). Wang et al. suggested that the amount of processed foods eaten correlates with the frequency and severity of asthma [29].

Another important finding from this study was that approximately 80% of children with respiratory allergies snacked between meals every day. Moreover, although all children with excess body mass consumed more snacks compared to normal-weight patients and reported low physical activity, asthmatics consumed snacks more frequently ($\chi^2 = 0.59$; $p = 0.04$) and were more likely to eat their last meal of the day 1 h before sleeping ($\chi^2 = 19.4$; $p = 0.001$). Similar results were seen in the PANACEA study, which showed that among a population of 700 Greek children 10–12 years old with a 23.7% prevalence of asthma symptoms, almost half the children reported salty snack consumption ≥1 times/week [41]. In the cited study, consumption of salty snacks >3 times/week (vs. never/rarely) was associated with a 4.8 times higher likelihood of having asthma symptoms, irrespective of potential confounders. The authors noted that the association of salty snack eating and asthma symptoms was more prominent in children who watched television or played video games >2 h/day [41].

Unlike other researchers, we studied the times of meals consumed and found, interestingly, that almost half of the children ate in the last hour before bedtime. This incorrect habit was more common in children with asthma symptoms. There are well-known factors that affect and exacerbate inflammation in the lower respiratory tract in asthmatics, such as infection or gastroesophageal reflux. Eating immediately before bed might have contributed to the formation of gastroesophageal reflux and bronchial hyperreactivity in the studied group of children with AR. This is also interesting because children with AR differed compared to asthmatics in lung function (FEV_1%pv), but not in nutritional status or other eating habits except for snacking and meals consumed less than 1 h before bedtime. Unfortunately, we did not study the symptoms of gastroesophageal reflux, and we, therefore, cannot form any specific conclusions.

Braithwaite et al. [31] postulated some possible mechanisms to explain the relationship between asthma and allergic disease and the consumption of fast food, which may involve higher concentrations of saturated fatty acids, trans fatty acids, sodium, carbohydrates, and sugar, as well as preservatives that may modulate immune reactions. Consumption of processed foods reduces the consumption of foods that are rich in protective nutrients, such as fruits and vegetables. A reduced intake of fruits and vegetables, which have antioxidative and anti-inflammatory properties, is likely to have an unfavorable impact on asthma prevalence/management [42]. Additionally, indications are that a diet poor in antioxidants is a key factor influencing the development of allergic diseases; a Western lifestyle and processed food consumption can also cause reduced exposure to microbial products and a changed microbiome, which are thus possible causes of the increase in allergic disease [43].

4.3. Physical Activity

In our study, children from both groups (AR and AA) in over 50% reported low physical activity. It is well known that a lack of exercise increases the risk of obesity. This was confirmed by research in the Phase 3 ISAAC trial, in which television viewing (5+ h/day vs. <1 h/day, $p < 0.001$) (the group with low physical activity) was statistically significantly associated with higher BMI in comparison to vigorous physical activity (3+ h/week vs. never, $p < 0.001$) (the group with high physical activity) in adolescents. The authors also suggested that current behaviors are more important than other factors such as birth weight, breastfeeding, current maternal or paternal smoking in early childhood in the development of obesity [24].

A few studies have shown a relationship between physical activity and allergy. In the ISAAC study, associations were found between vigorous physical activity and a sedentary lifestyle for 13-year-olds with allergic rhinoconjunctivitis. Mitchell et al. showed that several hours of TV viewing was associated with symptoms of current asthma in adolescents [24]. Similarly, studies indicate that physical activity could be protective against the development of asthma [44]. On the other hand, Byberg et al. found no association between physical activity and allergic rhinoconjunctivitis [45].

Our results do not contradict the association between pulmonary function and physical activity but show a correlation between physical activity level and BMI percentile in the whole study population (Spearman's $R = -0.19$; $p < 0.05$).

Our study provides two very important issues in the study of respiratory affections such as allergy and asthma. These are the fact that this is the first study on nutrition carried out in newly diagnosed AR teenagers, before any medication that could mislead any result and the fact that this is another study from a few existent about nutrition in respiratory allergy. The limitation of our study is the relatively small group of patients; therefore, a more accurate analysis was not possible, for example based on age or sex. This study is not generalizable to the Polish population because it was performed in a clinical sample of children. Although the relationship between incorrect dietary habits, low physical activity, and obesity in children with respiratory allergies is supported by our findings, no conclusions about causality can be made due to the cross-sectional design.

Further studies with large groups are necessary to determine the relationship between respiratory allergy, body weight, and diet.

5. Conclusions

The risk factors of obesity in allergic children were found to be snacking and low physical activity. Most children with respiratory allergies, especially asthmatics, reported incorrect eating habits such as snacking and eating before bedtime. A correlation between pulmonary function and body composition or dietary habits was not found.

Our study also indicated that in groups of children with respiratory allergies, there is a need for correction of diet and lifestyle. We suggest that early dietary correction may be helpful for children with allergic rhinitis and a high risk of asthma.

Author Contributions: E.W.: S.M., M.S. designed the study. E.W., S.M. collected and analysed the data. M.S., M.G.-N. and E.J. carried out independent internal peer review of the data. All authors agreed the final version of the manuscript submitted for publication.

References

1. McNeill, G.; Tagiyeva, N.; Aucott, L.; Russell, G.; Helms, P.J. Changes in the prevalence of asthma, eczema and hay fever in pre-pubertal children: A 40-year perspective. *Paediatr. Perinatal. Epidemiol.* **2009**, 23, 506–512. [CrossRef] [PubMed]

2. Masoli, M.; Fabian, D.; Holt, S.; Beasley, R. Global Initiative for Asthma (GINA) Program. Global burden of asthma developed for the Global Initiative for Asthma. *Allergy* **2004**, *59*, 469–478. [CrossRef] [PubMed]
3. Samoliński, B.; Sybilski, A.J.; Raciborski, F.; Tomaszewska, A.; Samelkowalik, P.; Walkiewicz, A.; Lusawa, A.; Borowicz, J.; Gutowskaślesik, J.; Trzpil, L.; et al. Prevalence of rhinitis in Polish population according to the ECAP (Epidemiology of Allergic Disorders in Poland) study. *Otolaryngol. Pol.* **2009**, *63*, 324–330. [CrossRef]
4. Bousquet, P.J.; Demoly, P.; Devillier, P.; Mesbah, K.; Bousquet, J. Impact of allergic rhinitis symptoms on quality of life in primary care. *Int. Arch. Allergy. Immunol.* **2013**, *160*, 393–400. [CrossRef]
5. Guerra, S.; Sherrill, D.L.; Martinez, F.D.; Barbee, R.A. Rhinitis is an independent risk factor for adult-onset asthma. *J. Allergy Clin. Immunol.* **2002**, *109*, 419–425. [CrossRef]
6. Bosquet, J.; Van Cauwenberge, P.; Khaltaev, N. ARIA Workshop Group. Allergic rhinitis and its impact on asthma. *J. Allergy Clin. Immunol.* **2001**, *108*, 147–334. [CrossRef]
7. Samoliński, B.; Raciborski, F.; Lipiec, A.; Tomaszewska, A.; Krzych-Fałta, E.; Nowicka, A. Epidemiology of allergic diseases in Poland. *Pol. J. Allergol.* **2014**, *1*, 10–18.
8. Nagel, G.; Weinmayr, G.; Kleiner, A.; Garcia-Marcos, L.; Strachan, D.P. Effect of diet on asthma and allergic sensitisation in the International Study on Allergies and Asthma in Childhood (ISAAC) phase two. *Thorax.* **2010**, *65*, 516–522. [CrossRef]
9. Rosenheck, R. Fast food consumption and increased caloric intake: A systematic review of a trajectory towards weight gain and obesity risk. *Obes. Rev.* **2008**, *9*, 535–547. [CrossRef]
10. Leynaert, B.; Neukirch, C.; Liard, R.; Bousquet, J.; Neukirch, F. Quality of life in allergic rhinitis and asthma: A population-based study of young adults. *Am. J. Respir. Crit. Care. Med.* **2000**, *162*, 1391–1396. [CrossRef]
11. Bernstein, J.A. Allergic and mixed rhinitis: Epidemiology and natural history. *Allergy Asthma Proc.* **2010**, *31*, 365–369. [CrossRef] [PubMed]
12. International Obesity Task Force. Prevalence of overweight and obesity in a number of countries (global prevalence database) [in:] European Union Public Health Information System 2007. Available online: http://www.euro.who.int/__data/assets/pdf_file/0005/96980/2.3.-Prevalence-of-overweight-and-obesity-EDITED_layouted_V3.pdf (accessed on 12 June 2018).
13. Oblacinska, A.; Wroclawska, M.; Woynarowska, B. Frequency of overweight and obesity in the school-age population in Poland and health care for pupils with these disorders. *Ped. Pol.* **1997**, *72*, 241–245.
14. Mazur, A.; Malecka-Tendera, E.; Lewin-Kowalik, J. Overweight and obesity in primary school children from the Podkarpatian Region. *Ped. Pol.* **2001**, *76*, 743–748.
15. Lipowicz, A.; Opuszalska, M.; Kolodziej, H.; Szklarska, A.; Bielicki, T. Secular trends in BMI and the prevalence of obesity in young Polish males from 1965 to 2010. *Eur. J. Public Health* **2015**, *25*, 279–282. [CrossRef]
16. De, A.; Rastogi, D. Association of pediatric obesity and asthma, pulmonary physiology, metabolic dysregulation, and atopy; and the role of weight management. *Expert Rev. Endocrinol. Metab.* **2019**, *14*, 335–349. [CrossRef]
17. Global Initiative for Asthma. Global Strategy for Asthma Management and Prevention. 2020. Available online: www.ginasthma.org (accessed on 3 April 2018).
18. Miller, M.R.; Crapo, R.; Hankinson, J.; Brusasco, V.; Burgos, F.; Casaburi, R.; Coates, A.; Enright, P.; van der Grinten, C.P.M.; Gustafsson, P.; et al. General consideration for lung function testing. *Eur. Respir. J.* **2005**, *26*, 153–161. [CrossRef]
19. Niedzwiedzka, E.; Wadolowska, L.; Kowalkowska, J. Reproducibility of a Non-Quantitative Food Frequency Questionnaire (62-Item FFQ-6) and PCA-Driven Dietary Pattern Identification in 13–21-Year-Old Females. *Nutrients* **2019**, *11*, 2183. [CrossRef]
20. Kułaga, Z.; Litwin, M.; Tkaczyk, M.; Palczewska, I.; Zajączkowska, M.; Zwolińska, D.; Krynicki, T.; Wasilewska, A.; Moczulska, A.; Morawiec-Knysak, A.; et al. Pan HPolish 2010 growth references for school-a-ged children and adolescents. *Eur. J. Pediatr.* **2011**, *170*, 599–609.
21. Stankiewicz, M.; Pieszko, M.; Sliwińska, A.; Małgorzewicz, S.; Wierucki, Ł.; Zdrojewski, T.; Wyrzykowski, B.; Łysiak-Szydlowska, W. Obesity and diet awareness among Polish children and adolescents in small towns and villages. *Cent. Eur. J. Public Health.* **2014**, *22*, 12–16. [CrossRef]
22. Chrzanowska, M.; Suder, A. Changes in central fatness and abdominal obesity in children and adolescents from Cracow, Poland 1983–2000. *Ann. Hum. Biol.* **2010**, *37*, 242–252. [CrossRef]

23. Forno, E.; Acosta-Pérez, E.; Brehm, J.; Han, YY.; Alvarez, M.; Colón-Semidey, A.; Canino, G.; Celedón, J. Obesity and adiposity indicators, asthma, and atopy in Puerto Rican children. *J. Aller. Clin. Immunol.* **2014**, *133*, 1308–1314. [CrossRef]
24. Mitchell, E.A.; Stewart, A.W.; Braithwaite, I.; Murphy, R.; Hancox, R.J.; Wall, C.; Beasley, R. ISAAC Phase Three Study Group. Factors associated with body mass index in children and adolescents: An international cross-sectional study. *PLoS ONE* **2018**, *2*, e0196221. [CrossRef]
25. Lang, J.E. Obesity, Nutrition, and Asthma in Children. *Ped. Allerg. Immunol. Pulmonol.* **2012**, *25*, 64–75. [CrossRef]
26. Papoutsakis, C.; Priftis, K.N.; Drakouli, M.; Prifti, S.; Konstantaki, E.; Chondronikola, M.; Antonogeorgos, G.; Matziou, V. Childhood overweight/obesity and asthma: Is there a link? A systematic review of recent epidemiologic evidence. *J. Acad. Nutr. Diet.* **2013**, *113*, 77–105. [CrossRef]
27. Han, Y.Y.; Forno, E.; Gogna, M.; Celedón, J. FAAAAI Obesity and rhinitis in a nationwide study of children and adults in the United States. *J. Allerg. Clin. Immunol.* **2016**, *137*, 1460–1465. [CrossRef]
28. Evans, E.W.; Koinis-Mitchell, D.; Kopel, S.J.; Jelalian, E. Lung Function, Dietary Intake, and Weight Status in Children with Persistent Asthma from Low-Income, Urban Communities. *Nutrients* **2019**, *3*, 2943. [CrossRef]
29. Wang, C.S.; Wang, J.; Zhang, X.; Zhang, L.; Zhang, H.P.; Wang, L.; Wood, L.G.; Wang, G. Systematic Review Free Access Is the consumption of fast foods associated with asthma or other allergic diseases? *Respirology* **2018**, *23*, 901–913. [CrossRef]
30. Wickens, K.; Barry, D.; Friezema, A.; Rhodius, R.; Bone, N.; Purdie, G.; Crane, J. Fast foods—Are they a risk factor for asthma? *Allergy* **2005**, *60*, 1537–1541. [CrossRef]
31. Braithwaite, I.; Stewart, A.; Hancox, R.J.; Beasley, R.; Murphy, R.; Mitchell, E.A. ISAAC Phase Three Study Group. Fast-food consumption and body mass index in children and adolescents: An international cross-sectional study. *BMJ Open* **2014**, *8*, 4.
32. Lawson, J.A.; Rennie, D.C.; Dosman, J.A.; Cammer, A.L.; Senthilselvan, A. Obesity, diet, and activity in relation to asthma and wheeze among rural dwelling children and adolescents. *J. Obes.* **2013**, *2013*, 315096. [CrossRef]
33. Mai, X.M.; Becker, A.B.; Liem, J.J.; Kozyrskyj, A.L. Fast foods consumption counters the protective effect of breastfeeding on asthma in children? *Clin. Exp. Allergy* **2009**, *39*, 556–561. [CrossRef] [PubMed]
34. Hijazi, N.; Abalkhail, B.; Seaton, A. Diet and childhood asthma in a society in transition a study in urban and rural Saudi Arabia. *Thorax* **2000**, *55*, 775–779. [CrossRef] [PubMed]
35. Kim, J.L.; Elfman, L.; Mi, Y.; Johansson, M.; Smedje, G.; Norbäck, D. Current asthma and respiratory symptoms among pupils in relation to dietary factors and allergens in the school environment. *Indoor Air.* **2005**, *15*, 170–182. [CrossRef] [PubMed]
36. Garcia-Marcos, L.; Canflanca, I.M.; Garrido, J.B.; Varela, A.L.; Garcia-Hernandez, G.; Grima, F.G.; Gonzalez-Diaz, C.; Carvajal-Urueña, I.; Arnedo-Pena, A.; Busquets-Monge, R.M.; et al. Relationship of asthma and rhinoconjunctivitis with obesity, exercise and Mediterranean diet in Spanish school children. *Thorax* **2007**, *62*, 503–508. [CrossRef] [PubMed]
37. Huang, S.L.; Lin, K.C.; Pan, W.H. Dietary factors associated with physician-diagnosed asthma and allergic rhinitis in teenagers: Analyses of the first nutrition and health survey in Taiwan. *Clin. Exp. Allergy* **2001**, *31*, 259–264. [CrossRef] [PubMed]
38. Takaoka, M.; Norback, D. Diet among Japanese female university students and asthmatic symptoms, infections, pollen and furry pet allergy. *Respir. Med.* **2008**, *102*, 1045–1054. [CrossRef]
39. Norbäck, D.; Zhao, Z.H.; Wang, Z.H.; Wieslander, G.; Mi, Y.H.; Zhang, Z. Asthma, eczema, and reports on pollen and cat allergy among pupils in Shanxi province, China. *Int. Arch. Occup. Environ. Health* **2007**, *80*, 207–216. [CrossRef]
40. Awasthi, S.; Kalra, E.; Roy, S. Prevalence and risk factors of asthma and wheeze in school-going children in Lucknow, North India. *Indian Pediatr.* **2004**, *41*, 1205–1210.
41. Arvaniti, F.; Priftis, K.N.; Papadimitriou, A.; Yiallouros, P.; Kapsokefalou, M.; Anthracopoulos, M.B.; Panagiotakos, D.B. Salty-Snack Eating, Television or Video-Game Viewing, and Asthma Symptoms among 10-to 12-Year-Old Children: The PANACEA Study. *J. Am. Diet. Assoc.* **2011**, *111*, 251–257. [CrossRef]
42. Wood, L.G.; Garg, M.L.; Gibson, P.G. A high-fat challenge increases airway inflammation and impairs bronchodilator recovery in asthma. *J. Allergy Clin. Immunol.* **2011**, *127*, 1133–1140. [CrossRef]

43. Weiland, S.K.; von Mutius, E.; Hüsing, A.; Asher, M.I. Intake of trans fatty acids and prevalence of childhood asthma and allergies in Europe. ISAAC Steering Committee. *Lancet* **1999**, *353*, 2040–2041. [CrossRef]
44. Eijkemans, M.; Mommers, M.M.; Draisma, J.; Thijs, C.; Martin, H. Physical Activity and Asthma: A Systematic Review and Meta-Analysis. *PLoS ONE* **2012**, *7*, e50775. [CrossRef] [PubMed]
45. Byberg, K.K.; Eide, G.E.; Forman, M.R.; Júlíusson, P.B.; Øymar, K. Body mass index and physical activity in early childhood are associated with atopic sensitization, atopic dermatitis and asthma in later childhood. *Clin. Trans. Allergy* **2016**, *6*, 33. [CrossRef] [PubMed]

3

The Infant Gut Microbiota and Risk of Asthma: The Effect of Maternal Nutrition during Pregnancy and Lactation

Naser A. Alsharairi

Heart, Mind & Body Research Group, Menzies Health Institute Queensland, Griffith University, Gold Coast 4215, Australia; naser.alsharairi@gmail.com

Abstract: Research has amply demonstrated that early life dysbiosis of the gut microbiota influences the propensity to develop asthma. The influence of maternal nutrition on infant gut microbiota is therefore of growing interest. However, a handful of prospective studies have examined the role of maternal dietary patterns during pregnancy in influencing the infant gut microbiota but did not assess whether this resulted in an increased risk of asthma later in life. The mechanisms involved in the process are also, thus far, poorly documented. There have also been few studies examining the effect of maternal dietary nutrient intake during lactation on the milk microbiota, the effect on the infant gut microbiota and, furthermore, the consequences for asthma development remain largely unknown. Therefore, the specific aim of this mini review is summarizing the current knowledge regarding the effect of maternal nutrition during pregnancy and lactation on the infant gut microbiota composition, and whether it has implications for asthma development.

Keywords: maternal diet; infant; gut microbiota; asthma; pregnancy; lactation

---

1. Introduction

Asthma is considered one of the most widespread chronic respiratory diseases of childhood, with hospitalization rates reportedly having increased for children under the age of 5 years over the last two decades [1]. The body of evidence around asthma development in young children suggests that genetic predisposition [2–4], environmental exposures [2,5] as well as the gut microbiome [6–9] have a strong influence.

The maternal gut microbiota promotes the microbiota colonization of the infant gut prior to birth in utero, after delivery and then through breastfeeding [10–12]. Gut microbial colonization during early life represents a critical window of offspring immune system development [13]. According to the sterile womb paradigm, the gut microbiota are transferred from mother to infant prior to or during delivery and breastfeeding via a vertical pathway, and from the environment after delivery via a horizontal pathway [14,15]. Early-life microbial dysbiosis of the gut has been linked to an increased risk of asthma in the first years of life [16–18]. Such a link is significantly modified by the mode of birth delivery, antibiotic exposure and maternal body mass index (BMI), asthma and stress [6,16,18–23]. However, pre- and postnatal pet exposure may influence the infant gut microbiota and the development of their immune systems, with a subsequent reduced risk of asthma [24].

The maternal diet has been found to be a significant factor that influences the gut microbiota and potentially the development of asthma in offspring [25]. There is apparently an additional value obtained from animal models in understanding the mechanisms by which maternal dietary patterns during pregnancy influence asthma development in offspring via the maternal gut microbiota and their metabolites [21,26,27]. However, our understanding of the aforementioned mechanisms is incomplete and further long-term studies in humans are needed. In addition, the mechanisms by which maternal dietary patterns and breast milk microbiota alter the offspring gut microbiota, which may in turn underlie asthma, remain underdeveloped. Indeed, the protective role of breastfeeding against asthma in childhood is still a controversial matter. This controversy arises because there are inconsistent results from previous studies [19,28]. Recently, the modulation of gut microbiota composition by probiotics and prebiotics during pregnancy and lactation has been proposed as a potential dietary strategy to reduce the risk of asthma in offspring. Despite evidence of alterations in maternal gut bacteria, a systematic review and meta-analysis of a randomized controlled trial (RCT) reported no benefit of probiotic supplements during pregnancy and early life for asthma or wheeze prevention in children [29]. Because of the low certainty of the evidence, the World Allergy Organization panel suggests not recommending prebiotic supplementation in both pregnant and lactating women for the prevention of asthma and allergic diseases in children [30].

The maternal gut microbiota progressively changes throughout pregnancy and significantly determines what is transmitted to the offspring and how the offspring gut microbiota eventually develops [31]. Diet is considered a major driver of the maternal gut microbiota changes [31] and therefore, in human studies, maternal dietary intake in gestation is associated with alterations in the offspring gut microbiota as well [32–34]. In particular, the type of dietary fat in the diet of pregnant mothers can negatively affect the trajectory of the offspring microbiota. It has been found that a high-fat maternal diet during gestation is associated with lower levels of the genera Bacteroides in the offspring gut [32].

Breastfeeding has a significant effect on the alterations in the gut microbiota following birth either by infant exposure to milk microbiota or by breast milk factors interacting with the maternal and infant gut microbiota such as human milk oligosaccharides (HMOs) [35]. The composition and diversity of breast milk microbiota are influenced by several maternal factors such as mode of delivery, gestational age, lactation stage, maternal BMI, mode of feeding and antibiotic exposure [36–45]. A few compelling studies have been undertaken which do indeed demonstrate that maternal dietary nutrient intake strongly influences breast milk microbiota. Further studies are needed to understand how maternal nutrition during pregnancy and lactation alter the infant gut microbiota, and whether this interaction increases the risk of asthma. Therefore, this mini review aims to summarize the existing evidence demonstrating the effect of maternal nutrition during pregnancy and lactation on the infant gut microbiota composition, and whether it influences asthma risk.

2. Gut Microbiota in Early Life and Its Relationship with Asthma Development

The first large wave of microbes to colonize the gut occurs following birth and the gut continues to acquire microbes during the transition between infancy and early childhood [12]. The early gut microbial colonization plays a significant role in the maturation of the metabolic, endocrine and immune systems [46]. The gut microbiota during the first three years of life has taxonomic and functional compositions different to that in adults, and the gut of some infant may exhibit lower microbial diversity than in others [47]. Following birth, the gut microbiota is predominantly colonized by Enterobacteriaceae and Staphylococcus genera [11]. During breastfeeding, the gut microbiota are dominated by Bifidobacterium genera which have the ability to metabolize HMOs [11,48]. HMOs are soluble complex carbohydrates and are thought to play a crucial role in increasing the abundance of Bifidobacteria which protect against pathogenic infection and alter bacteria-host interactions [42,49,50]. The time of weaning, the initiation of solid foods results in the establishment of microorganisms, represented by the genera Bacteroidetes and Firmicutes [11,51], species known to disassemble complex plant-derived polysaccharides [52]. The introduction of food items with protein and fiber contents (e.g., rye bread, meat, cheese, animal fat) increased the relative abundance of *Ruminococcaceae* and *Lachnospiraceae* spp. in the infant gut [53]. By around three years of age, the gut microbiota are colonized by microbial-enriched genes, most belong to the genera Prevotella, Veillonella, Ruminococcus,

Clostridium, Bacteroides and Firmicutes, species involved in carbohydrate metabolism, xenobiotic degradation and vitamin B synthesis [11,47].

There is strong evidence that early-life gut microbial exposure plays a significant role in the development of childhood asthma [17]. The link between the early life dysbiosis of the gut microbiota and the subsequent development of asthma has been well-established in large-cohort studies [16–18]. It has also become clear through findings from epidemiological studies and reviews that this link is conceivably influenced by a wide range of perinatal factors. These findings suggest that maternal asthma during pregnancy [18,23], pre-gestational BMI [23], delivery mode (vaginal, cesarean) [6,16,19,20], breastfeeding mothers with a history of atopic conditions [19], maternal stress [19,22] and antibiotic exposure [6,19,21] are considered the main modifiers of the infant gut microbiota contributing to the development of asthma.

Maternal diet has also been considered a key factor that influences asthma development in offspring through the maternal gut microbiota and its metabolites' modulating effects [25]. There are substantial animal mechanistic studies, which demonstrate that diet and microbial exposure during pregnancy influence asthma development in offspring [26]. However, our understanding at this point is still incomplete in human studies. Evidence in animal models demonstrates that the gut microbiome transferred through the placenta produces diverse metabolites, which act as significant mediators of fetal immune development [21]. Short-chain fatty acids (SCFAs), propionate, acetate and butyrate, are the main metabolites generated by the microbial fermentation of complex plant carbohydrates derived from microbiota-accessible carbohydrates (MACs), which represent the major energy sources for gut bacteria [21,27]. SCFAs influence T lymphocytes and dendritic cells through their binding to protein-coupled receptors and the direct inhibition of histone deacetylase, thereby promoting the differentiation of helperT cells (Th1, Th2). The Th2 asthmatic phenotype plays a pivotal role in increasing eosinophils, Immunoglobulin E (IgE) production, and the production of inflammatory cytokines. These cytokines enhance the allergic immune system and increase the risk of asthma in offspring [21,26]. Changes in dietary patterns during pregnancy may affect the microbial composition and diversity in the gut as well as the production of SCFAs [21]. A low-MAC diet is found to decrease bacterial diversity and SCFA production, which may hinder the functioning of regulatory T cells and lead to inhibited immunoglobulin A and G (IgA, IgG) production [27]. Data from human research has shown that a high maternal fiber intake during late pregnancy increases acetate (but not propionate or butyrate) levels in serum, which leads to a reduced risk of coughing and wheezing symptoms in the offspring's first year of life [54].

3. Breastfeeding as a Key Pillar of Asthma Prevention by Microbiota Shaping

Breastfeeding has a wide range of positive short-and long-term health benefits for mothers and infants, including a protective role against neurological disorders, cancers and obesity in infants and diabetes/cardiovascular risk in mothers [55]. Despite its known protective role, not all studies have reported a protection against childhood asthma [19,28]. Breast milk in its complex composition contains several bioactive components such as cytokines, immunoglobulins, chemokines, polyunsaturated fatty acids, eosinophil-derived granular proteins, antigens and polyamines that stimulate infant immune system development [28]. Since gut microbial dysbiosis in early life is found to be associated with asthma development [17], breast milk would be an optimal nutritional solution for modulating the infant gut microbiota, which may therefore reduce the long-term asthma risk. Breast milk has the potential to shape the gut microbiota after birth by exposure of the infant to the milk microbiota or by breast milk-modulating factors such as HMOs, which can affect microbiota growth and metabolism [35]. Breast milk is a source of probiotics (milk microbiota) and prebiotics (HMOs) which play a role in increasing the colonization of beneficial bacteria in the infant gut [50]. An analysis of breast milk using culture-dependent and independent techniques has revealed that lactic acid bacteria, *streptococci* and *staphylococci* spp. are the most abundant beneficial bacteria to the offspring gut [56]. Indeed, it remains unclear how the milk microbiota are established. An entero-mammary pathway has been proposed to explain the origin of bacteria in milk. This pathway involves bacterial translocation through the intestinal lumen by internalization in the maternal dendritic cells or macrophages, which is then taken up into the lactating mammary gland through blood/lymphatic circulation [56].

4. Search Methodology

The PUBMED/MEDLINE database was searched up to June 2020 to identify pertinent studies. Studies of potential interest published in English were selected for inclusion if they addressed the effect of maternal nutrition on the infant gut/milk microbiota composition, and/or their consequences on asthma development. Relevant articles were identified using the combination of the following search terms: (nutrition OR diet OR dietary pattern OR dietary quality) AND (gut microbiota OR milk microbiota) AND (pregnancy OR lactation). The search was limited to human studies. A total of 712 articles were assessed using the specified searches. As a result, six studies met the search criteria. The selected studies are provided in the following section and a summary is presented in Table 1.

Table 1. Alterations of infant gut and/or milk microbiota associated with maternal nutrition.

Design and Subject Characteristics.	Maternal Nutrition	To Indicate if Microbiota Changes are Seen in Infants' Gut or Milk Microbiota	Ref.
Prospective cohort study 81 pregnant women 82 women at delivery and 6-wk postpartum	High-fat diet	Third trimester of pregnancy = Enterococcus↑, Bacteroides↓ At delivery and beyond = Bacteroides↓	[32] [a]
Prospective cohort study 97 vaginal delivery 48 cesarean section delivery	Mediterranean (MED) Dairy Fish and seafood Fruit Red and processed meat	Vaginal delivery MED = Streptococcus↑, Clostridium↑, Bacteroides↓, *Escherichiacoli*↓, Ruminococcus↓ Dairy = Clostridium↑, Staphylococcus↑, *Lachnospiraceae*↓ Fish and seafood = Streptococcus↑, Bacteroides↓ Fruit = Clostridium↑, Bifidobacterium↓ Cesarean delivery MED = Enterococcus↑, *Lachnospiraceae*↑, *Escherichiacoli*↓, Streptococcus↓, Blautia↓ Dairy = *Enterobacteriaceae*↑, *Escherichiacoli*↑, Bifidobacterium↓, Pseudomonas↓, Bacteroides↓, Corynebacterium↓ Fish and seafood = Bacteroides↑, Clostridium↓, Streptococcus↓ Red and processed meat = Bifidobacterium↑, *Escherichiacoli*↑, Enterococcus↑	[33] [a]
Prospective cohort study 114 infants	Fish	Third trimester of pregnancy = Bifidobacterium↑	[34] [a]
Prospective cohort study 21 lactating women	Macro- and micronutrients	Energy and protein = Gemella↑ SFA and MUFA = Corynebacterium↓ Total carbohydrates, total disaccharides and lactose = Firmicutes↓ Insoluble fiber = Rothia↑ Pantothenic acid = Streptococcus↓ Riboflavin and calcium = Veillonella↑ Thiamine, niacin, folate, vitamin B-6 and chromium = Lactobacillus↓	[40] [b]
Cross-sectional study 94 lactating women	Nutrients	Pregnancy: vitamin C = Staphylococcus↑ Lactation (1-month post-partum): PUFA & linoleic acid = Bifidobacterium↑, sugars = Pseudomonas↓, vitamin B9 = Pseudomonas↑, Thiamine & vitamin B9 = Enterococcus↓	[57] [b]
Prospective cohort study 14 lactating women	High-fat diet	*Erysipelotrichaceae*↑, Roseburia↑	[58] [b]

[a] Studies suggest that maternal nutrition lead to a change in the infant gut microbiota. [b] Studies suggest that maternal nutrition lead to a change in the milk microbiota. ↑ reflects positive associations, ↓ reflects negative association.

5. Effect of Maternal Nutrition during Pregnancy and Lactation on Infant Gut and Milk Microbiota Composition

5.1. Maternal Nutrition during Pregnancy

The pregnancy period is marked by substantial immunological, metabolic and hormonal changes which appear to be significant factors in modulating the mother's gut microbiota composition and function [59]. The effect of maternal nutrition during pregnancy on infant gut microbiota composition alterations has been widely reported in animal models; however, evidence from cohort studies in humans is limited [59–61]. One study [32] reported associations between a maternal high-fat diet intake and the abundance of genera Bacteroides and Enterococcus in the infant gut. Another study [33] showed that the associations between maternal dietary patterns and the infant gut microbiota at 6 weeks postpartum differ according to the mode of birth delivery. In a recent study [34], consuming the recommended amount of fish was found to be associated with Bifidobacterium dominance in the infant gut.

5.2. Maternal Nutrition during Lactation

Maternal nutrition may influence the milk microbiota composition and diversity directly [40,57] or indirectly [43] through alterations in the maternal gut microbiota diversity. Few studies on the effects of maternal nutrition during lactation on the milk microbiota composition have been conducted. Research evidence has revealed that variations in maternal macro- and micronutrients intake impacted on the relative abundance of several bacterial taxa in milk 6 months postpartum [40]. A recent study [57] has demonstrated that maternal dietary nutrient intake influences the composition of milk microbiota, and such effect appears to be different between pregnancy and lactation. Another study [58] found that a maternal high-fat diet throughout breastfeeding altered both the milk microbiota and HMO. Collectively, these studies indicate that maternal nutrition may alter the microbial composition of breast milk. The mechanisms whereby maternal nutrition influences the milk microbiota are not yet fully understood. It is likely that both probiotic (bacteria in the diet) and nutrient intake influence the microbial composition present in the maternal gastrointestinal (GI) tract and these may enter the mammary glands through the entero-mammary route [62].

5.3. Effect Modification

Among the key factors worthy of explanation for associations between maternal nutrition and alterations in infant gut and breast milk microbiota is obesity. Previous studies have shown evidence indicating that obesity-associated maternal gut microbiota may alter the infant gut microbiota towards a state of dysbiosis and induce later-life obesity. In support of this fact, lower levels of *Bacteroides* spp. and *Bifidobacterium* spp. have been found to be associated with weight gain in obese infants compared with their normal weight counterparts [63–66]. In addition, a significantly less diverse microbiota in breast milk has been demonstrated in obese breastfeeding mothers, corroborating the conclusion that obesity influences the milk microbiota [36,40,43,62]. The abundance of the Bacteroides genera decreased significantly in milk produced by obese mothers [40], who consumed high-fat diets during pregnancy and lactation [32]. Obesity alters the maternal microbiota composition during pregnancy and lactation, and this may have a significant impact on asthma risk in the first years of life [63,67]. The immune system reacts to changes in microbiota composition, and gut microbiota depleted of *Proteobacteria* spp. in infants of mothers with obesity could result in alterations in immune profiles, leading to an increased risk of developing inflammatory diseases [67]. Infants born to obese mothers or fed a high-fat diet showed a disturbed gut microbiota that is not entirely corrected by offering a specific diet later by complementary feeding. This has profound clinical implications for maternal diet-induced alterations to the maternal gut microbiota which, in turn, could have a lasting impact on the infant gut microbiota composition, thus making children more susceptible to inflammatory diseases [65]. Further long-term human dietary interventions are needed to determine if specific changes in maternal dietary patterns during both pregnancy and lactation induce permanent alterations in the infant gut microbiota, and to delineate if this results in reduced risk of asthma later in life. A direct effect of maternal nutrition on the milk microbiota with subsequent development of asthma, and as a result of the influence of obesity, has not yet been uncovered. Given that milk microbiota are associated with obesity [36,40,43,62], a skewed microbial milk composition could be a potential factor contributing to shifts in the microbial composition of the infant gut, and might contribute to asthma. Therefore, understanding the effect of milk microbiota on obesity-related asthma could facilitate the development of new avenues for dietary interventions during both pregnancy and lactation to reduce the risk of asthma.

Maternal early life factors (mode of delivery, antibiotics use and mode of feeding) may also modify such association. Obesity interacting with maternal and early life factors may alter the gut/milk microbiota and increase the susceptibility of children to develop asthma later in life. Infants born by cesarean (C-section) are at an increased risk of food allergies [68], obesity [69] and asthma [70]. The breast milk of mothers who had delivered by elective C-section was associated with reduced relative abundances of beneficial microbes [36–39,44]. The use of antibiotics for C-section delivery increases the susceptibility to gut dysbiosis and obesity later in life [69]. Both prenatal and postnatal exposure to antibiotics increases the risk of asthma in childhood [6,19,21]. Mothers following elective C-section delivery without intrapartum antibiotic use exhibited significantly lower milk microbiota richness and diversity compared to mothers who used antibiotics and delivered vaginally [44].

Formula feeding is associated with a higher risk of obesity and asthma than breastfeeding [71,72]. Compared to breastfed infants, formula-fed infants are exposed to a mix of nutrients and a more complex form of carbohydrates, causing colonization with diverse gut microbes [14]. Infants who were fed exclusively formula/breastmilk supplemented with formula and born by C-section had a less diverse gut microbial community [73,74]. Infants who were not breastfed but who were exposed to antibiotics and born by C-section delivery displayed significantly decreased relative abundances of gut microbial taxa [75]. Exclusive breastfeeding over mixed feeding can potentially restore the gut microbiota dysbiosis of C-section born infants [76].

6. Conclusions

The maternal gut microbiota promotes the microbiota colonization of the infant gut throughout pregnancy and later in life. Therefore, it is likely that maternal gut microbiota during both pregnancy and lactation influences the infant gut microbiota via maternal nutrition. The exact mechanisms are yet to be fully understood, and further long-term follow-up studies of pregnancy and lactation cohorts are needed. While few prospective studies have found associations between maternal nutrition during pregnancy and alterations in the infant gut microbiota, no studies have found that such associations were related to an increased risk of asthma later in life. There is also a paucity of human data examining the associations between maternal dietary nutrient intake during lactation and alterations in milk microbiota composition. However, the effect of such associations on the infant gut microbiota and, furthermore, their consequences in relation to asthma, still remain unclear and require more comprehensive investigations.

This review suggests that maternal life factors (e.g., mode of delivery, antibiotics use and mode of feeding) may modify the associations between maternal nutrition and the infant gut/milk microbiota composition. Overall, maternal dietary patterns during both pregnancy and lactation influence maternal obesity, which directly influences infant gut/milk microbiota. Maternal nutrition may indirectly influence the infant gut/milk microbiota through maternal early life factors. These factors may affect maternal obesity and could directly alter the milk microbiota by influencing the infant gut microbiota. Further studies are needed to examine the potential modification effect caused by these factors in the association of maternal nutrition–infant gut microbiota with subsequent asthma development.

References

1. Ferrante, G.; La Grutta, S. The burden of pediatric asthma. *Front. Pediatr.* **2018**, *6*, 186. [CrossRef] [PubMed]
2. Subbarao, P.; Mandhane, P.J.; Sears, M.R. Asthma: Epidemiology, etiology and risk factors. *Can. Med. Assoc. J.* **2009**, *181*, 181–190. [CrossRef] [PubMed]
3. Thomsen, S.F. Genetics of asthma: An introduction for the clinician. *Eur. Clin. Respir. J.* **2015**, *16*, 2. [CrossRef] [PubMed]
4. Manti, S.; Marseglia, L.; D'Angelo, G. "Cumulative Stress": The effects of maternal and neonatal oxidative stress and oxidative stress-inducible genes on programming of atopy. *Oxid. Med. Cell. Longev.* **2016**, *2016*, 8651820. [CrossRef] [PubMed]
5. Dick, S.; Friend, A.; Dynes, K.; AlKandari, F.; Doust, E.; Cowie, H.; Ayres, J.G.; Turner, S. A systematic review of associations between environmental exposures and development of asthma in children aged up to 9 years. *BMJ Open* **2014**, *4*, e006554. [CrossRef]
6. Johnson, C.C.; Ownby, D.R. The infant gut bacterial microbiota and risk of pediatric asthma and allergic diseases. *Transl. Res.* **2017**, *179*, 60–70. [CrossRef]
7. Stiemsma, L.T.; Turvey, S.E. Asthma and the microbiome: Defining the critical window in early life. *Allergy Asthma Clin. Immunol.* **2017**, *13*, 3. [CrossRef]
8. Frati, F.; Salvatori, C.; Incorvaia, C.; Bellucci, A.; Di Cara, G.; Marcucci, F.; Esposito, S. The role of the microbiome in asthma: The Gut-Lung Axis. *Int. J. Mol. Sci.* **2018**, *20*, 123. [CrossRef]
9. Sokolowska, M.; Frei, R.; Lunjani, N.; Akdis, C.A.; O'Mahony, L. Microbiome and asthma. *Asthma Res. Pract.* **2018**, *4*, 1. [CrossRef]
10. Walker, R.W.; Clemente, J.C.; Peter, I.; Loos, R.J.F. The prenatal gut microbiome: Are we colonized with bacteria in utero? *Pediatr. Obes.* **2017**, *12*, 3–17. [CrossRef]
11. Tanaka, M.; Nakayama, J. Development of the gut microbiota in infancy and its impact on health in later life. *Allergol. Int.* **2017**, *66*, 515–522. [CrossRef] [PubMed]
12. McDonald, B.; D McCoy, K. Maternal microbiota in pregnancy and early life. *Science* **2019**, *365*, 984–985. [CrossRef] [PubMed]
13. Houghteling, P.D.; Walker, W.A. Why is initial bacterial colonization of the intestine important to infants' and children's health? *J. Pediatr. Gastroenterol. Nutr.* **2015**, *60*, 294–307. [CrossRef] [PubMed]
14. Milani, C.; Duranti, S.; Bottacin, F.; Casey, E.; Turroni, F.; Mahony, J.; Belzer, C.; Palacio, S.D.; Montes, S.A.; Mancabelli, L.; et al. The first microbial colonizers of the human Gut: Composition, activities, and health implications of the infant gut microbiota. *Microbiol. Mol. Biol. Rev.* **2017**, *81*, e00036-17. [CrossRef] [PubMed]
15. Perez-Muñoz, M.E.; Arrieta, M.C.; Ramer-Tait, A.E.; Walter, J. A critical assessment of the "sterile womb" and "in utero colonization" hypotheses: Implications for research on the pioneer infant microbiome. *Microbiome* **2017**, *5*, 48. [CrossRef] [PubMed]
16. Van Nimwegen, F.A.; Penders, J.; Stobberingh, E.E.; Postma, D.S.; Koppelman, G.H.; Kerkhof, M.; Reijmerink, N.E.; Dompeling, E.; Brandt, P.A.V.D.; Ferreira, I.; et al. Mode and place of delivery, gastrointestinal microbiota, and their influence on asthma and atopy. *J. Allergy Clin. Immunol.* **2011**, *128*, 948–955. [CrossRef]
17. Arrieta, M.C.; Stiemsma, L.T.; Dimitriu, P.A.; Thorson, L.; Russell, S.; Yurist-Doutsch, S.; Kuzeljevic, B.; Gold, M.J.; Britton, H.; Lefebvre, D.L.; et al. Early infancy microbial and metabolic alterations affect risk of childhood asthma. *Sci. Transl. Med.* **2015**, *7*, 307ra152. [CrossRef]
18. Stokholm, J.; Blaser, M.J.; Thorsen, J.; Rasmussen, M.A.; Waage, J.; Vinding, R.; Schoos, A.-M.M.; Kunøe, A.; Fink, N.R.; Chawes, B.L.; et al. Maturation of the gut microbiome and risk of asthma in childhood. *Nat. Commun.* **2018**, *9*, 141. [CrossRef]
19. Azad, M.B.; Kozyrskyj, A.L. Perinatal programming of asthma: The role of gut microbiota. *Clin. Dev. Immunol.* **2012**, *2012*, 932072. [CrossRef]
20. Sordillo, J.E.; Zhou, Y.; McGeachie, M.J.; Ziniti, J.; Lange, N.; Laranjo, N.; Savage, J.R.; Carey, V.; O'Connor, G.; Sandel, M.; et al. Factors influencing the infant gut microbiome at age 3–6months: Findings from the ethnically diverse Vitamin D Antenatal Asthma Reduction Trial (VDAART). *J. Allergy Clin. Immunol.* **2017**, *139*, 482–491.e14. [CrossRef]

21. Gray, L.E.; O'Hely, M.; Ranganathan, S.; Sly, P.D.; Vuillermin, P. The maternal diet, gut bacteria, and bacterial metabolites during pregnancy influence offspring asthma. *Front. Immunol.* **2017**, *8*, 365. [CrossRef] [PubMed]
22. Douros, K.; Moustaki, M.; Tsabouri, S.; Papadopoulou, A.; Papadopoulos, M.; Priftis, K.N. Prenatal maternal stress and the risk of asthma in children. *Front. Pediatr.* **2017**, *5*, 202. [CrossRef] [PubMed]
23. Koleva, P.T.; Tun, H.M.; Konya, T.; Guttman, D.S.; Becker, A.B.; Mandhane, P.J.; E Turvey, S.; Subbarao, P.; Sears, M.R.; Scott, J.A.; et al. Sex-specific impact of asthma during pregnancy on infant gut microbiota. *Eur. Respir. J.* **2017**, *50*, 1700280. [CrossRef]
24. Tun, H.M.; Konya, T.; Takaro, T.K. Exposure to household furry pets influences the gut microbiota of infant at 3-4 months following various birth scenarios. *Microbiome* **2017**, *5*, 40. [CrossRef] [PubMed]
25. Neerven, R.J.J.V.; Savelkoul, H. Nutrition and allergic diseases. *Nutrients* **2017**, *9*, 762. [CrossRef] [PubMed]
26. Vuillermin, P.J.; Macia, L.; Nanan, R.; Tang, M.L.; Collier, F.; Brix, S. The maternal microbiome during pregnancy and allergic disease in the offspring. *Semin. Immunopathol.* **2017**, *39*, 669–675. [CrossRef]
27. Daïen, C.I.; Pinget, G.V.; Tan, J.K.; Macia, L. Detrimental impact of microbiota-accessible carbohydrate-deprived diet on gut and immune homeostasis: An overview. *Front. Immunol.* **2017**, *8*, 548. [CrossRef]
28. Oddy, W.H. Breastfeeding, childhood asthma, and allergic disease. *Ann. Nutr. Metab.* **2017**, *70*, 26–36. [CrossRef]
29. Azad, M.B.; Coneys, J.G.; Kozyrskyj, A.L.; Field, C.J.; Ramsey, C.D.; Becker, A.B.; Friesen, C.; Abou-Setta, A.M.; Zarychanski, R. Probiotic supplementation during pregnancy or infancy for the prevention of asthma and wheeze: A systematic review and meta-analysis. *Br. Med. J.* **2013**, *347*, f6471. [CrossRef]
30. Cuello-Garcia, C.A.; Fiocchi, A.; Pawankar, R.; Yepes-Nuñez, J.J.; Morgano, G.P.; Zhang, Y.; Ahn, K.; Al-Hammadi, S.; Agarwal, A.; Gandhi, S.; et al. World Allergy Organization-McMaster University Guidelines for Allergic Disease Prevention (GLAD-P): Prebiotics. *World Allergy Organ. J.* **2016**, *9*, 10. [CrossRef]
31. Valentine, G.; Chu, D.M.; Stewart, C.J.; Aagaard, K.M. Relationships between perinatal interventions, maternal-infant microbiomes, and neonatal outcomes. *Clin. Perinatol.* **2018**, *45*, 339–355. [CrossRef] [PubMed]
32. Chu, D.M.; Antony, K.M.; Ma, J.; Prince, A.L.; Showalter, L.; Moller, M.; Aagaard, K.M. The early infant gut microbiome varies in association with a maternal high-fat diet. *Genome Med.* **2016**, *8*, 77. [CrossRef] [PubMed]
33. Lundgren, S.N.; Madan, J.C.; Emond, J.A.; Morrison, H.G.; Christensen, B.C.; Karagas, M.R.; Hoen, A.G. Maternal diet during pregnancy is related with the infant stool microbiome in a delivery mode-dependent manner. *Microbiome* **2018**, *6*, 109. [CrossRef] [PubMed]
34. Simione, M.; Harshman, S.G.; Castro, I.; Linnemann, R.; Roche, B.; Ajami, N.J.; Petrosino, J.F.; Raspini, B.; Portale, S.; A Camargo, C.; et al. Maternal fish consumption in pregnancy is associated with a *Bifidobacterium*-dominant microbiome profile in infants. *Curr. Dev. Nutr.* **2020**, *4*, nzz133. [CrossRef]
35. Van den Elsen, L.W.J.; Garssen, J.; Burcelin, R.; Verhasselt, V. Shaping the gut microbiota by breastfeeding: The gateway to allergy prevention? *Front. Pediatr.* **2019**, *7*, 47. [CrossRef]
36. Cabrera-Rubio, R.; Collado, M.C.; Laitinen, K.; Salminen, S.; Isolauri, E.; Miras, A.D.; Jackson, R.N.; Jackson, S.N.; Goldstone, A.; Olbers, T.; et al. The human milk microbiome changes over lactation and is shaped by maternal weight and mode of delivery. *Am. J. Clin. Nutr.* **2012**, *96*, 544–551. [CrossRef]
37. Khodayar-Pardo, P.; Mira-Pascual, L.; Collado, M.C.; Martínez-Costa, C. Impact of lactation stage, gestational age and mode of delivery on breast milk microbiota. *J. Perinatol.* **2014**, *34*, 599–605. [CrossRef]
38. Kumar, H.; du Toit, E.; Kulkarni, A.; Aakko, J.; Linderborg, K.M.; Zhang, Y.; Nicol, M.P.; Isolauri, E.; Yang, B.; Collado, M.C.; et al. Distinct patterns in human milk microbiota and fatty acid profiles across specific geographic locations. *Front. Microbiol.* **2016**, *7*, 1619. [CrossRef]
39. Gomez-Gallego, C.; Garcia-Mantrana, I.; Salminen, S.; Collado, M.C. The human milk microbiome and factors influencing its composition and activity. *Semin. Fetal Neonatal Med.* **2016**, *21*, 400–405. [CrossRef]
40. Williams, J.E.; Carrothers, J.M.; Lackey, K.A.; Beatty, N.F.; A York, M.; Brooker, S.L.; Shafii, B.; Price, W.J.; Settles, M.L.; A McGuire, M.; et al. Human milk microbial community structure is relatively stable and related to variations in macronutrient and micronutrient intakes in healthy lactating women. *J. Nutr.* **2017**, *147*, 1739–1748.

41. Li, S.W.; Watanabe, K.; Hsu, C.C.; Chao, S.H.; Yang, Z.-H.; Lin, Y.-J.; Chen, C.-C.; Cao, Y.-M.; Huang, H.-C.; Chang, C.-H.; et al. Bacterial composition and diversity in breast milk samples from mothers living in Taiwan and Mainland China. *Front. Microbiol.* **2017** *8*, 965. [CrossRef] [PubMed]
42. Le Doare, K.; Holder, B.; Bassett, A.; Pannaraj, P.S. Mother's milk: A purposeful contribution to the development of the infant microbiota and immunity. *Front. Immunol.* **2018**, *9*, 361. [CrossRef] [PubMed]
43. Moossavi, S.; Sepehri, S.; Robertson, B.; Bode, L.; Goruk, S.; Field, C.J.; Lix, L.M.; De Souza, R.J.; Becker, A.B.; Mandhane, P.J.; et al. Composition and variation of the human milk microbiota are influenced by maternal and early-life factors. *Cell Host Microbe* **2019**, *25*, 324–335. [CrossRef] [PubMed]
44. Hermansson, H.; Kumar, H.; Collado, M.C.; Salminen, S.; Isolauri, E.; Rautava, S. Breast milk microbiota is shaped by mode of delivery and intrapartum antibiotic exposure. *Front. Nutr.* **2019**, *6*, 4. [CrossRef]
45. Ding, M.; Qi, C.; Yang, Z.; Jiang, S.; Bi, Y.; Lai, J.; Sun, J.; Yang, Z. Geographical location specific composition of cultured microbiota and Lactobacillus occurrence in human breast milk in China. *Food Funct.* **2019**, *10*, 554–564. [CrossRef] [PubMed]
46. Robertson, R.C.; Manges, A.R.; Finlay, B.B.; Prendergast, A.J. The human microbiome and child growth—First 1000 days and beyond. *Trends Microbiol.* **2019**, *27*, 131–147. [CrossRef]
47. Derrien, M.; Alvarez, A.S.; de Vos, W.M. The gut microbiota in the first decade of life. *Trends Microbiol.* **2019**, *27*, 997–1010. [CrossRef]
48. Thomson, P.; Medina, D.A.; Garrido, D. Human milk oligosaccharides and infant gut bifidobacteria: Molecular strategies for their utilization. *Food Microbiol.* **2018**, *75*, 37–46. [CrossRef]
49. Musilova, S.; Rada, V.; Vlkova, E.; Bunesova, V. Beneficial effects of human milk oligosaccharides on gut microbiota. *Benef. Microbes* **2014**, *5*, 273–283. [CrossRef]
50. Moossavi, S.; Miliku, K.; Sepehri, S.; Khafipour, E.; Azad, M.B. The prebiotic and probiotic properties of human milk: Implications for infant immune development and pediatric asthma. *Front. Pediatr.* **2018**, *6*, 197. [CrossRef]
51. Koenig, J.E.; Spor, A.; Scalfone, N.; Fricker, A.D.; Stombaugh, J.; Knight, R.D.; Angenent, L.T.; Ley, R.E. Succession of microbial consortia in the developing infant gut microbiome. *Proc. Natl. Acad. Sci. USA* **2011**, *108*, 4578–4585. [CrossRef] [PubMed]
52. Flint, H.J.; Scott, K.P.; Duncan, S.H.; Louis, P.; Damiano-Forano, E. Microbial degradation of complex carbohydrates in the gut. *Gut Microbes* **2012**, *3*, 289–306. [CrossRef] [PubMed]
53. Laursen, M.F.; Bahl, M.I.; Michaelsen, K.F.; Licht, T.R. First Foods and Gut Microbes. *Front. Microbiol.* **2017**, *8*, 356. [CrossRef] [PubMed]
54. Thorburn, A.N.; McKenzie, C.I.; Shen, S.; Stanley, D.; Macia, L.; Mason, L.J.; Roberts, L.K.; Wong, C.H.Y.; Shim, R.; Robert, R.; et al. Evidence that asthma is a developmental origin disease influenced by maternal diet and bacterial metabolites. *Nat. Commun.* **2015**, *6*, 7320. [CrossRef] [PubMed]
55. Dieterich, C.M.; Felice, J.P.; O'Sullivan, E.; Rasmussen, K.M. Breastfeeding and health outcomes for the mother-infant dyad. *Pediatr. Clin.* **2013**, *60*, 31–48. [CrossRef] [PubMed]
56. Fernández, L.; Langa, S.; Martín, V.; Maldonado, A.; Jiménez, E.; Martín, R.; Rodríguez, J.M. The human milk microbiota: Origin and potential roles in health and disease. *Pharmacol. Res.* **2013**, *69*, 1–10. [CrossRef] [PubMed]
57. Padilha, M.; Danneskiold-Samsøe, N.B.; Brejnrod, A.; Hoffmann, C.; Cabral, V.P.; Iaucci, J.D.M.; Sales, C.H.; Fisberg, R.M.; Cortez, R.V.; Brix, S.; et al. The human milk microbiota is modulated by maternal diet. *Microorganisms* **2019**, *7*, 502. [CrossRef]
58. Meyer, K.M.; Mohammad, M.; Bode, L.; Chu, D.M.; Ma, J.; Haymond, M.; Aagaard, K. 20: Maternal diet structures the breast milk microbiome in association with human milk oligosaccharides and gut-associated bacteria. *Am. J. Obstet. Gynecol.* **2017**, *216*, S15. [CrossRef]
59. Edwards, S.M.; Cunningham, S.A.; Dunlop, A.L.; Corwin, E.J. The maternal gut microbiome during pregnancy. *MCN Am. J. Matern. Child Nurs.* **2017**, *42*, 310–317. [CrossRef]
60. García-Mantrana, I.; Bertua, B.; Martínez-Costa, C.; Collado, M.C. Perinatal nutrition: How to take care of the gut microbiota? *Clin. Nutr. Exp.* **2016**, *6*, 3–16. [CrossRef]
61. Chu, D.M.; Meyer, K.M.; Prince, A.L.; Aagaard, K.M. Impact of maternal nutrition in pregnancy and lactation on offspring gut microbial composition and function. *Gut Microbes* **2016**, *7*, 459–470. [CrossRef] [PubMed]
62. Demmelmair, H.; Jiménez, E.; Collado, M.C.; Salminen, S.; McGuire, M.K. Maternal and perinatal factors associated with the human milk microbiome. *Curr. Dev. Nutr.* **2020**, *4*, nzaa027. [CrossRef] [PubMed]

63. Mesa, M.D.; Loureiro, B.; Iglesia, I.; Fernandez Gonzalez, S.; Olivé, E.L.; Garcia-Algar, O.; Solana, M.J.; Perez, M.J.C.; Sainz, T.; Martinez, L.; et al. The evolving microbiome from pregnancy to early infancy: A comprehensive review. *Nutrients* **2020**, *12*, 133. [CrossRef] [PubMed]
64. Koleva, P.T.; Bridgman, S.L.; Kozyrskyj, A.L. The infant gut microbiome: Evidence for obesity risk and dietary intervention. *Nutrients* **2015**, *7*, 2237–2260. [CrossRef] [PubMed]
65. Mulligan, C.M.; Friedman, J.E. Maternal modifiers of the infant gut microbiota: Metabolic consequences. *J. Endocrinol.* **2017**, *235*, R1–R12. [CrossRef]
66. Soderborg, T.K.; Clark, S.E.; Mulligan, C.E.; Janssen, R.C.; Babcock, L.; Ir, D.; Young, B.; Krebs, N.; Lemas, D.J.; Johnson, L.K.; et al. The gut microbiota in infants of obese mothers increases inflammation and susceptibility to NAFLD. *Nat. Commun.* **2018**, *9*, 4462. [CrossRef]
67. Friedman, J.E. The maternal microbiome: Cause or consequence of obesity risk in the next generation? *Obesity* **2017**, *25*, 497–498. [CrossRef]
68. Mitselou, N.; Hallberg, J.; Stephansson, O.; Almqvist, C.; Melén, E.; Ludvigsson, J.F. Cesarean delivery, preterm birth, and risk of food allergy: Nationwide Swedish cohort study of more than 1 million children. *J. Allergy Clin. Immunol.* **2018**, *142*, 1510–1514.e2. [CrossRef]
69. Mueller, N.T.; Whyatt, R.; Hoepner, L.; Oberfield, S.; Dominguez-Bello, M.G.; Widen, E.M.; Hassoun, A.; Perera, F.; Rundle, A. Prenatal exposure to antibiotics, Cesarean section and risk of childhood obesity. *Int. J. Obes.* **2015**, *39*, 665–670. [CrossRef]
70. Loo, E.X.L.; Sim, J.Z.T.; Loy, S.L.; Goh, A.; Chan, Y.H.; Tan, K.H.; Yap, F.; Gluckman, P.D.; Godfrey, K.M.; Van Bever, H.; et al. Associations between caesarean delivery and allergic outcomes: Results from the GUSTO study. *Ann. Allergy Asthma Immunol.* **2017**, *118*, 636–638. [CrossRef]
71. Appleton, J.; Russell, C.G.; Laws, R. Infant formula feeding practices associated with rapid weight gain: A systematic review. *Matern. Child Nutr.* **2018**, *14*, e12602. [CrossRef] [PubMed]
72. Miliku, K.; Azad, M.B. Breastfeeding and the developmental origins of asthma: Current evidence, possible mechanisms, and future research priorities. *Nutrients* **2018**, *10*, 995. [CrossRef] [PubMed]
73. Azad, M.B.; Konya, T.; Maughan, H. Gut microbiota of healthy Canadian infants: Profiles by mode of delivery and infant diet at 4 months. *Can. Med. Assoc. J.* **2013**, *185*, 385–394. [CrossRef] [PubMed]
74. Madan, J.C.; Hoen, A.G.; Lundgrenc, S.N.; Farzan, S.F.; Cottingham, K.L.; Morrison, H.G.; Sogin, M.L.; Li, H.; Moore, J.H.; Karagas, M.R. Effects of Cesarean delivery and formula supplementation on the intestinal microbiome of six-week old infants. *JAMA Pediatr.* **2016**, *170*, 212–219. [CrossRef] [PubMed]
75. Yasmin, F.; Tun, H.M.; Konya, T.B. Cesarean section, formula feeding, and infant antibiotic exposure: Separate and combined impacts on gut microbial changes in later infancy. *Front. Pediatr.* **2017**, *5*, 200. [CrossRef] [PubMed]
76. Liu, Y.; Qin, S.; Song, Y.; Feng, Y.; Lv, N.; Xue, Y.; Liu, F.; Wang, S.; Zhu, B.-L.; Ma, J.; et al. The perturbation of infant gut microbiota caused by cesarean delivery is partially restored by exclusive breastfeeding. *Front. Microbiol.* **2019**, *10*, 598. [CrossRef]

4

Human Milk and Allergic Diseases: An Unsolved Puzzle

Daniel Munblit [1,2,3,*,†], Diego G. Peroni [3,4,†], Alba Boix-Amorós [3,5,†], Peter S. Hsu [3,6,†], Belinda Van't Land [7,8,†], Melvin C. L. Gay [3,9,†], Anastasia Kolotilina [2], Chrysanthi Skevaki [3,10], Robert J. Boyle [1,3,†], Maria Carmen Collado [3,5,†], Johan Garssen [7,11,†], Donna T. Geddes [3,9,†], Ralph Nanan [12,†], Carolyn Slupsky [13,†], Ganesa Wegienka [3,14,15,†], Anita L. Kozyrskyj [16,†] and John O. Warner [1,3,17,†]

1 Department of Paediatrics, Imperial College London, London W2 1NY, UK; r.boyle@nhs.net (R.J.B.); j.o.warner@imperial.ac.uk (J.O.W.)
2 Faculty of Pediatrics, I.M. Sechenov First Moscow State Medical University, 119991 Moscow, Russia; aikolotilina@yandex.ru
3 The In-FLAME Global Network, an Affiliate of the World Universities Network (WUN), West New York, NJ 07093, USA; diego.peroni@unipi.it (D.G.P.); albaboix90@gmail.com (A.B.-A.); peter.hsu@health.nsw.gov.au (P.S.H.); melvin.gay@uwa.edu.au (M.C.L.G.); Chrysanthi.Skevaki@uk-gm.de (C.S.); mcolam@iata.csic.es (M.C.C.); Donna.Geddes@uwa.edu.au (D.T.G.); gwegien1@hfhs.org (G.W.)
4 Department of Clinical and Experimental Medicine, Section of Paediatrics, University of Pisa, 56126 Pisa, Italy
5 Institute of Agrochemistry and Food Technology, National Research Council (IATA-CSIC), 46980 Valencia, Spain
6 Allergy and Immunology, The Kids Research Institute, The Children's Hospital at Westmead, Sydney, NSW 2145, Australia
7 Nutricia Research, 3584 CT Utrecht, The Netherlands; Belinda.vantland@danone.com (B.V.L.); johan.garssen@danone.com (J.G.)
8 Department of Paediatric Immunology, Wilhelmina Children's Hospital, University Medical Centre Utrecht, 3584 EA Utrecht, The Netherlands
9 School of Molecular Sciences, The University of Western Australia, Perth, WA 6009, Australia
10 Institute of Laboratory Medicine and Pathobiochemistry, Molecular Diagnostics, Philipps University Marburg, University Hospital Giessen and Marburg GmbH Baldingerstr, 35043 Marburg, Germany
11 Utrecht Institute for Pharmaceutical Sciences, Faculty of Science, Utrecht University, 3584 CG Utrecht, The Netherlands
12 Charles Perkins Centre Nepean, University of Sydney, Sydney, NSW 2747, Australia; ralph.nanan@sydney.edu.au
13 Department of Nutrition, University of California, Davis, CA 95616-5270, USA; cslupsky@ucdavis.edu
14 Department of Public Health Sciences, Henry Ford Health System, Detroit, MI 48202, USA
15 Center for Urban Responses to Environmental Stressors, Detroit, MI 48202, USA
16 Department of Pediatrics, University of Alberta, Edmonton, AB T6G 1C9, Canada; kozyrsky@ualberta.ca
17 National Institute for Health Research, Collaboration for Leadership in Applied Health Research and Care for NW London, London SW10 9NH, UK
* Correspondence: daniel.munblit08@imperial.ac.uk
† All authors contributed equally to this work.

Abstract: There is conflicting evidence on the protective role of breastfeeding in relation to the development of allergic sensitisation and allergic disease. Studies vary in methodology and definition of outcomes, which lead to considerable heterogeneity. Human milk composition varies both within and between individuals, which may partially explain conflicting data. It is known that human milk composition is very complex and contains variable levels of immune active molecules, oligosaccharides, metabolites, vitamins and other nutrients and microbial content. Existing evidence suggests that modulation of human breast milk composition has potential for preventing allergic diseases in early life. In this review, we discuss associations between breastfeeding/human milk composition and allergy development.

Keywords: breastfeeding; human milk; allergy; allergic diseases; oligosaccharides; microbiome; cytokines; thymus

---

1. Introduction

Over the last few decades there has been a worldwide steady increase in the prevalence of allergic diseases [1]. Commensurate with a decrease in infectious diseases, allergy has become a considerable health/economic burden, most notably in relatively more affluent countries [2]. However, similar trends are starting to be seen in the developing world [3]. Explanations for this virtual allergy pandemic are not entirely clear but the "hygiene hypothesis" [4] remains the most widely quoted theory, explaining allergic disease rise as a mutually counter-regulatory interaction between the immune response to infection and that associated with allergy. Urban affluent lifestyles have been associated with significantly reduced infant exposure to bacterial infection and an altered commensal microbiome leading to a default allergic pattern of immune responses to common environmental ostensibly harmless antigens/allergens. Earlier birth order and/or fewer number of siblings, late or no attendance in day care facilities, and reduced exposure to pets [5] are among factors most commonly associated with allergic disease development. The apparent importance of rural environment exposure has been demonstrated in the study by Sozanska and co-authors [6], showing dramatic changes in community lifestyle leads to increased risk of allergy development. The accession of Poland to the European Union and changes in agricultural policies have resulted in an increase in prevalence of allergic diseases over an eight-year period. Within this timeframe, population contact with domestic animals and unpasteurised milk consumption has significantly declined while allergy rates have risen.

Although the "hygiene hypothesis" provides a mechanistically credible explanation for the rise in allergy prevalence, other societal factors have been brought forward, such as dramatic changes in dietary preferences over the past few decades. The less frequent consumption of fresh fruit, vegetables and fish has lowered fibre intake, and altered omega-3 and omega-6 polyunsaturated fatty acid (PUFA) ratios. Other environmental factors include lack of ultraviolet exposure leading to vitamin D insufficiency, greater exposure to air pollutants such as volatile organic compounds, diesel particulates and ozone, and even, increased exposure to chemical contaminants from packaged foods. Allergy is therefore, perceived as a "modern malady" prompting clinicians, researchers and policy makers around the globe to search for effective primary prevention [7]. Preventative strategies are particularly important for children at high risk of allergy development [8,9], with one or both parents being allergic [10]. It is suggested that the "window of opportunity" for allergy prevention is somewhere within the timeframe between conception and the first six months after birth [7,11,12]. As virtually all association studies do not discriminate between exposures of the mother during pregnancy, and/or lactation, or those directly affecting the infant, it is not possible to attribute a more exact timing of the "window". It is perhaps more likely that a sequence of events during pregnancy and the early months of life combine to alter the risk of allergic sensitization and subsequent disease.

Human milk (HM) should be the main source of nutrition during a critical period of metabolic and immune programming, driven in part by its effects on intestinal function. Accumulated data suggests that a wide range of bioactive factors: such as proteins, polyunsaturated fatty acids, oligosaccharides, microbial content, metabolites, and micronutrients [13] present in HM can influence the infant's gut immune maturation. Chronic allergic diseases are linked with the altered functioning of the innate and adaptive immune systems [14] and evidence suggests that it can be influenced using interventional strategies [15]. Recent research shows that various maternal exposures, such as immunisation, dietary patterns, vitamin D, ω-3 fatty acids and/or probiotics, may influence HM composition and thereby affect infant health. HM composition varies over time from delivery, within and between women, and even within the same feed, which may in part, explain some of the conflicting results of general observational studies regarding the provision of breastfeeding. Although HM constituents will be critical in influencing a range of other aspects of breastfeeding, such as its "exclusivity", the close physical contact during nursing and time of weaning may also have important implications for health and development. However, results are inconsistent between studies, and there is no clear understanding of the pathways linking the intervention with effects on HM composition and health outcomes.

This review summarises existing evidence on breastfeeding and human milk composition in relation to allergic disease development.

2. Breastfeeding and Immunological Outcomes

Many aspects of breastfeeding can potentially influence its health effects [16]. These include duration of breastfeeding, maternal diet during lactation [17], and age at complementary food introduction [18–20], which can all differentially affect how breastfeeding may act on child health and immune development. Breastfeeding alters a child's gut microbiome and subsequent immune development [21,22] and influences risk of respiratory infections through maternal antibody transfer [21]. It also impacts childhood nutrient intake such as vitamin D. The latter nutrient has been of particular interest because there are vitamin D receptors on many immune active cells and most notably on regulatory T-cells. Insufficiency is associated with reduced T-cell regulation of immune hyper-sensitive responses [23]. Data from some studies suggests that breastfeeding may impact immune organ functioning, with a difference in thymus involution seen between breastfed and formula fed children (discussed in more detail in Section 2.3).

It is well established that breastfeeding confers protection against both short-term adverse outcomes including reduced morbidity and mortality from neonatal infections) and long-term events including reduction in blood pressure, type 2 diabetes, increased IQ and better educational achievements in later life (even when adjusted for family socio-economic status [24]) [25]. A World Health Organisation (WHO) report suggests that there is a lower long term morbidity from gastrointestinal and allergic diseases in infants who were exclusively breastfed for 6 months in comparison to non-breastfed children [26]. Moreover, breastfeeding seems to play an important role at a time of complementary food introduction. Thus, during introduction of gluten into the infant diet it may reduce the risk of coeliac disease, suggesting important interactions between BM components, dietary antigens, and gut associated lymphoid tissue (GALT) [27]. However, this protective effect on coeliac disease remains uncertain, as studies have produced conflicting evidence [28]. Similar associations of reduced allergy in infants who have continued being breastfed during weaning have been reported [29]. Based on these data, current UNICEF and WHO recommendations are "every infant should be exclusively breastfed for the first six months of life, with continued breastfeeding for up to two years or longer" [30].

Despite some high-quality research, there is conflicting evidence on the protective role of breastfeeding in relation to many non-communicable diseases, including immunological (allergic and autoimmune) outcomes. It has been hypothesised that the mixed results may be in part due to variations in HM composition as it is known to contain a large variety of immune active components [13] which are present in differing concentrations [31]. Which factors are able to provide sufficient influence on short and long-term health outcomes in infants is still a matter of discussion, despite a number of studies attempting to address this question.

2.1. *Importance of Breastfeeding Duration*

When evaluating the relationship between breastfeeding duration and health outcomes it is important to have clear definitions for breastfeeding duration. It is usually defined as total breastfeeding duration, the time between birth and complete cessation of breastfeeding; while exclusive breastfeeding duration is the time between birth and first introduction of a non-breastmilk feed. Feeding expressed breastmilk, fresh or frozen, by bottle, and use of donor breastmilk, given directly or fresh or frozen by bottle, are variably included within these definitions of total or exclusive breastfeeding, depending on the focus of the research study. Use of the term exclusive breastfeeding is problematic in that it combines two separate interventions—timing of first solid ('complementary') food introduction, and use of a breastmilk substitute (formula milk). In general the evidence that early formula milk introduction is not optimal for development of infants health is stronger than the evidence that early complementary food introduction causes harm. It also depends on the type of allergy developed and exposure of allergens involved. This discrepancy has been highlighted by recent data showing that early complementary food introduction has defined health benefits—recent studies show that the phenomenon of oral tolerance induction, known for over 100 years to occur in animal experiments, also occurs in humans [7,29,32–34]. Oral tolerance occurs when early and sustained feeding of a food antigen reduces risk for developing food allergy to that antigen. This phenomenon has been shown to occur in humans for the two most common food allergies affecting young children: egg and peanut allergy [34]. However it is important to underline that tolerance development was only demonstrated in the per protocol and not ITT group in the latter study and further research is needed to make definitive conclusions.

This first sign that early introduction of complementary foods may be beneficial to infant health, suggests that future studies will need to more clearly distinguish timing of infant formula introduction and timing of complementary food introduction when evaluating relationships between exclusive breastfeeding duration and allergic disease risk.

2.2. Breastfeeding and Allergic Diseases

At the beginning of the last century, Grulee and Sanford suspected a link between HM substitute feeding and a higher incidence of eczema [35]. Since then many prospective and retrospective observational studies have tested breastfeeding associations with the onset of allergic disease, providing mixed results for eczema [19–21,36–49] sensitisation [21,37,42,46–58] and asthma [19–21,36,42,47,48,59–66]. Messages culminating from these studies range from a protective effect of breastfeeding [67], to a higher risk of atopy [68], or no significant effect [69]. Despite the conflicting evidence, several clinical societies have made recommendations regarding the duration and type of breastfeeding. As mentioned above, the WHO recommends exclusive breast feeding for at least 6 months in all infants with continued breastfeeding up to 2 years or longer if a mother wishes to do so [30].

The first efforts to systematically review existing evidence on breastfeeding associations with the selected eczema [70] and asthma [71], were made by Gdalevich and Mimouni two decades ago. Later, additional systematic reviews and meta-analyses were undertaken, assessing worldwide evidence [26,72,73], or focusing on data from developed countries [74]. The main challenge in the meta-analyses of these data was significant heterogeneity in the definitions of breastfeeding, which are not always consistent with WHO recommendations, and in phenotyping of for health outcomes. In the most recent systematic review which was published just two years ago [75], Lodge and colleagues reported on 4 different definitions of eczema, food allergy and asthma, and 3 definitions of allergic rhinitis used across studies [75], with differing breastfeeding exclusiveness and duration creating even more uncertainty.

Assessment of breastfeeding's potential to prevent allergic disease in observational studies is not an easy task as several factors, such as socioeconomic status, positive allergy family history, early exposure to pets and timing of solid food introduction, alongside variations in HM composition, are all sources of bias. Prospective randomised studies are needed to provide solid evidence of causal relationships, however such studies would be unethical. The sole large randomized controlled trial used an innovative approach in a country with a very low breast feeding rate and investigators randomised mothers to a breast feeding promotion group or continued standard practice. The intervention significantly increased breast feeding rates and facilitated evaluation of the breastfeeding associations with health outcomes in Belarus [76]. There was a reduced risk of early eczema (Odds Ratio (OR) 0.54, 95% CI 0.31–0.95) with breastfeeding but no long-term protection against eczema, allergic rhinitis and asthma at 6.5 years of age, despite the long duration and exclusivity of breastfeeding observed in this trial [77]. However, the extent to which WHO recommendations delayed introduction of non-milk food sources at a critical period where tolerance induction may be important to prevent allergy is uncertain [78].

2.2.1. Eczema

Most of the studies assessing breastfeeding impact on eczema development come from the cross-sectional studies or birth cohorts. The major weakness of collected data is related to a long retrospective recall period and lack of adjustment for potential confounding factors, such as allergy family history [75]. Authors of The International Study of Asthma and Allergies in Childhood (ISAAC), a large observational study assessing more than two hundred thousand children worldwide, failed to find evidence of a breastfeeding protective effect on eczema development at 6–7 years of age (OR 1.05, 95% CI 0.97–1.12), but reported some protection against severe eczema (OR 0.79, 95% CI 0.66–0.95) [79]. Outcomes of a systematic review and meta-analysis, covering literature up to 2014, suggested that children below 2 years of age who were exclusively breastfed for more than 3–4 months were are at lower risk (OR 0.74, 95% CI 0.57–0.97) of eczema development; however, this protective effect was no longer evident after the age of 2 (OR 1.07, 95% CI 0.98–1.16) [75]. The authors highlighted a potential high risk of bias from smaller studies showing more significant protective effects.

2.2.2. Food Allergy

Studies assessing the association between breastfeeding and food allergy contribute conflicting results, with some cohort studies reporting a reduced risk of food allergy development in a general population [80,81] and in high risk children [82], with others suggesting a greater risk after breastfeeding [83,84]. The most recent meta-analysis showed no statistically significant association between breastfeeding and food allergy development (OR 1.02, 95% CI 0.88–1.18). Assessment of food allergy is not straightforward in the context of a clinical trial, as the gold standard for confirming the diagnosis is the double-blind food challenge, which is not always a viable option for study participants. In many studies, a combination of a clinical history and skin prick test (SPT) or serum IgE testing is used as surrogate markers of a diagnosis of food allergy with inevitable high heterogeneity. Hence, the primary goal for future research should be harmonization of the outcome definition [75]. Recent clinical trials showing benefits in early food introduction (from 3 to 4 months of age), in parallel with breastfeeding, may indicate a worthwhile strategy to decrease risks of food allergy development. This has been driven by recent studies, such as the Learning Early About Peanut Allergy (LEAP) and Enquiring About Tolerance (EAT) trials [29,33], suggesting that in some children, early introduction (before child age 6 months) of peanut and/or egg protein reduces the risk of allergy to these foods [7].

2.2.3. Asthma

More than 15 years ago, Gdalevich and Mimouni reported a link between breastfeeding and lowered asthma prevalence in children (OR 0.70, 95% CI 0.60–0.81) [71]. This association has been further confirmed in two subsequent meta-analyses (OR 0.78, 95% CI 0.74–0.84] [73] and OR 0.88, 95% CI 0.82–0.95 [75]). Biological plausibility or coherence in published evidence for a role of breastfeeding in protecting against asthma development includes its demonstrated benefit in reducing the number of respiratory tract infections in early infancy, especially among infants in middle- and low-income countries [75]. In addition, exclusive breastfeeding reduces the duration of hospital admission, risk of respiratory failure and the requirement for supplemental oxygen in infants hospitalized with bronchiolitis [85,86]. Some of the described protective effects may be mediated through an antiviral mechanism or non-specific enhancement/maturation of the infant immune system.

However, there is significant heterogeneity (study design, outcome definition, country development) between studies reporting an inverse association between breastfeeding infants and asthma development. Some of the differences can be explained by variations in the definitions for breastfeeding exclusivity and duration, and methods to diagnose asthma in children [87]. It is known that many infants who wheeze in the first years of life do not develop asthma in later life [88], but wheeze is often used as the diagnostic marker of asthma. There are several notable large prospective birth cohorts, such as Avon Longitudinal Study of Parents and Children (ALSPAC) [50], Prevention and Incidence of Asthma and Mite Allergy (PIAMA) [89] and the cross-sectional International Study of Asthma and Allergies in Childhood (ISAAC) [90] study, with data from these studies considered of higher quality [75]. The protective effects of breastfeeding on asthma are more apparent in recent studies, perhaps due to improvements in methodology [73,75]. It is worth noting that subgroup analysis shows a greater protective effect of breastfeeding in middle to low income countries where allergy is less common [75]. It seems likely that the major effect is on respiratory infection induced wheeze rather than atopic asthma. Future studies will need to phenotype and endotype asthma more precisely.

2.3. Breastfeeding, Thymus and Immunity

The thymus is an essential organ for generation of T cell immunity and tolerance. Lymphoid progenitors from the bone marrow migrate to the thymus, where a series of stringent positive and negative selection processes take place [91]. These processes are important for the production of functional T cells, which are able to recognize and respond to foreign/microbial antigens presented by the MHC in the periphery, but also Foxp3+ regulatory T (Treg) cells, which mediate immune tolerance to self and a variety of self and foreign antigens [92]. Not surprisingly, thymic aplasia as seen in DiGeorge syndrome is associated with immune deficiency and immune dysregulation [93]. Furthermore, in all vertebrates the thymus naturally shrinks in size with age. This process of thymic involution is poorly understood to date [94] but impacts directly on thymic output [95].

Thymic size can also be influenced by a variety of factors. Prenatally, maternal factors such as preeclampsia has been associated with reduced thymic diameter [96], although the mechanism and the consequences of this need to be further investigated. Postnatally, various events such as acute stress are known to reduce the thymic size [97].

Breastfeeding on the other hand, has been associated with increased thymic size. At 4 months of age, the thymus size (as assessed by ultrasound) in exclusively breast-fed infants was more than double the size of formula fed infants, an effect that persisted at least until 10 months of age [98]. A further study revealed that persistent breast feeding between 8 and 10 months also correlated with increased thymus size in a "dose dependent" manner [99]. Although the immune implication of this remains unclear, a subsequent study showed a correlation between breast feeding and peripheral CD4 and CD8 T cell counts and proportion [100]. The importance of thymic tissue for T cell immunity is further supported by a study showing that partial or total thymectomy in infants undergoing cardiac surgery was associated with lower T cell numbers and immunoglobulin levels later in life [101]. The mechanism by which breastfeeding may influence thymus size is unclear. However, one study conducted in rural Gambia suggested that the reduced thymic size and output in exclusively breastfed infants born in the "hungry season" compared to "harvest season" was associated with reduced Interleukin 7 (IL7) levels in the breast milk [102]. As IL7 is critical for thymopoiesis [103], it seems plausible that this cytokine may influence thymic size. However, other breast milk cytokines and metabolic components need to be considered as well.

In addition, breast milk is known to shape the infant's gut microbiome [104]. The gut microbiome is the main source of bacterial metabolites such as short chain fatty acids, which have been shown to play a central role in T cell development and differentiation [105]. Hence, a mechanistic explanation implicating a beneficial role of breastfeeding on the infant's gut microbiome may be an alternative explanation for enhanced thymic size in breastfed infants.

Overall, evidence suggests that breastfeeding influences thymic size. However, evidence is lacking regarding the mechanism and the immune impact of this observation. Future longitudinal cohort studies are required to address this. These studies should include good measures of thymic output such as assays of T cell receptor excision circles (TREC) and thorough immune phenotyping of T cell subsets, gut microbiome profiling as well as good clinical data on immune outcomes.

3. Human Milk Composition and Allergy

Human milk is the earliest and should be the only source of nutrition during first few months of life, a crucial period for infant immune system development and metabolic programming for lifelong health and development. Many biologically active components are found in HM, and there is some evidence, arising from the studies in humans, suggesting maternal exposures can change both HM composition and subsequent infant health outcomes [78,106–108].

3.1. Human Milk Immunological Composition

Variations in breast milk immune composition (and the infant's response to HM immune constituents) may also explain some of the conflicting results of studies evaluating whether prolonged exclusive breast-feeding can prevent allergic disease [109,110]. Human milk is a "soup" full of immune active factors, including leukocytes (polymorphonuclear neutrophils, monocytes/macrophages, lymphocytes), which potentially may influence immunological outcomes in infancy and early childhood. It contains over 250 potentially immunologically active proteins, including a wide variety of cytokines, inflammatory mediators, signalling molecules, and soluble receptors [13], as well as prebiotic oligosaccharides: polyunsaturated fatty acids (PUFAs) [111]: and a diverse microbiome [112], all of which are involved in complex interactions which could influence immune outcomes.

Colostrum (early human milk, produced during the first days of life) is very rich in immunologically active molecules that are present in much higher concentrations than mature HM [106,113–116]. The levels of growth factors in colostrum decline very rapidly, which may be partially explained by increasing dilution, as in the first days of life the infant's volume requirements are low [116]. As HM matures, the relative concentrations of the immunologically active molecules decrease as the volume and nutritional requirements of the infant increase.

There is only limited literature on the relationship between maternal diet (including intervention trials), human milk immunological composition, and allergy development [117,118]. The main studies are summarised in Tables 1 and 2.

Table 1. Maternal dietary interventions and human milk immunological composition.

Study	Intervention	Time of HM Collection Postpartum	HM Composition Changes
		Fish Oil and Fresh Fish	
Hawkes 2001 [119]	Fish oil supplementation	5 weeks	no significant influence on TGF-β1 and TGF-β2
Dunstan 2004 [120]	Fish oil supplementation	3 days	no significant influence on IgA and sCD14 levels
Urwin 2012 [121]	Farmed salmon supplementation	1, 5 and 28 days	no significant influence on TGF-β1, TGF-β2 and sCD14
		Probiotics	
Bottcher 2008 [122]	Probiotic supplementation (*L. reuteri*)	3 days and 1 month	↓ TGF-β2 and ↑ IL-10 (*borderline significance*) in 3 day samples no difference in IgA, SIgA, TGF-β1, TNF, sCD14 in 1 month samples
Prescott 2008 [123]	Probiotic supplementation (*L. rhamnosus* or *B. lactis*)	7 days	↑ TGF-β1 in HM from *B. lactis* group no significant influence on IL6, IL10, IL13, IFN-γ, TNF-α, sCD14, total IgA
Boyle 2011 [124]	Probiotic supplementation (*L. rhamnosus*)	7 and 28 days	↓ sCD14 and IgA levels in HM from *L. rhamnosus GG* group no significant influence of on TGF-β1

Table 1. *Cont.*

Study	Intervention	Time of HM Collection Postpartum	HM Composition Changes
Hoppu 2012 [125]	Diet and Probiotic supplementation (*L. rhamnosus* and *B. lactis*)	colostrum (after birth) and 1 month	↑ IL-2, IL-4, IL10 TNF-α and total *n*-3 fatty acids in probiotic group no significant influence on IFN-γ and IL6
Kuitunen 2012 [126]	Probiotic supplementation (A combination of 2 species of *L. rhamnosus, B. breve and P. freudenreichii*)	0–3 days and 3 months	↑ IL-10 and ↓ casein IgA antibodies in probiotics group
Savilahti 2015 [127]	Probiotic supplementation (A combination of 2 species of *L. rhamnosus, B. breve and P. freudenreichii*)	0–3 days and 3 months	no significant influence on sCD14, HBD2 and HNP1–3
		Other Interventions	
Linnamaa 2013 [128]	Blackcurrant seed oil	after delivery and 3 months	↑ IFN-γ and ↓ IL-4 in blackcurrant seed oil group no significant influence on IL-5, IL-10, IL-12 and TNF levels
Nikniaz 2013 [129]	Synbiotic	3 and 4 months	↑ IgA and TGF-β2 in synbiotic group no significant influence on TGF-β1

"↑"—stands for increased levels of a particular factor and "↓"—stands for decreased levels of a particular factor.

Table 2. Human milk immunological composition and allergy development.

Study	Allergic Outcomes Assessed	Relationship between Human Milk Composition and Outcomes	
		Human Milk Composition Factors	***Outcome of Influence***
Kalliomaki 1999 [130]	Eczema (up to 12 months)	↑ TGF-β1 and TGF-β2 (colostrum)	higher post weaning-onset atopic disease
Jones 2002 [131]	Eczema (up to 6 months)	↓ sCD14 (3 months HM)	higher eczema incidence at 6 months of age
Bottcher 2003 [132]	Allergic sensitisation (up to 2 years) Salivary IgA (up to 2 years) Eczema (up to 2 years)	IL-4, IL-5, IL-6, IL-8, IL-10, IL-13, IL-16, IFN-γ, TGF-β1, TGF-β2, RANTES, eotaxin or SIgA (colostrum and 1 month HM)	no significant influence on atopy and/or allergy
Oddy 2003 [133]	Asthma-like symptoms (up to 12 months)	↑ TGF-β1 (2 weeks HM) TNF-α, sCD14 and IL10 (2 weeks HM)	lower risk of wheeze in infancy no significant association with infant wheeze
Savilahti 2005 [134]	Allergic sensitisation (up to 4 years) Eczema (up to 4 years)	↓ IgA casein antibodies and sCD14 (colostrum)	higher incidence of atopy development
Snijders 2006 [135]	Eczema (up to 12 months) Allergic sensitisation (up to 2 years) Wheezing (up to 2 years)	TGF-β1, IL-10, IL-12 and sCD14 (1 month HM)	no significant influence on any of the atopic manifestations
Bottcher 2008 [122]	Allergic sensitisation (up to 2 years) Eczema (up to 2 years)	↓ TGF-β2 (colostrum)	lower incidence of sensitisation during the first 2 years of life a trend of protective effect on eczema development
Kuitunen 2012 [126]	Allergic diseases (up to 5 years) Eczema (up to 5 years) Allergic sensitisation (up to 2 years)	↑ TGF-β2 (3 month HM) IL-10 and TGF-β2 (3 month HM)	higher risk of allergic disease and eczema at 2 years of age no significant association with allergic outcomes at 2 and 5 years of age
Soto-Ramirez 2012 [136]	Asthma-like symptoms (up to 12 months)	infants in the highest quartile of IL-5 and IL-13 (2 weeks HM)	higher risk of asthma-like symptoms development
Ismail 2013 [137]	Eczema (up to 12 months) Allergic sensitisation (up to 12 months)	TGF-β1, sCD14, total IgA (7 and 28 days HM)	no significant association with any of the atopic manifestations

Table 2. *Cont.*

Study	Allergic Outcomes Assessed	Relationship between Human Milk Composition and Outcomes	
		Human Milk Composition Factors	*Outcome of Influence*
Orivuori 2014 [138]	Eczema (up to 4 years) Asthma (up to 6 years) Allergic sensitisation (up to 6 years)	↑ sIgA (2 months HM) TGF-β1 (2 months HM) sIgA (2 months HM)	lower eczema incidence up to the age of 2 years no significant association with the outcomes no significant association with atopy or asthma up to the age of 6
Savilahti 2015 [127]	Allergic diseases (up to 5 years)	↑ sCD14 (3 months HM)	higher incidence of allergic sensitisation and eczema
Jepsen 2016 [58]	Eczema (up to 3 years) Recurrent wheeze (up to 3 years)	↑ IL-1β (1 month HM) CXCL10, TNF-α, CCL2, CCL4, CCL5, CCL17, CCL22, CCL26, TSLP, IL17, CXCL1, CXCL8, TGF-β1 (1 month HM)	lower eczema incidence up to the age of 3 years no significant association with eczema or wheeze
Munblit 2017 [139]	Eczema-like symptoms (up to 6 months) Wheeze (up to 6 months) Food allergy parental-reported (up to 6 months)	↑ TGF-β2 (1 month HM) detectable IL-13 (colostrum) detectable IL-13 (1 month HM) HGF, TGF-β1, TGF-β3, IL-2, IL-4, IL-5, IL-10, IFN-γ, IL-12 (colostrum and 1 month HM)	higher risk of eczema lower risk of food allergy lower risk of eczema no significant association with eczema, wheeze or food allergy

"↑"—stands for increased levels of a particular factor and "↓"—stands for decreased levels of a particular factor

3.1.1. Immune Composition and Allergy

Among the immunological markers assessed in HM, TGF-β is probably the most studied to date. The systematic review by Oddy and Rosales assessed relationships between TGF-β in human milk and immunological outcomes in infants and children [140]. Two-thirds the studies selected for this review found an association between higher TGF-β1 or TGF-β2 levels in colostrum or mature milk and reduced risk of atopic outcomes in the infant. The authors suggested that TGF-β found in human milk may play a role in homeostasis maintenance in the intestine, regulating inflammation and subsequently promoting oral tolerance which may reduce the risk of allergy development [140].

A few studies focused on eczema, found increased TGF-β1 and/or TGF-β2 in HM associated with this skin disease onset in infants [122,126,130,139]. However, contrasting results of other studies do not allow final conclusions on the influence of TGF-β on eczema development [132,135,137,138]. Oddy and co-authors reported increased TGF-β1 levels in breast milk to have some protective effect against wheeze development in infancy [133] but this conflicts with two other large cohort studies [135,138]. As it is assumed that TGF-β has biological relevance and is active in the infant gut [141], these results suggest that TGF-β plays an important role and may be a missing component of progression from allergic sensitisation to allergy disease in early life, but inconsistency in results prevents us from making any definitive statements. Differences in the outcomes can be affected by the stage of lactation when samples were collected.

Another immune active molecule that is of interest is soluble CD14, a bacterial pattern recognition receptor for cell wall components such as lipopolysaccharide. It is primarily expressed on the surface of monocytes, macrophages and neutrophils as membrane CD14 [142,143] but is also found in HM in its soluble form—sCD14. In all the studies levels of sCD14 in HM were very high as this immune active molecule is amongst those immune factors actively excreted into HM. CD14 may play an important role, providing protection against subsequent allergy manifestation [144–146]. More than a decade ago, Jones and co-authors showed that low sCD14 levels in mature milk were associated with eczema development [131] and then Savilahti reported similar trends for colostrum [134]. Later studies, however, failed to reproduce these results and did not report any protective effect of this soluble receptor on eczema [135,137]. The conflict between the outcomes of the studies may be a consequence of a difference in CD14 genotype with breastfeeding being associated with a decreased risk of atopic sensitisation in children with a CT/CC genotype [52]. We now recognise eczema as a consequence of genetically determined skin barrier defects with allergy being a likely secondary outcome. Phenotyping and genotyping eczema in relation to breast feeding therefore becomes a priority.

There is a general agreement between studies suggesting that levels of other human milk immune active molecules, cytokines in particular, are not associated with atopy and/or allergy development in early life [126,132,135,137]. The only outlying results come from the recent paper by Jepsen and co-authors, suggesting that high levels of IL1β in mature milk are associated with lower risk of eczema by the age of 3 [58] and Jarvinen et al. showing that networks of pro-inflammatory and regulatory cytokines in HM are associated with tolerance to cow's milk [147]. As many cytokines exist in very low concentrations in HM, the sensitivity of the assays is critical and many studies report a high proportion of undetectable levels in their samples [58,148,149]. This may explain lack of conclusive data on HM cytokines association with immunological outcomes. Furthermore, if there are only trace levels of these mediators they are unlikely to have significant biological activity. Future studies will need to assess biological activity alongside assays of concentrations.

Most of the studies were aimed at allergic sensitisation, eczema, early wheezing and/or asthma and allergic rhinitis development as the main phenotypic outcomes which allow for some comparison. However, significant methodological heterogeneity between the studies, especially with regards to the stage of HM collection and outcome definitions, are the main obstacles on the way to any meta-analysis of up to date data in this field. Despite these difficulties it is apparent that certain factors of interest in HM may play a role in allergic sensitisation and/or allergy prevention. The most promising HM components are TGF-β, sCD14, and particularly their relationship with HM oligosaccharides (HMOs) and microbiome, interactions which have not been extensively studied and may represent a prime area for future research. In view of the large number of potentially immune-active constituents in breast milk, investigation of only a limited range of constituents may well produce conflicting results. There is a lack of studies, attempting to assess HM as a whole, rather than focusing on single components. In other words, the "soup" is likely more important than individual ingredients.

3.1.2. Potential for Immunological Composition Alteration via Dietary Interventions

Given the observations discussed above there is the intriguing possibility for interventions which modify maternal immunity to impact infant immune responses and allergic disease in offspring [131,134]. With the development of the 'hygiene hypothesis' many focused their research on the protective effects of environmental exposures during pregnancy and early life, during a period of time when infant gut colonization and maturation of the immune system takes place. Despite a number of birth-cohort studies, the ability to change human milk composition remains a "grey area" in existing knowledge and more hypothesis driven research is required before large population intervention trials can begin.

Existing data provides evidence that HM composition is highly variable within the same individual and between women. It has been shown that maternal lifestyle (dietary habits, physical activity, place of residence) can have a significant influence on HM biologically active components [106–108,116]. These findings have motivated a number of intervention trials aiming to prevent allergy development in early infancy.

There are many trials of probiotic administration, as single-entity products of a specific strain or mixtures, in the prevention of allergy development, with cumulative meta-analytic evidence suggesting some protection against eczema [150]. Prescott et al. observed higher levels of TGF-β1 and IgA in human milk of mothers receiving B. lactis HN019 probiotics, and higher IgA levels alone in those receiving *L. Rhamnosus* HN001. In contrast probiotic supplementation did not seem to have an effect on the rest of BM immunological profile (IL-13, IFN-γ, IL-6, TNF-a, IL-10 and sCD14) [123]. Two other studies of probiotic use during pregnancy reported no effect on TGF-β levels in HM [124,151] and they were in opposition to findings by Rautava and co-authors [152]. Heterogeneity of methods again confounds attempts at meta-analysis.

Another potential intervention approach is the use of prebiotics. Prebiotics are non-digestible food components that may confer benefit by providing the substrates for normal bacterial growth the gut. It is more common now to see prebiotics added to formula milk. It is unclear whether prebiotics are capable of modifying HM composition or influencing subsequent allergy development in both high risk and general populations [153].

PUFAs (e.g., ω-3 and ω-6 fatty acids) are an essential part of HM composition and, as a logical investigation, researchers have attempted to influence PUFA levels in HM by means of intervention, selecting fish oil or whole fish as a main source of PUFA. Some of these studies also evaluated HM immunological composition. Data from several intervention trials showed no apparent evidence for the impact of fish consumption on immune active molecules in HM [119–121]. Another source rich in ω-3 and ω-6 fatty acids is blackcurrant seed oil. A Finnish study reported lower levels of IL-4 and increased IFN-γ in HM following black currant seed oil consumption, with no differences in IL-5, IL-10, IL-12 and TNF levels, in comparison to an olive oil fed group [128].

Overall, there is some evidence that probiotic [123,124,152] administration to pregnant and lactating women, or a diet with a high fish intake [121] alters breast milk immune composition. Although the specific changes identified are not always correlated with clinical outcomes, maternal supplementation during pregnancy and lactation to enhance human milk "quality" may have a beneficial influence on health outcomes, and modulation of breast milk composition is one possible mechanism [154] (see Table 2).

3.2. *Human Milk Oligosaccharides*

3.2.1. The Fascinating Complexity of Human Milk Oligosaccharides

Unique to HM is the complexity and abundance of HMOs consisting of both short-chain as well as long-chain oligosaccharide structures in a unique ratio based on molecular size (roughly 9:1 respectively). Together with specific metabolites derived from bacterial fermentation, the HMOs play a key role in microbiome development and building a healthy immune system, creating a fit and resilient immune system in early and later life [155]. It is important to realize that the complex HMO composition is determined by genetic polymorphisms and activity of the secretor fucosyltransferase2 gene (FUT2), the *Lewis* gene (FUT3), and is regulated by glycosyl-transferases within the mammary gland. Differences in genetically determined glycosyl-transferase patterns affect HMO amount and composition between mothers and during lactation [156]. The presence or absence of α1,2-linked fucosylated epitopes in secretions, including saliva and milk, defines secretor and non-secretors respectively. Consequently, the secretor-phenotype distribution differs among populations [157,158]. The provision of secretor type related complex mixtures of HMOs, have been associated with a direct protection against infections [159] and may be linked to a reduction in allergic disease incidence in breast-fed infants later in life [46].

The basic HMO structure is fucosylated and/or sialylated, resulting in respectively neutral and acidic oligosaccharide structures within short- as well as long-chain structures. In addition to the inter-individual genetic variation, the total HMO concentration varies during lactation which normally provides the optimal needs over time. Colostrum contains approximately 20–25 g/L HMOs, whereas mature HM has declining HMO concentrations to 5–15 g/L [160,161]. 2′-Fucosyllactose (2′-FL) is a disaccharide which is thought to be the most abundant oligosaccharide with a concentration ranging from 0.06 to 4.65 g/L [157,158]. Each HMO is structurally unique and effects of individual structures may not be universal to all HMOs, therefore understanding the balanced complex mixture is of considerable importance.

Although the protective capacity of HM against infections within infants is clearly observed, the possible benefit for the prevention of immune related disorders such as allergy remains controversial [135,162,163]. Any discordance between the early developmental requirements for an infant's immune development and the dynamic nature of HM constituents may possibly contribute to the development of allergic diseases [162]. Whether observed effects are derived from direct interaction with immune cells or indirectly through the alterations in microbiome composition and change in derivatives thereof remains unknown. It is clear however, that the microbiota composition and activity can have an influence on the development of allergy, more specifically regulatory T cell development is strongly influenced by the microbial composition, and therefore subject to modulation by dietary intervention and specific oligosaccharides [164–166]. Several studies have shown that the composition of the gut microbiome differs significantly between those with allergy and/or allergic disease and those without [167–171]. How a microbiome composition becomes dysbiotic and thereby leads to the development of immune related disorders such as allergy is hitherto not fully understood; however, it is thought that early-life ecological succession of mucosal colonization occurs concomitantly with development, expansion, and education of the mucosal immune system [172]. Indeed, gnotobiotic mouse studies have demonstrated that there is a critical window of time for immune development, after which intestinal immune development cannot be fully achieved [173–175].

3.2.2. Shaping the Microbial Balance in Early Life

The question of how optimal early-life microbial ecological succession occurs is a topic of intense interest. Once HMOs are formed, only those bacteria that possess the necessary enzymes (incl. glycosyl hydrolases) can cleave and utilize these oligosaccharides [176]. Members of the *Bacteroidaceae* and *Bifidobacteriaceae* families have been shown to consume HMOs, including several *Bifidobacteria* which have the sialidases and glycosidases necessary to internalize and catabolize HMOs [177–181]. What this means is that for breast-fed infants, *bifidobacteria* have the capability to preferentially colonize the infant GI tract by the third month of life [177]. In addition, it was recently shown in a mouse study that the combination of *B. infantis* with HMO decreased GI inflammation and permeability [182]. Other mouse studies revealed that oral administration of *Bifidobacteria* is able to modulate inflammation associated with allergy [171,183,184]. However, the total HM oligosaccharide composition is likely to be very important and it should be realized that individual oligosaccharides in HM might have their own unique function on microbes, immune cells and epithelial cells.

Given that maternal secretor status impacts the bifidobacterial community structure of the infant gut [185], it can be hypothesized that a combination of HMOs with specific bacteria are able to modulate gut immunity and gut integrity. Additional roles of fucosylated and sialyated HMOs are related to the common structural motifs they share with glycans on the gut epithelia that are known receptors for pathogens. It is thought that HMOs competitively interact with pathogens, preventing adhesion and biofilm formation on the gut epithelium [186–188]. Together with their ability to only be fermented by specific bacteria, HMOs therefore play an important role in shaping early gut microbial succession. The nature of this succession, and exactly how different oligosaccharides function in this context, are questions that remain to be elucidated.

As previously discussed, there have been conflicting reports regarding the relationship between breastfeeding and development of allergy [19,117,189,190], and it may be that it is the combination of oligosaccharides and bacteria that shape immunity. Indeed, it was recently reported that infants born by caesarean section with a high risk of allergies had a lower risk of IgE-associated eczema at 2 years, but this association was not observed at 5 years [46]. In addition, prebiotic oligosaccharides together with *Bifidobacteria* have recently shown in caesarean-delivered infants to be able to modulate the microbial composition which was associated with the emulation of the gut physiological environment observed in vaginally delivered infants [191,192]. Moreover, epidemiological studies have frequently shown that there is a clear associational link between perinatal factors, such as breastfeeding, caesarean delivery, and antibiotic use, and the programming of intestinal inflammatory disorders. However, more work needs to be done to fully understand how HMOs and allergy development are related.

3.2.3. HMOs Are Directly Involved in Early Life Immune Development

How the complete mixture of and/or specific HM oligosaccharides are able to beneficially regulate gut microbiota composition, maintain gut integrity, and most importantly, enhance mucosal immunity to establish a balanced immune development is not completely understood. Because of the multiple different structures within authentic HMOs, several distinct receptors and pathways are thought to play an important role within the direct immune modulating role of HMOs. Direct interaction has recently been shown (by using glycan microarray technology) between glycan-binding proteins expressed on the epithelial cells and cells of the innate immune system to specific HMOs. For instance, 2′-Fucosyllactose and 3-fucosyllactose were shown to bind human DC-SIGN (Dendritic cell-specific intercellular adhesion molecule-3-grabbing non-integrin), a C-type lectin receptor present on the surface of both macrophages and dendritic cells. Moreover, the involvement of a set of glycan binding receptors including the C-type lectin receptors and Toll-like receptors (TLR) has been identified [193–195]. The direct binding of 2′FL to human DC-SIGN has been shown to be fucose-specific and DC-SIGN signaling seems to be influenced, leading to alteration in pro-inflammatory cytokine response in a TLR specific fashion [196,197]. In addition, it has long been known that human galectins expressed by intestinal epithelial cells also interact with oligosaccharides [198]. However, the exact mechanisms of how HMOs are able to alter the biological function of these human cells are still unknown.

Only a few limited studies have focused on the immune-modulatory effects of individual HMOs within infants and in animal studies, and have suggested anti-inflammatory and immune regulatory potential, but the mechanism by which specific HMOs may influence the risk for allergy development is currently not known [199]. Supplementation of the diet with 2′FL or 6′SL did not show any effect on the levels of allergen specific Immunoglobulin (Ig)E or IgG1 in sensitized or challenged mice. Dietary supplementation with specific oligosaccharides providing some of the functional benefits of HMOs, have been shown to reduce the risk of developing allergies in infants [200,201]. Recent data suggest that the onset of IgE-associated allergic manifestations, (but only in infants with a high hereditary risk for allergies and born by C-section) might be associated with FUT2-dependent oligosaccharide composition in breast milk consumed by these infants [46]. These mechanisms collectively include but may not be limited to the pathogen decoy capacity of specific HMOs, the prebiotic effect on the microbiome composition, the modulation of the SCFA production which in turn supports the barrier integrity and/or through direct immune modulatory functions [202]. However, further clinical studies are needed to support either one of these mechanisms to identify the full potential of HMOs within the early life immune development.

Within the last few years an interesting increase in understanding and knowledge regarding the presence and effects of HMOs and composition has been achieved. Consequently, with expansion of these studies and progress in biotechnology, the potential of adding HMOs to the complex mixture of prebiotic oligosaccharides in infant formulas are increasing. However, in order to decide which to add, in which concentration, composition and combination to prevent and treat allergy development in early life, as well as later in life, clearly needs additional study.

3.3. Human Milk Microbiota

Early microbial colonization is essential for infant's metabolic and immunological development [203]. Cumulative evidence suggests a direct link between microbial colonization and the risk of non-communicable diseases in later life, including allergies [204,205]. After birth, the transfer of microbiota continues during lactation, and is considered to be the cause of differences in gut microbiota between exclusively breastfed and formula fed infants during the first months of life [206]. In the recent years the presence of a HM microbiome has been confirmed, with a variety of microbes and their associated genes and antigens transmitted to the infant during breastfeeding [112]. Available data show that HM contains approximately 10^3–10^5 viable bacteria per mL [207,208].

Initially, the presence of microbes in human milk was evaluated by use of culture-dependent techniques and isolates belonged to *Staphylococcus*, *Streptococcus*, and *Lactobacillus* and *Bifidobacterium* species, which have been used as probiotics in intervention trials [209]. With the development and application of culture-independent techniques including next-generation sequencing, it has become clear that HM contains a much more diverse variety of bacteria, including other lactic acid bacteria, such as *Enterococcus, Lactococcus* and *Weissella*; typical inhabitants of the oral cavity, such as *Veillonella* and *Prevotella;* bacteria usually found in the skin, like *Propionibacterium,* and other Gram negatives, e.g., *Pseudomonas*, etc., [112,210–212]. In a recent systematic review, a core of predominant organisms was described, which includes *Staphylococcus, Streptococcus* and *Propionibacterium* [213]. These genera are universally predominant in human milk, regardless of different potential confounding factors, such as sampling, geographic location or analytical methods [213].

There is still scarce information about the influence of environmental and perinatal factors on HM microbiota composition [214]. Some studies reported that geographical location [112,204,206,215], delivery mode [207,208], maternal body mass index (BMI) [211,216] or antibiotic intake [217] would have an impact on HM microbiota. However, others did not find similar effect with regards to other perinatal factors [218]. Furthermore, an imbalance in the normal bacterial composition of HM can lead to the overgrowth of specific opportunistic pathogens and lead to mammary infection, such as lactational mastitis [219,220].

The origin of HM bacteria is currently unknown. A number of hypotheses have been proposed: (1) human milk microbiota could derive from the mother's skin, and the infant's oral cavity during suckling; (2) an internal route, the "entero-mammary pathway" has been proposed and suggests that bacteria from maternal gut could be taken up by immune cells and transported via blood stream or lymphatic system to the mammary gland [221]; (3) specific microbes were detected in the human breast tissue, which may also supply microorganisms to the milk [222,223].

Human milk microbes hypothesised to play a key role as early gut colonizers, likely contribute to the immune system development and maturation [224,225]. Alterations or divergent antibodies/microbiota transferred via HM may affect an infant's immune development. Lower proportions in the *Bifidobacterium* genus have been observed in HM from allergic mothers [226]. The gut microbiome from allergic children also differs from non-allergic in composition and diversity [226]. Recently, altered immune responses towards gut microbiota were observed as early as 1 month postpartum, in exclusively breastfed children who subsequently developed allergies [227]. Relationships between HM components (HMOs, fatty acids, immunological constituents, etc.) and allergy development in infants have been recently receiving increased attention [46,60,139,228–230]. Several studies reported that allergic disease and asthma are less common in children exposed to unpasteurized cow's milk (CM), which is a source of viable microorganisms [231]. Therefore, bacterial communities of HM could also be taking part in the protection of infants against allergic diseases, acting as a natural probiotic, and this requires further elucidation. However, unpasteurized CM also contains many immune active constituents with close sequence homology to those found in HM. These could also potentially explain the benefits of raw CM. Existing data suggests that some *Lactobacillus* and *Bifidobacterium* strains have been linked to allergy protection, in particular against eczema [150]. It is worth noting, however, that eczema is not synonymous to allergy, as discussed in other sections of the manuscript. This highlights a need in precision of outcome definitions alongside pheno- and endo-typing infant outcomes. As these genera can be found in HM, it is, therefore, plausible that their transfer to the infant during breastfeeding could provide immunological protection, although more work is needed to confirm this link.

The potential protective effect of HM bacteria against allergic diseases development has not been properly studied and future research should also investigate HM bacterial recognition by the immune system. Better knowledge would help to understand the importance of maternal transference of altered immune responses towards microbiota during breastfeeding, and their potential influence on allergy development during infancy. However, it is rather difficult to establish causal relationships between HM microbiome and its role in protection against allergic diseases. It is impossible to rule out the probability of an epi-phenomenon, and future research should tackle cause-effect relationships. Further analysis based on state-of-the-art, next-generation sequencing methods will be crucial in understanding the association between bacterial diversity inherited through breastfeeding and an infant's potential allergy development.

In clinical trials, oral administration of bacterial strains to lactating mothers showed modulatory effects both on human milk composition and on the infant's gut. It was shown that *Lactobacillus reuteri* intake led to its detection in the mother's milk and infant faeces [210]. Similarly, another study studied the effect of supplementation with *L. rhamnosus* to reduce the risk of allergy development when given to women during pregnancy and lactation [232]. Probiotic intake during pregnancy and lactation also induced specific changes in the infant *Bifidobacterium* colonization and influenced HM microbiota composition compared with those receiving placebo [233]. Recently, the effects of perinatal probiotic supplementation on the HM composition have been reinforced, leading to changes in its microbiota, including *Bifidobacterium* and *Lactobacillus* sp., and also functional components of HM, such as oligosaccharides (HMO) and lactoferrin [234].

Protective effects of certain *Lactobacillus* and *Bifidobacterium* strains on eczema development have been previously reported [235,236]. Their ability to provide protection against other allergic diseases has also been described, although results are conflicting and existing evidence does not support their use for allergy prevention. The beneficial effect on eczema has been proved [150], but the causality is still unclear. As eczema is a consequence of a skin barrier defect, the possibility of protection due to direct effects of short-chain fatty acids on skin rather than immune modulation cannot be excluded. If strong relationships between specific HM microorganisms and allergic diseases are further confirmed, prebiotics and probiotics could be used to improve HM composition and infant microbiota modulation.

3.4. Human Milk Micronutrients

While breastfeeding is recommended as the sole source of infant nutrition up to 6 months of age by WHO [237], there are caveats that an adequate maternal diet is required in conjunction with sufficient volumes of milk that can be transferred to the infant [237]. Lactating women and infants have a greater physiological demand for micronutrients and are therefore at higher risk of adverse consequences with insufficiency. Despite HM containing a multitude of micronutrients that are the infant's sole source in early life, comprehensive methodical research has not been carried out in this area [238]. Further, many HM micronutrients differ between women, such as Vitamin A and group B vitamins, which are influenced by maternal dietary intake (Table 3). Owing to this variation and the limited number of studies that often use small participant numbers, frequently suffer from lack of control for stage of lactation, fail to record maternal supplementation, and have inconsistent sampling, robust reference ranges for HM micronutrients do not exist. To add fuel to the fire, various methods have been employed such as microbiology and radioisotope dilution with the recent addition of chromatography, coupled with UV, fluorometric and mass spectrometry detection making comparisons even more challenging. Only recently has there been a concerted effort to shed light on questions such as variation within feeding, circadian rhythms and the impact of maternal supplementation. This lack of research likely explains conflicting results and has subsequently hampered the determination of recommended daily intakes for infants [239]. The other potential explanation is failure to consider the timing of deficiencies. Transfer of nutrients to the foetus during pregnancy is likely equally, if not more important, than HM composition. During the first trimester of pregnancy, programming of growth trajectories will have a profound effect on foetal and infant requirements for micronutrients. Keeping in mind the "Developmental Origins of Health and Disease" (DOHaD) hypothesis, which suggests fetal developmental 'plasticity' and discordance between intra- and extra-uterine exposures produces the greatest adverse effects [240].

Table 3. Human milk micronutrients known to be influenced by maternal diet. The range of mean concentrations is given for mature milk. Reference [241]—"Handbook of Milk Composition" summarises milk composition up to approximately 1993.

Component Affected by Maternal Diet	Concentration	Component Unaffected by Maternal Diet	Concentration
Fat Soluble Vitamins			
K	0.12–0.98 ug/dL [241–243]	Tocopherol (vit E)	207–366 ug/dL [244–246]
D	0.008–0.62 ug/dL [242,246–248]		
Retinol (Vit. A) *	40–485 μg/L [242,245,249]		
Water Soluble Vitamins			
Thiamin (vit B-1)	21.1–228 ug/L [249–251]	Folate	53–133 ug/L [241,252,253]
Riboflavin (vit B-2)	0.03–0.35 mg/L [249,251]		
Niacin (vit B-3)	68.7–260 ug/L [251,254]		
Vit B-6	0.06–0.31 mg/L [241,249,251,255]		
Cobalamin (vit B-12)	85–970 ng/L [249,255,256]		
Ascorbic acid (vit C)	35–105 mg/L [241,246,249]		
Pantothenic acid (vit B-5)	2.0–2.5 mg/L [241,251]		
Choline	144–258 mg/L [241,257]		
Minerals			
Selenium	3–60 ng/mL [241,249,258,259]	Zinc	0.68–12 ug/mL [241,245,260–262]
Iodine	9–250 ug/L [241,249,263–265]	Copper	0.006–0.5 ug/mL [241,245,253]
		Iron	0.3–0.9 ug/mL [245,262,266]
		Calcium	259–300 mg/L [241,245,262]
		Phosphorus	130–170 mg/L [241,245,262]
		Magnesium	30.5–31.4 mg/L [241,245]
		Sodium	111–300 mg/L [241,245,262]
		Potassium	380–630 mg/L [241,245,262]
		Chromium	0.15–0.8 ng/mL [241,247,253]
		Chloride	453–690 mg/L [241,262]
		Manganese	0.33–125 ng/mL [241,245,253,262]

* Vit.—Vitamin.

3.4.1. Vitamin A

A number of HM vitamins are influenced by maternal diet including vitamin A, which plays a major role in both growth and immune function. In a small study of lactating Bangladeshi women ($n = 18$) intensive sampling showed that the most appropriate sample should be taken from a pumped volume from a full breast and that there was a small but significant circadian variation that disappeared when milk fat was accounted for. Further, vitamin A content increased significantly with acute supplementation [254]. Vitamin deficiencies in the infant included adverse outcomes such as severe respiratory and gastrointestinal infections, as well as increased morbidity and mortality [267]. In a mouse model, maternal supplementation during lactation prevented allergic airway inflammation and had a protective effect on oral tolerance induction [268]. This finding is consistent with a meta-analysis of human studies that shows dietary intake of vitamin A to have either a beneficial association in asthma prevention or no association [269]. In contrast, direct neonatal supplementation in human neonates appears to increase the risk of atopy and wheezing, particularly in females [270]. It is speculated that HM borne vitamin A reduces allergy via promotion of intestinal crypt development and a reduction of gut permeability without impacting the digestion of milk [16,268]. Future studies will serve to shed light on the protective mechanisms of HMvitamin A.

3.4.2. B Vitamins

In general, group B vitamins concentration of HM is also strongly related to maternal intake and levels respond to dietary supplementation [271,272]. Levels of HM B vitamins are based on samples from women in established lactation, as thiamin, vitamin B-6, and folate are lower, and vitamin B-12 higher in the first few weeks of lactation (transitional milk) [272], whereas, in established lactation the levels of all B vitamins remain relatively stable [246]. Importantly, maternal depletion impacts infant status to varying degrees depending on the vitamin and the levels of the vitamin. Further, complicating the picture is the lack of global documentation on the prevalence of HM vitamin B deficiency.

Studies investigating relationships between vitamin B and infant allergy are also scant with one study showing no relationship between wheeze or eczema in infants (16–24 months) and maternal intake of folate, vitamin B12, vitamin B6, and vitamin B2 during pregnancy [273].

3.4.3. Vitamin D

Vitamin D is a steroid hormone produced by skin exposure to ultraviolet light and has many important roles such as maintaining bone health via the regulation of calcium and phosphorus absorption. It also plays a role in the innate and adaptive immune system. Due to the ubiquitous reduction in the time spent outdoors, maternal HM concentrations of vitamin D (25-Hydroxyvitamin D) are often deficient. Since HM vitamin D levels are positively related to maternal serum concentrations [274–276] there are serious concerns regarding the vitamin D status of exclusively breastfed infants, evidenced by a resurgence in the diagnosis of rickets [277]. Maternal daily vitamin D supplementation of 400–2000 IU of vitamin D/day increases HM concentrations and subsequently infant 25-Hydroxyvitamin D status [278]. Hence, the current recommendations of the American Academy of Pediatrics is that all breastfed infants be supplemented with 400 IU/day of oral vitamin D from birth [279].

It is not clear whether vitamin D intake during pregnancy and lactation lowers the risk of infant allergies. In a number of studies, high maternal vitamin D levels have been associated with increased risk of eczema, asthma, food allergy or sensitization to food allergens [280–282] while others report reduced risk of allergic outcomes [269,283–286] or no relationship [286–288]. An interesting study on a large Finnish cohort found that maternal vitamin D intake from food was associated with reduced risk of cow's milk allergy (CMA) while supplementation of both vitamin D and folic acid was associated with increased risk of CMA [289]; however, it is likely that other lifestyle factors have contributed to this finding. Comparisons of these studies are limited due to differences in study design, methodologies, supplementation, time of measurements, along with a lack of information regarding lactation. The other issue is the reported non-linear relationship between allergy outcomes in relation to vitamin D levels with very low and very high levels increasing the risks. The optimal level for immunological health is still to be defined and this may well differ dependent on stage in pregnancy and the age of the infant. Supplementation of lactating women and monitoring of their infants for allergy has yet to be carried out and may yield different results as seen with vitamin A. Hence, due to the limited and conflicting evidence, the World Allergy Organization has not recommended supplementing women in pregnancy or lactation as an allergy preventative strategy [290].

3.4.4. Iron

Iron levels in HM are relatively low (0.3 mg/L), but this micronutrient is highly bio-available to the infant with absorption rates ranging between 16% and 50%, which is higher than that available from formula feeds [291]. The reported prevalence of iron deficient anemia is <2% up to 6 months and 2–3% between 6 and 9 months in European infants [291]. Therefore, infant supplementation is generally not recommended in the first 6 months of life with the exception of infants of diabetic mothers and low birth weight infants that have low iron stores [266,292]. However, it is recommended that the first complementary foods are rich in iron [293]. A recent study has found as many as a third of healthy fully breastfed infants are iron deficient or have iron deficiency anaemia at 5 months of age [294]. Supplementation of breastfed infants (1–6 months) with 7.5 mg per day of ferrous sulfate resulted in higher haemoglobin concentration and higher mean corpuscular volume at 6 months of age than those not supplemented [295]. Better visual acuity and greater Bayley Mental and Psychomotor Developmental Indices were also recorded at 13 months in supplemented infants. Thus, the American Academy of Paediatrics recommends that exclusively breastfed term infants and those receiving more than half of their daily feeds as breast milk be supplemented with oral iron at 1 mg/kg per day from 4 months of age [296].

Adequate iron is essential for both normal infant neurodevelopment [266] and immune protection yet is the most common global micronutrient deficiency worldwide [297] with infants and children at high risk due to the high demand for rapid growth. Very few studies have investigated the relationship of infant iron status and immunological outcomes with one case-control study showing no difference in infant status with respect to eczema [298].

3.4.5. Zinc

Infants and children have high requirements for zinc due to rapid growth and tissue synthesis. Zinc deficiency is not uncommon (>20%) particularly in infants/children less than 5 years of age [299,300]. Symptoms of zinc deficiency include growth retardation, altered immune function and gastrointestinal effects such as diarrhea. Those infants/children at highest risk are those consuming a combination of breast milk and a predominantly plant-based diet of low zinc content as well as prematurity and low birth weight. [301]. HM zinc content is not related to maternal zinc status and in developed settings, zinc intake from HM is considered adequate provided the mother is able to generate enough milk for her infant [301]. However, infant zinc supplementation is often indicated in low resources settings and those where complementary foods are low in zinc [301].

Again, research into the relationship between infant zinc intake during lactation and allergy is scarce. Of note a case control study has shown that zinc status is lower in those infants with eczema compared to their matched controls [298], which is more likely a direct effect on skin barrier rather than immune responses.

3.4.6. Summary

Micronutrients are important part of the HM composition, but there is a only small body of evidence that their intake during early life may be related to allergy. In order to establish firm relationships future research will need to consider sampling and measurement methods of HM. This includes importance of adjustment for timing—pregnancy vs. lactation; foetal and infant growth trajectories; and includes better clinical outcome definition. It is also possible to measure dose (rather than concentration) by employing methods such as test weighing [302] to further improve the quality of subsequent studies.

3.5. The New Frontier: Human Milk Glycoproteins and Metabolites

Metabolomics is one of the newest "omics" sciences which has been integrated into HM study using a top-down systems biology approach to explore and unravel the genetic-environment-health paradigm [303]. Metabolomics, or the study of metabolites, is useful to elucidate the complex interactions of HM constituents, and to understand the physiological state of HM in various stages of lactation [304] and in response to infection. Metabolomics, together with other the "omics" such as proteomics and glycomics and genomics can enable us to understand this complex and dynamic relationship. Several complementary analytical platforms such as nuclear magnetic resonance (NMR), capillary electrophoresis (CE), liquid or gas chromatography (LC or GC) coupled with mass spectrometry (MS) have been used to profile the composition of HM [305,306]. Recent study by Andreas et al. has identified 710 metabolites in HM using various modified extraction methods, such as Folch extraction and single-phase extraction using methanol and methyl *tert*-butyl ether (MTBE) [305].

Besides characterizing the HM metabolome, temporal changes in metabolites across stages of lactation can be tracked to demonstrate the adaptation of breasts to meet the nutritional and developmental requirements of the growing infant. Using LC- and GC-MS methods, Villasenor et al. reported increases in several fatty acids such as linoleic and oleic acid, from the first to the fourth week postpartum in full-term infants, while cholesterol, fucose and α-tocopherol levels declined [306]. In NMR-based analyses, Wu et al. reported decreases to phosphocholine and glycerol-phosphocholine concentrations after the first month of lactation that coincided with an elevation in levels of choline, a compound essential for the neonate's growth and neuronal development [307]. Whereas, Sundekilde et al. characterized and compared 51 metabolites including HMOs, in preterm and full-term milk up to 100-days post-partum [304,308]. Lacto-*N*-difucohexaose I, 3′-sialyllactose and 6′-sialyllactose were identified to be higher in preterm milk compared to term milk [304]; these HMOs have been implicated in the onset of necrotizing enterocolitis in rat pups [309] and infants [310]. Recent studies have revealed strong associations between HM metabolites (including HMOs) and the microbiota of the infant's gut [311]; this content was covered in earlier sections of this review.

The hygiene hypotheses have expanded our understanding of how allergic disease originates during infancy. Equally important and likely in response to our microbial environment is the role of breastfeeding in promoting tolerance to antigens and subsequently reducing the incidence of allergy and asthma [312,313]. This protection is potentially related to bioactive compounds such as secretory immunoglobulin A (sIgA) and TGF-β, present in colostrum and mature human milk that provide protection during the time when the infant's own immune responses are immature. TGF-β is discussed in the earlier sections of this review and this section will focus on a few constituents of HM in relation to infant infection and inflammation as follows: 2 glycoproteins, secretory immunoglobulin A, and lactoferrin, and low molecular weight compounds such as lactose, choline and anti-inflammatory short-chain fatty acids. Increasingly, we are appreciating the anti-infective and anti-inflammatory roles of HM microbiota to directly influence the infant's gut microbiome, and of HMOs which drive the growth of microbes to shape gut immunity. These interactions between HM metabolites, the gut microbiome and allergic disease are reviewed in more detail by Kumari and Kozyrskyj [314] and Julia et al. [315]. The expanded role for antimicrobial proteins/peptides in HM, as breakdown products of lactoferrin, will only be briefly mentioned in this section.

3.5.1. Secretory Immunoglobulin A (sIgA)

Secretory Immunoglobulun A (sIgA) is the principal immunoglobulin on human mucosal surfaces which blocks microorganisms and toxins from attaching to mucosal epithelial cells. While oral administration of monoclonal antigen-specific IgA prevents infection with bacterial and viral pathogens, in its natural polyclonal state, non-specific sIgA protects against gastrointestinal and respiratory infections [316]. In colostrum, levels of non-specific sIgA reaching 12 g/L are not uncommon, and they decrease to 1 g/L in mature milk [317]. The HM transfer of sIgA from mother to an infant provides protection against infection by binding pathogens and stimulating gut microbes until the infant immune system takes over to produce sufficient sIgA levels [318]. It also has an important role in the development of oral tolerance to gut microbiota. Fecal sIgA concentrations reach a peak of 4.5 mg/g feces at 1 month of age in exclusively breastfed infants (fed some formula immediately after birth); they decline to 1.5 mg/g of feces at 5 months of age where they remain for the duration of infancy [319]. In exclusively formula-fed infants, however, fecal sIgA concentrations peak at 1.5 mg/g feces, drop to 1 mg/g feces at 3 months, then reach comparable levels to breastfed infants at 9 months of age. Much higher sIgA levels have been observed 1 week after birth with exclusive breastfeeding [320]. Low levels of non-specific faecal IgA in infants were among the first associated with a higher risk of allergy [321].

The production of intestinal IgA commences around 1 month after birth when low levels of fecal sIgA can be detected in non-breastfed infants [322]. Hence, sIgA in colostrum has been likened to an immune booster, a beneficial attribute that varies by maternal characteristics and can be impacted by medical intervention. Residual country variation in colostrum sIgA levels has been reported, even after accounting for collection time, and maternal parity, smoking, fruit and fish consumption, and allergen sensitization [323]. Cesarean delivery was independently associated with reduced sIgA colostrum levels in this study. Breakey et al. reported lower HM sIgA levels in time periods before and after respiratory or gastrointestinal infections in 8-month old infants of a traditional population living in rural Argentina [324].

As evident by the presence of fecal IgA in exclusively formula-fed infants, full-term infants produce substantial levels of their own IgA within 3 months after birth [325]. However, the highest IgA levels are seen in exclusively breastfed infants and they increase in direct proportion to the "dose" of HM (exclusive, partial versus no breastfeeding) provided to the infant. At this age, the likelihood of *C. difficile* colonization in gut microbiota was reduced by 75% among infants with fecal IgA levels [326] in the highest tertile, independent of parity, birth mode and breastfeeding status. While *C. difficile* presence in the infant gut is not uncommon, it is a marker for lowered colonization resistance to pathogenic bacteria and has been found to be associated with future allergic disease [327,328]. Hence, BM and infant sIgA have an important role in reducing *C. difficile* colonization. Furthermore, infant fecal IgA levels are noted to be inversely associated with infant serum levels of IgE and lower binding of IgA to *Bacteroides* species increases risk for asthma at age 7 [227,321].

3.5.2. Lactoferrrin

Lactoferrin is a large molecular weight glycoprotein that is also present in colostrum and transition milk, and at higher levels than in mature milk [329]. Lactoferrin participates in host defense against microbial pathogens by binding bacterial membranes, binding iron and making it less available for microbial growth, down-regulating tumor necrosis factor-alpha (TNF-α) and interleukin-1β (IL-1β) production, and stimulating the maturation of lymphocytes [330]. Peptide breakdown products of lactoferrin have specific direct antibacterial and antifungal activity.

Higher lactoferrin levels were seen in HM preceding and following an infectious episode in the rural infants of the Breakey et al. study [324]. Since this association with infection was in the opposite direction to that seen for sIgA secretion in the same infants, the study authors proposed that lactoferrin "responds" to an infection. Lactoferrin is detected in infant feces. Mastromarino et al. found fecal *bifidobacteria* and *lactobacilli* concentrations in newborns to be positively correlated with fecal lactoferrin levels soon after delivery [329]. Due to reported associations between child atopy with reduced and not elevated *lactobacillus* abundance in the infant gut [331], it is interesting that Zhang et al. found eczema and atopic sensitization at 6 months (but not later) to be more likely in infants of mothers with higher HM levels of lactoferrin at 6 weeks after birth [332]. Upper respiratory tract infections were less likely when children were 1 or 2 years of age with higher HM lactoferrin. Clearly, the interactions between anti-infective and anti-inflammatory effects of this HM protein are complex and require further study.

3.5.3. Low Molecular Weight Metabolites

Milk Fatty Acids

Milk lipids are principal macronutrients in HM and account for over 50 % of the infant energy daily intake requirements. Polyunsaturated fatty acids (PUFAs), more specifically the omega-3 (ω-3) fatty acids: docosahexaenoic (DHA) and eicosapentaenoic (EPA), have been shown to have anti-inflammatory effects in chronic inflammatory diseases, such as asthma [333]. Several specialized pro-resolving mediators such as resolvin and protectin, are synthesized from ω-3 fatty acids by lipoxygenase and cyclooxygenase in Th2-cytokine-stimulated macrophages and airway epithelial cells of human and murine origin [334,335]. These mediators have anti-inflammatory properties and demonstrated suppressive effects on allergic asthma [336].

More recently, the short-chain fatty acids (SCFAs), acetate, butyrate and propionate, have gained interest as mediators of allergic inflammations. They are produced by gut microbes and are used as an energy source by gut epithelial cells (colonocytes) and after absorption, by the liver for gluconeogenesis [314]. Increasingly, inflammation is being viewed as a by-product of the metabolic activity of gut microbiota from evidence that SCFAs are altered in children who are or become overweight or atopic. New evidence shows that maternal SCFA levels during pregnancy can directly impact the health of infants. Thorburn et al. observed that when a high-fibre diet was consumed during pregnancy, maternal serum acetate (but not other SCFA) levels were higher [337]. Lower serum levels of acetate during pregnancy were associated with wheeze in infants. In a follow-up murine model experiment, feeding dams acetate during pregnancy and the immediate postpartum period reduced the development of allergic airway inflammation in offspring.

SCFAs are the first metabolites produced by the gut microbiota of newborns, with synthesis increasing rapidly after birth [338]. In the few published studies, total SCFA levels are elevated in the gut of formula-fed versus breastfed infants born at term gestation, yet relative to other SCFA, acetate levels are highest with exclusive breastfeeding [314,339]. Since microbiota have been detected in HM and breastfeeding influences SCFA levels in infants, it is quite plausible that HM contains SCFA. In our pilot comparison of HM across 5 countries, butyrate and acetate were detected by NMR spectroscopy in HM collected 1 month after vaginal delivery in women who had not received antibiotics. Tan et al. have observed a reduction in food allergy and total serum IgE levels in mice treated with acetate and butyrate, but not propionate in drinking water [340]. This protection against food allergy was not observed in the absence of gut microbiota, suggesting that in addition to SCFAs, a cascade of other signaling molecules are required to prevent sensitization to food antigens [341].

Choline

Choline is a component of the non-protein nitrogen in human milk and is an important metabolite for lipid synthesis and in the neurodevelopment of the infant [342]. The circulatory concentration of free choline, phosphocholine, glycerophosphocholine in breastfed infants is positively correlated with the choline contents of consumed HM [343]. Ozarda et al. has demonstrated that the water-soluble choline content of early HM at 1 to 3 days postpartum was positively associated with maternal serum C-reactive protein (CRP) levels [344]. Since serum CRP is typically elevated during active infection or acute severe inflammatory processes [345,346], the Ozarda study suggests that HM choline content is a response to low-grade inflammation in the nursing mother. In fact, higher intake of dietary choline in adults has been independently associated with a reduction in inflammatory markers, namely with lowered levels of serum CRP, interleukin-6 (IL-6) and tumour necrosis factor-α (TNF-α) [347], although the exact cause of this association remains unclear. Of interest, in the Ozarda et al. study, both HM levels of choline and serum CRP were higher after caesarean versus vaginal delivery, differences which could not be attributed to the weight, height or body-mass index of breastfeeding women [344]. It is of particular interest considering known notable associations between delivery by C-section and increased risk of allergic diseases development [348].

Lactose

Lactose is the main component of the carbohydrate portion of HM and induces innate immunity by up-regulating gastrointestinal antimicrobial peptides that protect the infant's gut against pathogens and regulate gut microbial homeostasis [349]. As such, the lactose concentration in HM increases after closure of the tight junctions at the initiation of lactation [350]. Before the infant can absorb lactose for energy use, it is broken down to glucose and galactose by β-galactosidase lactase in the small intestine [351]. Infant lactose intolerance is not common, as lactase is tightly regulated in infant and is then progressively down regulated in most children by 2 to 3 years of age [317]. As lactase activity decreases, the lactose moiety remains intact and then reaches the large intestine, where it is metabolized by gut microbes. This fermentation process produces hydrogen, methane, carbon dioxide and lactate [352], molecules which have the potential to cause bloating, abdominal cramps, nausea and symptoms typical of lactose intolerance. This lactose-lactase system is suggested to act as a biological timer, controlling birth spacing in human and eventual weaning. Noteworthy is that lactase deficiency is more prominent in those of Asian, South American and African descent [317]. However, there is no high-quality research providing a link between the lactose and allergic diseases development.

4. Breastfeeding/Human Milk Research Unmet Needs

Hitherto in this state-of-the-art review two predominant approaches were presented in the field of breastfeeding and HM research, with some studies assessing the impact of breastfeeding on health outcomes, while others testing putative associations between HM composition and the development of non-communicable disease in general, and allergy in particular. There is an evident lack of studies combining both, which therefore does not elaborate on the reasons for breastfeeding being beneficial in some children, with no effect, or even conferring a higher risk of allergy development, in the others. Furthermore, each field of study had its own methodologic challenges.

We pointed out that various methods of quantifying breastfeeding (exclusive breastfeeding versus supplementation, feeding duration categorization), differences in assessing outcomes (self-report versus clinical measures), and the timing of outcome assessment have all contributed to the inconsistent results of association studies and intervention trials. In addition, the role of breastfeeding may vary in importance depending on characteristics of the infant, such as age and mode of delivery. When comparing the impact of breastfeeding on gut microbiota in neonates versus infants, Levin et al. reported greater variance in microbial composition explained by breastfeeding at 6 months than at 1 month of age [353]. Before 3 months of age, the impact of caesarean section (CS) on gut microbial composition has been found to be stronger than breastfeeding [353,354] and to be independent of breastfeeding status [353,355]. On the other hand, findings from the Canadian Healthy Infant Longitudinal Development birth cohort suggest that early breastfeeding may modify intrapartum antibiotic prophylaxis and CS-associated dysbiosis of the gut microbiome later in infancy [355]. Hence, in addition to correctly applying breastfeeding definitions, separating ante- from postnatal influences, better phenotyping allergy outcomes and utilizing "big data" to study the impact of clusters of HM components, assessment of infant subgroups is required for a more precise recommendations to be made about breastfeeding according to maternal characteristics (i.e., asthmatic status, allergic history, parity, etc.) and delivery mode.

We have also shown that HM has a very complex composition, consisting of a wide range of immunologically active markers, oligosaccharides, live microorganisms, micronutrients, metabolites and many other bioactive compounds. Human milk composition is dynamic and variable. Early milk is particularly rich in its constituents and they undergo rapid change during the very first days of life. Country differences are also apparent, but not fully explainable at this stage, indicating that women living in different geographic locations may have distinct human milk profiles. The impact of HM composition on allergic disease development in children is still a matter of discussion as studies continue to produce conflicting results. In view of the vast number of crucial components in human milk, investigation of a single or limited range of constituents may well lead to confusing outcomes. An appealing thesis is that lactating women can be characterized according to specific and individual constituents of their milk, called "lactotypes". Future studies should investigate the possibility of a lactotype phenotype in a large number of nursing women by analyzing human milk for multiple constituents at a time and looking for associations with a variety of immunologic phenotype and outcomes (Figure 1).

Methodological differences in the detection of constituents are also a major issue in HM studies, which makes it challenging for meta-analyses to be undertaken. HM composition comparisons between populations or countries should consider strict harmonisation of sampling, storage and analysis protocols, especially for the timing of sampling, and the collection of samples from lactating women with similar characteristics. Such studies would reduce variations caused by differences between populations and between sampling methods, although variation in storage time of milk samples could not be controlled in this way.

There are number of unmet research needs in breastfeeding and HM research (Box 1) which have arisen during the development of this manuscript and should be addressed in the future research. Addressing these needs would lead to a better understanding of the links between breastfeeding/HM composition and allergic disease development in infancy and childhood.

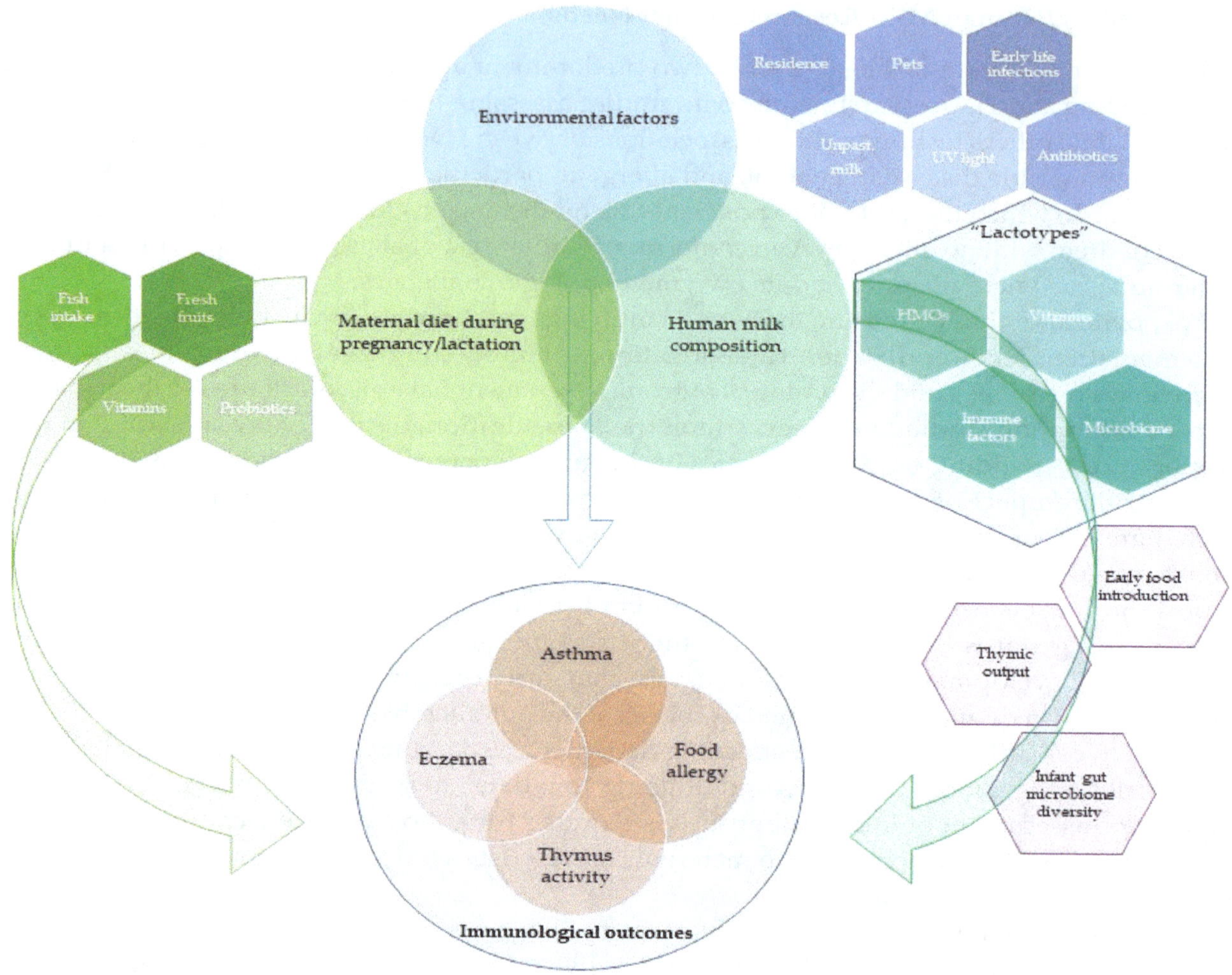

Figure 1. Maternal, environmental and human milk composition factors influence on immunological outcomes in child.

Box 1. Unmet research needs in breastfeeding and human milk research.

- Large and well-standardised studies of HM composition (integrated data on immune markers, HMOs, PUFAs, microbiome and metabolites), defining lactotypes and assessing variation between women residing in different countries
- Application of omics approaches (metabolomics, proteomics, genomics, etc.) to highlight the most important components of HM in relation to allergic diseases
- Studies evaluating biological activity of a specific components within HM
- Randomised trials of breastfeeding interventions with long-term follow-up for allergic disease development
- Randomised trials of early weaning (3–4 months) using different dietary approaches
- Large cohort studies which combine assessments of breastfeeding influence on allergy development with the constituent analysis of HM samples
- Development of a new intervention strategies for HM composition modification and indirect preventative effect on allergy prevention
- Relevance of a geographical location/lifestyle/diet and its' influence on the composition of human milk should be assessed in more detail and research should account for these important confounders

As evidence accumulates from HM research, it will address some of these gaps to better inform policy makers, clinicians and nursing mothers. Future studies must continue to apply sound methodological approaches [356], as well as to incorporate new technologies and bring a "patient-centered" individualised approach to their application. Emerging laboratory and analytical methods will facilitate the inclusion of data on the human milk microbiome and metabolome as likely mechanistically important components of breastfeeding and these findings must be investigated for their roles in the developmental origins of health and disease (DOHAD) [154]. As allergic sensitization and allergy associated diseases are increasingly common and constitute the commonest group of common conditions afflicting young people, they provide the best opportunity to investigate DOHAD hypotheses.

5. Conclusions

Allergic diseases such as eczema, food allergy and asthma are the commonest chronic diseases of childhood in many countries, and there is evidence that early life events, such as variations in breastfeeding patterns, maternal diet, environmental and microbial exposures may be important in their development. There remain a number of hurdles to overcome before we come to a clear understanding on how to translate these associations into clinical practice because association is not synonymous with cause and effect. The possibility that interventions which modify maternal immunity can impact infant immune responses by changing HM composition is in part supported by associations between HM composition and immunological outcomes.

Complexity and variability in human milk composition (and known infant's response to many of HM constituents) may also explain some of the conflicting results of studies evaluating the effect of prolonged exclusive breastfeeding and the prevention of allergic disease development. Future research needs to account for different environmental exposures and use systematic methodologies to characterize variations in human milk composition in relation to well-defined clinical and immune outcomes during childhood. Statistical approaches using cluster analysis should be implemented more frequently, in order to define the role of lactotypes, consisting of immune active molecules, PUFA's, microbiome composition. Understanding the relationship between HM composition and development of non-communicable diseases, and particularly allergy, may allow us to establish a new paradigm in allergy prevention research—namely modulation of HM composition via maternal dietary and other interventions, in order to promote healthy infant immune development.

Acknowledgments: R.J.B. is supported by a National Institute for Health Research Biomedical Research Centre (BRC). Both J.O.W. and R.J.B. have received research grant income from Danone in relation to studies of the value of prebiotics in allergy prevention, and Airsonette to evaluate Temperature-controlled laminar airflow for asthma. J.O.W. is on a Danone, UCB and Airsonette scientific advisory board and both J.O.W. and R.J.B. have given paid lectures for the companies. D.M. has received consultancy payment from Dairy Goat Co-Operative (NZ) Ltd. and has given paid lectures for the MSD. D.T.G. receives an unrestricted research grant from Medela AG and has received travel funding and support for lectures. J.O.W. is supported by the NIHR CLAHRC for NW London and is its Early years theme lead. The views expressed in this paper are those of the authors and not the NIHR or Department of Health.

Author Contributions: Authors D.M., D.G.P., D.T.G., A.L.K. and J.O.W. designed this review paper and organized the literature papers. D.M., D.G.P., A.L.K. and J.O.W. revised the manuscript. All authors edited and contributed to drafts of the manuscript. Authors contributed most to the following sections of the manuscript: breastfeeding and immunological outcomes—D.M., A.K., C.S., R.J.B., G.W., D.G.P., J.O.W., P.S.H. and R.N.; immune composition—D.M., R.J.B. and J.O.W.; oligosaccharides—B.V.L., C.S. and J.G.; microbiota—A.B.-A. and M.C.C.; micronutrients—D.T.G. and M.C.L.G.; metabolomics—A.L.K. and M.C.L.G. All authors approved the final form of the manuscript.

References

1. Asher, M.I.; Montefort, S.; Bjorksten, B.; Lai, C.K.; Strachan, D.P.; Weiland, S.K.; Williams, H.; ISAAC Phase Three Study Group. Worldwide time trends in the prevalence of symptoms of asthma, allergic rhinoconjunctivitis, and eczema in childhood: Isaac phases one and three repeat multicountry cross-sectional surveys. *Lancet* **2006**, *368*, 733–743. [CrossRef]

2. Williams, H.; Robertson, C.; Stewart, A.; Ait-Khaled, N.; Anabwani, G.; Anderson, R.; Asher, I.; Beasley, R.; Bjorksten, B.; Burr, M.; et al. Worldwide variations in the prevalence of symptoms of atopic eczema in the international study of asthma and allergies in childhood. *J. Allergy Clin. Immunol.* **1999**, *103*, 125–138. [CrossRef]
3. Kung, S.J.; Steenhoff, A.P.; Gray, C. Food allergy in africa: Myth or reality? *Clin. Rev. Allergy Immunol.* **2014**, *46*, 241–249. [CrossRef] [PubMed]
4. Strachan, D.P. Hay fever, hygiene, and household size. *BMJ* **1989**, *299*, 1259–1260. [CrossRef] [PubMed]
5. Strachan, D.P. Family size, infection and atopy: The first decade of the "hygiene hypothesis". *Thorax* **2000**, *55*, S2–S10. [CrossRef] [PubMed]
6. Sozanska, B.; Blaszczyk, M.; Pearce, N.; Cullinan, P. Atopy and allergic respiratory disease in rural poland before and after accession to the european union. *J. Allergy Clin. Immunol.* **2014**, *133*, 1347–1353. [CrossRef] [PubMed]
7. Du Toit, G.; Tsakok, T.; Lack, S.; Lack, G. Prevention of food allergy. *J. Allergy Clin. Immunol.* **2016**, *137*, 998–1010. [CrossRef] [PubMed]
8. Greer, F.R.; Sicherer, S.H.; Burks, A.W.; American Academy of Pediatrics Committee on Nutrition; American Academy of Pediatrics Section on Allergy and Immunology. Effects of early nutritional interventions on the development of atopic disease in infants and children: The role of maternal dietary restriction, breastfeeding, timing of introduction of complementary foods, and hydrolyzed formulas. *Pediatrics* **2008**, *121*, 183–191. [CrossRef] [PubMed]
9. Host, A.; Halken, S.; Muraro, A.; Dreborg, S.; Niggemann, B.; Aalberse, R.; Arshad, S.H.; von Berg, A.; Carlsen, K.H.; Duschen, K.; et al. Dietary prevention of allergic diseases in infants and small children. *Pediatr. Allergy Immunol.* **2008**, *19*, 1–4. [CrossRef] [PubMed]
10. Kjellman, N.I. Prediction and prevention of atopic allergy. *Allergy* **1998**, *53*, 67–71. [CrossRef] [PubMed]
11. Muraro, A.; Halken, S.; Arshad, S.H.; Beyer, K.; Dubois, A.E.; Du Toit, G.; Eigenmann, P.A.; Grimshaw, K.E.; Hoest, A.; Lack, G.; et al. Eaaci food allergy and anaphylaxis guidelines. Primary prevention of food allergy. *Allergy* **2014**, *69*, 590–601. [CrossRef] [PubMed]
12. Prescott, S.L.; Tang, M.L.; Australasian Society of Clinical Immunology and Allergy. The australasian society of clinical immunology and allergy position statement: Summary of allergy prevention in children. *Med. J. Aust.* **2005**, *182*, 464–467. [PubMed]
13. D'Alessandro, A.; Scaloni, A.; Zolla, L. Human milk proteins: An interactomics and updated functional overview. *J. Proteome Res.* **2010**, *9*, 3339–3373. [CrossRef] [PubMed]
14. Holtzman, M.J. Asthma as a chronic disease of the innate and adaptive immune systems responding to viruses and allergens. *J. Clin. Investig.* **2012**, *122*, 2741–2748. [CrossRef] [PubMed]
15. Yan, F.; Polk, D.B. Probiotics and immune health. *Curr. Opin. Gastroenterol.* **2011**, *27*, 496–501. [CrossRef] [PubMed]
16. Munblit, D.; Verhasselt, V. Allergy prevention by breastfeeding: Possible mechanisms and evidence from human cohorts. *Curr. Opin. Allergy Clin. Immunol.* **2016**, *16*, 427–433. [CrossRef] [PubMed]
17. Lumia, M.; Luukkainen, P.; Kaila, M.; Tapanainen, H.; Takkinen, H.M.; Prasad, M.; Niinisto, S.; Nwaru, B.I.; Kenward, M.G.; Ilonen, J.; et al. Maternal dietary fat and fatty acid intake during lactation and the risk of asthma in the offspring. *Acta Paediatr.* **2012**, *101*, e337–e343. [CrossRef] [PubMed]
18. Joseph, C.L.; Ownby, D.R.; Havstad, S.L.; Woodcroft, K.J.; Wegienka, G.; MacKechnie, H.; Zoratti, E.; Peterson, E.L.; Johnson, C.C. Early complementary feeding and risk of food sensitization in a birth cohort. *J. Allergy Clin. Immunol.* **2011**, *127*, 1203–1210. [CrossRef] [PubMed]
19. Nwaru, B.I.; Craig, L.C.; Allan, K.; Prabhu, N.; Turner, S.W.; McNeill, G.; Erkkola, M.; Seaton, A.; Devereux, G. Breastfeeding and introduction of complementary foods during infancy in relation to the risk of asthma and atopic diseases up to 10 years. *Clin. Exp. Allergy* **2013**, *43*, 1263–1273. [CrossRef] [PubMed]
20. Nwaru, B.I.; Takkinen, H.M.; Niemela, O.; Kaila, M.; Erkkola, M.; Ahonen, S.; Haapala, A.M.; Kenward, M.G.; Pekkanen, J.; Lahesmaa, R.; et al. Timing of infant feeding in relation to childhood asthma and allergic diseases. *J. Allergy Clin. Immunol.* **2013**, *131*, 78–86. [CrossRef] [PubMed]
21. Matheson, M.C.; Allen, K.J.; Tang, M.L. Understanding the evidence for and against the role of breastfeeding in allergy prevention. *Clin. Exp. Allergy* **2012**, *42*, 827–851. [CrossRef] [PubMed]

22. Azad, M.B.; Becker, A.B.; Guttman, D.S.; Sears, M.R.; Scott, J.A.; Kozyrskyj, A.L.; Canadian Healthy Infant Longitudinal Development Study, I. Gut microbiota diversity and atopic disease: Does breast-feeding play a role? *J. Allergy Clin. Immunol.* **2013**, *131*, 247–248. [CrossRef] [PubMed]
23. Prietl, B.; Treiber, G.; Pieber, T.R.; Amrein, K. Vitamin d and immune function. *Nutrients* **2013**, *5*, 2502–2521. [CrossRef] [PubMed]
24. Victora, C.G.; Horta, B.L.; Loret de Mola, C.; Quevedo, L.; Pinheiro, R.T.; Gigante, D.P.; Goncalves, H.; Barros, F.C. Association between breastfeeding and intelligence, educational attainment, and income at 30 years of age: A prospective birth cohort study from brazil. *Lancet Glob. Health* **2015**, *3*, e199–e205. [CrossRef]
25. Victora, C.G.; Bahl, R.; Barros, A.J.; Franca, G.V.; Horton, S.; Krasevec, J.; Murch, S.; Sankar, M.J.; Walker, N.; Rollins, N.C.; et al. Breastfeeding in the 21st century: Epidemiology, mechanisms, and lifelong effect. *Lancet* **2016**, *387*, 475–490. [CrossRef]
26. Horta, B.; Bahl, R.; Martines, J.; Victoria, C.G. *Evidence of the Long-Term Effects of Breastfeeding: Systematic Reviews and Meta-Analysis*; WHO: Geneva, Switzerland, 2007.
27. Akobeng, A.K.; Ramanan, A.V.; Buchan, I.; Heller, R.F. Effect of breast feeding on risk of coeliac disease: A systematic review and meta-analysis of observational studies. *Arch. Dis. Child.* **2006**, *91*, 39–43. [CrossRef] [PubMed]
28. Vriezinga, S.L.; Auricchio, R.; Bravi, E.; Castillejo, G.; Chmielewska, A.; Crespo Escobar, P.; Kolacek, S.; Koletzko, S.; Korponay-Szabo, I.R.; Mummert, E.; et al. Randomized feeding intervention in infants at high risk for celiac disease. *N. Engl. J. Med.* **2014**, *371*, 1304–1315. [CrossRef] [PubMed]
29. Perkin, M.R.; Logan, K.; Tseng, A.; Raji, B.; Ayis, S.; Peacock, J.; Brough, H.; Marrs, T.; Radulovic, S.; Craven, J.; et al. Randomized trial of introduction of allergenic foods in breast-fed infants. *N. Engl. J. Med.* **2016**, *374*, 1733–1743. [CrossRef] [PubMed]
30. WHO. *Global Strategy for Infant and Young Child Feeding, the Optimal Duration of Exclusive Breastfeeding*; World Health Organization: Geneva, Switzerland, 2001.
31. Agarwal, S.; Karmaus, W.; Davis, S.; Gangur, V. Immune markers in breast milk and fetal and maternal body fluids: A systematic review of perinatal concentrations. *J. Hum. Lact.* **2011**, *27*, 171–186. [CrossRef] [PubMed]
32. Wells, H.G.; Osborne, T.B. The biological reactions of the vegetable proteins: Anaphylaxis. *J. Infect. Dis.* **1911**, *8*, 66–124. [CrossRef]
33. Du Toit, G.; Roberts, G.; Sayre, P.H.; Bahnson, H.T.; Radulovic, S.; Santos, A.F.; Brough, H.A.; Phippard, D.; Basting, M.; Feeney, M.; et al. Randomized trial of peanut consumption in infants at risk for peanut allergy. *N. Engl. J. Med.* **2015**, *372*, 803–813. [CrossRef] [PubMed]
34. Ierodiakonou, D.; Garcia-Larsen, V.; Logan, A.; Groome, A.; Cunha, S.; Chivinge, J.; Robinson, Z.; Geoghegan, N.; Jarrold, K.; Reeves, T.; et al. Timing of allergenic food introduction to the infant diet and risk of allergic or autoimmune disease: A systematic review and meta-analysis. *J. Am. Med. Assoc.* **2016**, *316*, 1181–1192. [CrossRef] [PubMed]
35. Grulee, C.; Sanford, H. The influence of breast and artificial feeding on infantile eczema. *J. Pediatr.* **1936**, *9*, 223–225. [CrossRef]
36. Lowe, A.J.; Thien, F.C.; Stoney, R.M.; Bennett, C.M.; Hosking, C.S.; Hill, D.J.; Carlin, J.B.; Abramson, M.J.; Dharmage, S.C. Associations between fatty acids in colostrum and breast milk and risk of allergic disease. *Clin. Exp. Allergy* **2008**, *38*, 1745–1751. [CrossRef] [PubMed]
37. Wijga, A.H.; van Houwelingen, A.C.; Kerkhof, M.; Tabak, C.; de Jongste, J.C.; Gerritsen, J.; Boshuizen, H.; Brunekreef, B.; Smit, H.A. Breast milk fatty acids and allergic disease in preschool children: The prevention and incidence of asthma and mite allergy birth cohort study. *J. Allergy Clin. Immunol.* **2006**, *117*, 440–447. [CrossRef] [PubMed]
38. Oddy, W.H.; Pal, S.; Kusel, M.M.; Vine, D.; de Klerk, N.H.; Hartmann, P.; Holt, P.G.; Sly, P.D.; Burton, P.R.; Stanley, F.J.; et al. Atopy, eczema and breast milk fatty acids in a high-risk cohort of children followed from birth to 5 yr. *Pediatr. Allergy Immunol.* **2006**, *17*, 4–10. [CrossRef] [PubMed]
39. Patel, R.; Oken, E.; Bogdanovich, N.; Matush, L.; Sevkovskaya, Z.; Chalmers, B.; Hodnett, E.D.; Vilchuck, K.; Kramer, M.S.; Martin, R.M. Cohort profile: The promotion of breastfeeding intervention trial (probit). *Int. J. Epidemiol.* **2013**, *43*, 679–690. [CrossRef] [PubMed]

40. Flohr, C.; Nagel, G.; Weinmayr, G.; Kleiner, A.; Strachan, D.P.; Williams, H.C.; ISAAC Phase Three Study Group. Lack of evidence for a protective effect of prolonged breastfeeding on childhood eczema: Lessons from the international study of asthma and allergies in childhood (isaac) phase two. *Br. J. Dermatol.* **2011**, *165*, 1280–1289. [CrossRef] [PubMed]
41. Giwercman, C.; Halkjaer, L.B.; Jensen, S.M.; Bonnelykke, K.; Lauritzen, L.; Bisgaard, H. Increased risk of eczema but reduced risk of early wheezy disorder from exclusive breast-feeding in high-risk infants. *J. Allergy Clin. Immunol.* **2010**, *125*, 866–871. [CrossRef] [PubMed]
42. Lee, M.T.; Wu, C.C.; Ou, C.Y.; Chang, J.C.; Liu, C.A.; Wang, C.L.; Chuang, H.; Kuo, H.C.; Hsu, T.Y.; Chen, C.P.; et al. A prospective birth cohort study of different risk factors for development of allergic diseases in offspring of non-atopic parents. *Oncotarget* **2017**, *8*, 10858–10870. [CrossRef] [PubMed]
43. Lee, K.S.; Rha, Y.H.; Oh, I.H.; Choi, Y.S.; Kim, Y.E.; Choi, S.H. Does breast-feeding relate to development of atopic dermatitis in young korean children? Based on the fourth and fifth korea national health and nutrition examination survey 2007–2012. *Allergy Asthma Immunol. Res.* **2017**, *9*, 307–313. [CrossRef] [PubMed]
44. Taylor-Robinson, D.C.; Williams, H.; Pearce, A.; Law, C.; Hope, S. Do early-life exposures explain why more advantaged children get eczema? Findings from the u.K. Millennium cohort study. *Br. J. Dermatol.* **2016**, *174*, 569–578. [CrossRef] [PubMed]
45. Draaisma, E.; Garcia-Marcos, L.; Mallol, J.; Sole, D.; Perez-Fernandez, V.; Brand, P.L.; Group, E.S. A multinational study to compare prevalence of atopic dermatitis in the first year of life. *Pediatr. Allergy Immunol.* **2015**, *26*, 359–366. [CrossRef] [PubMed]
46. Sprenger, N.; Odenwald, H.; Kukkonen, A.K.; Kuitunen, M.; Savilahti, E.; Kunz, C. Fut2-dependent breast milk oligosaccharides and allergy at 2 and 5 years of age in infants with high hereditary allergy risk. *Eur. J. Nutr.* **2017**, *56*, 1293–1301. [CrossRef] [PubMed]
47. Jelding-Dannemand, E.; Malby Schoos, A.M.; Bisgaard, H. Breast-feeding does not protect against allergic sensitization in early childhood and allergy-associated disease at age 7 years. *J. Allergy Clin. Immunol.* **2015**, *136*, 1302–1308. [CrossRef] [PubMed]
48. Elbert, N.J.; van Meel, E.R.; den Dekker, H.T.; de Jong, N.W.; Nijsten, T.E.C.; Jaddoe, V.W.V.; de Jongste, J.C.; Pasmans, S.; Duijts, L. Duration and exclusiveness of breastfeeding and risk of childhood atopic diseases. *Allergy* **2017**. [CrossRef] [PubMed]
49. Bion, V.; Lockett, G.A.; Soto-Ramirez, N.; Zhang, H.; Venter, C.; Karmaus, W.; Holloway, J.W.; Arshad, S.H. Evaluating the efficacy of breastfeeding guidelines on long-term outcomes for allergic disease. *Allergy* **2016**, *71*, 661–670. [CrossRef] [PubMed]
50. Elliott, L.; Henderson, J.; Northstone, K.; Chiu, G.Y.; Dunson, D.; London, S.J. Prospective study of breast-feeding in relation to wheeze, atopy, and bronchial hyperresponsiveness in the avon longitudinal study of parents and children (alspac). *J. Allergy Clin. Immunol.* **2008**, *122*, 49–54. [CrossRef] [PubMed]
51. Friedman, N.J.; Zeiger, R.S. The role of breast-feeding in the development of allergies and asthma. *J. Allergy Clin. Immunol.* **2005**, *115*, 1238–1248. [CrossRef] [PubMed]
52. Lee, S.Y.; Kang, M.J.; Kwon, J.W.; Park, K.S.; Hong, S.J. Breastfeeding might have protective effects on atopy in children with the cd14c-159t ct/cc genotype. *Allergy Asthma Immunol. Res.* **2013**, *5*, 239–241. [CrossRef] [PubMed]
53. Sakihara, T.; Sugiura, S.; Ito, K. The ingestion of cow's milk formula in the first 3 months of life prevents the development of cow's milk allergy. *Asia Pac. Allergy* **2016**, *6*, 207–212. [CrossRef] [PubMed]
54. Onizawa, Y.; Noguchi, E.; Okada, M.; Sumazaki, R.; Hayashi, D. The association of the delayed introduction of cow's milk with ige-mediated cow's milk allergies. *J. Allergy Clin. Immunol. Pract.* **2016**, *4*, 481–488. [CrossRef] [PubMed]
55. Warstedt, K.; Furuhjelm, C.; Falth-Magnusson, K.; Fageras, M.; Duchen, K. High levels of omega-3 fatty acids in milk from omega-3 fatty acid-supplemented mothers are related to less immunoglobulin e-associated disease in infancy. *Acta Paediatr.* **2016**, *105*, 1337–1347. [CrossRef] [PubMed]
56. Liao, S.L.; Lai, S.H.; Yeh, K.W.; Huang, Y.L.; Yao, T.C.; Tsai, M.H.; Hua, M.C.; Huang, J.L.; Study, P.C. Exclusive breastfeeding is associated with reduced cow's milk sensitization in early childhood. *Pediatr. Allergy Immunol.* **2014**, *25*, 456–461. [CrossRef] [PubMed]
57. Tran, M.M.; Lefebvre, D.L.; Dai, D.; Dharma, C.; Subbarao, P.; Lou, W.; Azad, M.B.; Becker, A.B.; Mandhane, P.J.; Turvey, S.E.; et al. Timing of food introduction and development of food sensitization in a prospective birth cohort. *Pediatr. Allergy Immunol.* **2017**, *28*, 471–477. [CrossRef] [PubMed]

58. Jepsen, A.A.; Chawes, B.L.; Carson, C.G.; Schoos, A.M.; Thysen, A.H.; Waage, J.; Brix, S.; Bisgaard, H. High breast milk il-1beta level is associated with reduced risk of childhood eczema. *Clin. Exp. Allergy* **2016**, *46*, 1344–1354. [CrossRef] [PubMed]
59. Van Meel, E.R.; de Jong, M.; Elbert, N.J.; den Dekker, H.T.; Reiss, I.K.; de Jongste, J.C.; Jaddoe, V.W.V.; Duijts, L. Duration and exclusiveness of breastfeeding and school-age lung function and asthma. *Ann. Allergy Asthma Immunol.* **2017**, *119*, 21–26. [CrossRef] [PubMed]
60. Logan, C.A.; Brandt, S.; Wabitsch, M.; Brenner, H.; Wiens, F.; Stahl, B.; Marosvolgyi, T.; Decsi, T.; Rothenbacher, D.; Genuneit, J. New approach shows no association between maternal milk fatty acid composition and childhood wheeze or asthma. *Allergy* **2017**, *72*, 1374–1383. [CrossRef] [PubMed]
61. Azad, M.B.; Vehling, L.; Lu, Z.; Dai, D.; Subbarao, P.; Becker, A.B.; Mandhane, P.J.; Turvey, S.E.; Lefebvre, D.L.; Sears, M.R.; et al. Breastfeeding, maternal asthma and wheezing in the first year of life: A longitudinal birth cohort study. *Eur. Respir. J.* **2017**, *49*, 1602019. [CrossRef] [PubMed]
62. North, M.L.; Brook, J.R.; Lee, E.Y.; Omana, V.; Daniel, N.M.; Steacy, L.M.; Evans, G.J.; Diamond, M.L.; Ellis, A.K. The kingston allergy birth cohort: Exploring parentally reported respiratory outcomes through the lens of the exposome. *Ann. Allergy Asthma Immunol.* **2017**, *118*, 465–473. [CrossRef] [PubMed]
63. Kashanian, M.; Mohtashami, S.S.; Bemanian, M.H.; Moosavi, S.A.J.; Moradi Lakeh, M. Evaluation of the associations between childhood asthma and prenatal and perinatal factors. *Int. J. Gynaecol. Obstet.* **2017**, *137*, 290–294. [CrossRef] [PubMed]
64. Oh, S.; Du, R.; Zeiger, A.M.; McGarry, M.E.; Hu, D.; Thakur, N.; Pino-Yanes, M.; Galanter, J.M.; Farber, H.J.; Eng, C.; et al. Breastfeeding associated with higher lung function in african american youths with asthma. *J. Asthma* **2016**. [CrossRef] [PubMed]
65. Arif, A.A.; Racine, E.F. Does longer duration of breastfeeding prevent childhood asthma in low-income families? *J. Asthma* **2016**, 1–6. [CrossRef] [PubMed]
66. Den Dekker, H.T.; Sonnenschein-van der Voort, A.M.; Jaddoe, V.W.; Reiss, I.K.; de Jongste, J.C.; Duijts, L. Breastfeeding and asthma outcomes at the age of 6 years. The generation r study. *Pediatr. Allergy Immunol.* **2016**, *27*, 486–492. [CrossRef] [PubMed]
67. Kull, I.; Wickman, M.; Lilja, G.; Nordvall, S.L.; Pershagen, G. Breast feeding and allergic diseases in infants—A prospective birth cohort study. *Arch. Dis. Child.* **2002**, *87*, 478–481. [CrossRef] [PubMed]
68. Matheson, M.C.; Erbas, B.; Balasuriya, A.; Jenkins, M.A.; Wharton, C.L.; Tang, M.L.; Abramson, M.J.; Walters, E.H.; Hopper, J.L.; Dharmage, S.C. Breast-feeding and atopic disease: A cohort study from childhood to middle age. *J. Allergy Clin. Immunol.* **2007**, *120*, 1051–1057. [CrossRef] [PubMed]
69. Burgess, S.W.; Dakin, C.J.; O'Callaghan, M.J. Breastfeeding does not increase the risk of asthma at 14 years. *Pediatrics* **2006**, *117*, e787–e792. [CrossRef] [PubMed]
70. Gdalevich, M.; Mimouni, D.; David, M.; Mimouni, M. Breast-feeding and the onset of atopic dermatitis in childhood: A systematic review and meta-analysis of prospective studies. *J. Am. Acad. Dermatol.* **2001**, *45*, 520–527. [CrossRef] [PubMed]
71. Gdalevich, M.; Mimouni, D.; Mimouni, M. Breast-feeding and the risk of bronchial asthma in childhood: A systematic review with meta-analysis of prospective studies. *J. Pediatr.* **2001**, *139*, 261–266. [CrossRef] [PubMed]
72. Horta, B.; Victora, C. *Long-Term Effects of Breastfeeding: A Systematic Review*; WHO: Geneva, Switzerland, 2013.
73. Dogaru, C.M.; Nyffenegger, D.; Pescatore, A.M.; Spycher, B.D.; Kuehni, C.E. Breastfeeding and childhood asthma: Systematic review and meta-analysis. *Am. J. Epidemiol.* **2014**, *179*, 1153–1167. [CrossRef] [PubMed]
74. Ip, S.; Chung, M.; Raman, G.; Chew, P.; Magula, N.; DeVine, D.; Trikalinos, T.; Lau, J. Breastfeeding and maternal and infant health outcomes in developed countries. *Evid. Rep. Technol. Assess.* **2007**, *153*, 1–186.
75. Lodge, C.J.; Tan, D.J.; Lau, M.X.; Dai, X.; Tham, R.; Lowe, A.J.; Bowatte, G.; Allen, K.J.; Dharmage, S.C. Breastfeeding and asthma and allergies: A systematic review and meta-analysis. *Acta Paediatr.* **2015**, *104*, 38–53. [CrossRef] [PubMed]
76. Kramer, M.S.; Chalmers, B.; Hodnett, E.D.; Sevkovskaya, Z.; Dzikovich, I.; Shapiro, S.; Collet, J.P.; Vanilovich, I.; Mezen, I.; Ducruet, T.; et al. Promotion of breastfeeding intervention trial (probit): A randomized trial in the republic of belarus. *J. Am. Med. Assoc.* **2001**, *285*, 413–420. [CrossRef]
77. Kramer, M.S.; Matush, L.; Vanilovich, I.; Platt, R.; Bogdanovich, N.; Sevkovskaya, Z.; Dzikovich, I.; Shishko, G.; Mazer, B.; Promotion of Breastfeeding Intervention Trial Study Group. Effect of prolonged

and exclusive breast feeding on risk of allergy and asthma: Cluster randomised trial. *BMJ* **2007**, *335*, 815. [CrossRef] [PubMed]
78. Tomicic, S.; Johansson, G.; Voor, T.; Bjorksten, B.; Bottcher, M.F.; Jenmalm, M.C. Breast milk cytokine and iga composition differ in estonian and swedish mothers-relationship to microbial pressure and infant allergy. *Pediatr. Res.* **2010**, *68*, 330–334. [CrossRef] [PubMed]
79. Bjorksten, B.; Ait-Khaled, N.; Innes Asher, M.; Clayton, T.O.; Robertson, C.; ISAAC Phase Three Study Group. Global analysis of breast feeding and risk of symptoms of asthma, rhinoconjunctivitis and eczema in 6–7 year old children: Isaac phase three. *Allergol. Immunopathol.* **2011**, *39*, 318–325. [CrossRef] [PubMed]
80. Saarinen, U.M.; Kajosaari, M. Breastfeeding as prophylaxis against atopic disease: Prospective follow-up study until 17 years old. *Lancet* **1995**, *346*, 1065–1069. [CrossRef]
81. Kull, I.; Melen, E.; Alm, J.; Hallberg, J.; Svartengren, M.; van Hage, M.; Pershagen, G.; Wickman, M.; Bergstrom, A. Breast-feeding in relation to asthma, lung function, and sensitization in young schoolchildren. *J. Allergy Clin. Immunol.* **2010**, *125*, 1013–1019. [CrossRef] [PubMed]
82. Lucas, A.; Brooke, O.G.; Morley, R.; Cole, T.J.; Bamford, M.F. Early diet of preterm infants and development of allergic or atopic disease: Randomised prospective study. *BMJ* **1990**, *300*, 837–840. [CrossRef] [PubMed]
83. Pesonen, M.; Kallio, M.J.; Ranki, A.; Siimes, M.A. Prolonged exclusive breastfeeding is associated with increased atopic dermatitis: A prospective follow-up study of unselected healthy newborns from birth to age 20 years. *Clin. Exp. Allergy* **2006**, *36*, 1011–1018. [CrossRef] [PubMed]
84. Mihrshahi, S.; Ampon, R.; Webb, K.; Almqvist, C.; Kemp, A.S.; Hector, D.; Marks, G.B.; Team, C. The association between infant feeding practices and subsequent atopy among children with a family history of asthma. *Clin. Exp. Allergy* **2007**, *37*, 671–679. [CrossRef] [PubMed]
85. Nishimura, T.; Suzue, J.; Kaji, H. Breastfeeding reduces the severity of respiratory syncytial virus infection among young infants: A multi-center prospective study. *Pediatr. Int.* **2009**, *51*, 812–816. [CrossRef] [PubMed]
86. Dixon, D.L.; Griggs, K.M.; Forsyth, K.D.; Bersten, A.D. Lower interleukin-8 levels in airway aspirates from breastfed infants with acute bronchiolitis. *Pediatr. Allergy Immunol.* **2010**, *21*, e691–e696. [CrossRef] [PubMed]
87. Brew, B.K.; Allen, C.W.; Toelle, B.G.; Marks, G.B. Systematic review and meta-analysis investigating breast feeding and childhood wheezing illness. *Paediatr. Perinat. Epidemiol.* **2011**, *25*, 507–518. [CrossRef] [PubMed]
88. De Benedictis, F.M.; Bush, A. Infantile wheeze: Rethinking dogma. *Arch. Dis. Child.* **2017**, *102*, 371–375. [CrossRef] [PubMed]
89. Scholtens, S.; Wijga, A.H.; Brunekreef, B.; Kerkhof, M.; Hoekstra, M.O.; Gerritsen, J.; Aalberse, R.; de Jongste, J.C.; Smit, H.A. Breast feeding, parental allergy and asthma in children followed for 8 years. The piama birth cohort study. *Thorax* **2009**, *64*, 604–609. [CrossRef] [PubMed]
90. Nagel, G.; Buchele, G.; Weinmayr, G.; Bjorksten, B.; Chen, Y.Z.; Wang, H.; Nystad, W.; Saraclar, Y.; Braback, L.; Batlles-Garrido, J.; et al. Effect of breastfeeding on asthma, lung function and bronchial hyperreactivity in isaac phase ii. *Eur. Respir. J.* **2009**, *33*, 993–1002. [CrossRef] [PubMed]
91. Klein, L.; Kyewski, B.; Allen, P.M.; Hogquist, K.A. Positive and negative selection of the t cell repertoire: What thymocytes see (and don't see). *Nat. Rev. Immunol.* **2014**, *14*, 377–391. [CrossRef] [PubMed]
92. Sakaguchi, S. Naturally arising foxp3-expressing cd25+cd4+ regulatory t cells in immunological tolerance to self and non-self. *Nat. Immunol.* **2005**, *6*, 345–352. [CrossRef] [PubMed]
93. McLean-Tooke, A.; Spickett, G.P.; Gennery, A.R. Immunodeficiency and autoimmunity in 22q11.2 deletion syndrome. *Scand. J. Immunol.* **2007**, *66*, 1–7. [CrossRef] [PubMed]
94. Shanley, D.P.; Aw, D.; Manley, N.R.; Palmer, D.B. An evolutionary perspective on the mechanisms of immunosenescence. *Trends Immunol.* **2009**, *30*, 374–381. [CrossRef] [PubMed]
95. Lynch, H.E.; Goldberg, G.L.; Chidgey, A.; Van den Brink, M.R.; Boyd, R.; Sempowski, G.D. Thymic involution and immune reconstitution. *Trends Immunol.* **2009**, *30*, 366–373. [CrossRef] [PubMed]
96. Mohamed, N.; Eviston, D.P.; Quinton, A.E.; Benzie, R.J.; Kirby, A.C.; Peek, M.J.; Nanan, R.K. Smaller fetal thymuses in pre-eclampsia: A prospective cross-sectional study. *Ultrasound Obstet. Gynecol.* **2011**, *37*, 410–415. [CrossRef] [PubMed]
97. Dominguez-Gerpe, L.; Rey-Mendez, M. Evolution of the thymus size in response to physiological and random events throughout life. *Microsc. Res. Tech.* **2003**, *62*, 464–476. [CrossRef] [PubMed]
98. Hasselbalch, H.; Jeppesen, D.L.; Engelmann, M.D.; Michaelsen, K.F.; Nielsen, M.B. Decreased thymus size in formula-fed infants compared with breastfed infants. *Acta Paediatr.* **1996**, *85*, 1029–1032. [CrossRef] [PubMed]

99. Hasselbalch, H.; Engelmann, M.D.; Ersboll, A.K.; Jeppesen, D.L.; Fleischer-Michaelsen, K. Breast-feeding influences thymic size in late infancy. *Eur. J. Pediatr.* **1999**, *158*, 964–967. [CrossRef] [PubMed]
100. Jeppesen, D.L.; Hasselbalch, H.; Lisse, I.M.; Ersboll, A.K.; Engelmann, M.D. T-lymphocyte subsets, thymic size and breastfeeding in infancy. *Pediatr. Allergy Immunol.* **2004**, *15*, 127–132. [CrossRef] [PubMed]
101. Eysteinsdottir, J.H.; Freysdottir, J.; Haraldsson, A.; Stefansdottir, J.; Skaftadottir, I.; Helgason, H.; Ogmundsdottir, H.M. The influence of partial or total thymectomy during open heart surgery in infants on the immune function later in life. *Clin. Exp. Immunol.* **2004**, *136*, 349–355. [CrossRef] [PubMed]
102. Ngom, P.T.; Collinson, A.C.; Pido-Lopez, J.; Henson, S.M.; Prentice, A.M.; Aspinall, R. Improved thymic function in exclusively breastfed infants is associated with higher interleukin 7 concentrations in their mothers' breast milk. *Am. J. Clin. Nutr.* **2004**, *80*, 722–728. [PubMed]
103. Candeias, S.; Muegge, K.; Durum, S.K. Il-7 receptor and vdj recombination: Trophic versus mechanistic actions. *Immunity* **1997**, *6*, 501–508. [CrossRef] [PubMed]
104. Pannaraj, P.S.; Li, F.; Cerini, C.; Bender, J.M.; Yang, S.; Rollie, A.; Adisetiyo, H.; Zabih, S.; Lincez, P.J.; Bittinger, K.; et al. Association between breast milk bacterial communities and establishment and development of the infant gut microbiome. *JAMA Pediatr.* **2017**, *171*, 647–654. [CrossRef] [PubMed]
105. Rooks, M.G.; Garrett, W.S. Gut microbiota, metabolites and host immunity. *Nat. Rev. Immunol.* **2016**, *16*, 341–352. [CrossRef] [PubMed]
106. Peroni, D.G.; Pescollderungg, L.; Piacentini, G.L.; Rigotti, E.; Maselli, M.; Watschinger, K.; Piazza, M.; Pigozzi, R.; Boner, A.L. Immune regulatory cytokines in the milk of lactating women from farming and urban environments. *Pediatr. Allergy Immunol.* **2010**, *21*, 977–982. [CrossRef] [PubMed]
107. Amoudruz, P.; Holmlund, U.; Schollin, J.; Sverremark-Ekstrom, E.; Montgomery, S.M. Maternal country of birth and previous pregnancies are associated with breast milk characteristics. *Pediatr. Allergy Immunol.* **2009**, *20*, 19–29. [CrossRef] [PubMed]
108. Holmlund, U.; Amoudruz, P.; Johansson, M.A.; Haileselassie, Y.; Ongoiba, A.; Kayentao, K.; Traore, B.; Doumbo, S.; Schollin, J.; Doumbo, O.; et al. Maternal country of origin, breast milk characteristics and potential influences on immunity in offspring. *Clin. Exp. Immunol.* **2010**, *162*, 500–509. [CrossRef] [PubMed]
109. Hong, X.; Wang, G.; Liu, X.; Kumar, R.; Tsai, H.J.; Arguelles, L.; Hao, K.; Pearson, C.; Ortiz, K.; Bonzagni, A.; et al. Gene polymorphisms, breast-feeding, and development of food sensitization in early childhood. *J. Allergy Clin. Immunol.* **2011**, *128*, 374–381. [CrossRef] [PubMed]
110. Kramer, M.S.; Kakuma, R. Optimal duration of exclusive breastfeeding. *Cochrane Database Syst. Rev.* **2012**, *8*, CD003517.
111. Koletzko, B.; Lien, E.; Agostoni, C.; Bohles, H.; Campoy, C.; Cetin, I.; Decsi, T.; Dudenhausen, J.W.; Dupont, C.; Forsyth, S.; et al. The roles of long-chain polyunsaturated fatty acids in pregnancy, lactation and infancy: Review of current knowledge and consensus recommendations. *J. Perinat. Med.* **2008**, *36*, 5–14. [CrossRef] [PubMed]
112. Hunt, K.M.; Foster, J.A.; Forney, L.J.; Schutte, U.M.; Beck, D.L.; Abdo, Z.; Fox, L.K.; Williams, J.E.; McGuire, M.K.; McGuire, M.A. Characterization of the diversity and temporal stability of bacterial communities in human milk. *PLoS ONE* **2011**, *6*, e21313. [CrossRef] [PubMed]
113. Takahata, Y.; Takada, H.; Nomura, A.; Ohshima, K.; Nakayama, H.; Tsuda, T.; Nakano, H.; Hara, T. Interleukin-18 in human milk. *Pediatr. Res.* **2001**, *50*, 268–272. [CrossRef] [PubMed]
114. Ustundag, B.; Yilmaz, E.; Dogan, Y.; Akarsu, S.; Canatan, H.; Halifeoglu, I.; Cikim, G.; Aygun, A.D. Levels of cytokines (il-1beta, il-2, il-6, il-8, tnf-alpha) and trace elements (zn, cu) in breast milk from mothers of preterm and term infants. *Mediat. Inflamm.* **2005**, *2005*, 331–336. [CrossRef] [PubMed]
115. Rigotti, E.; Piacentini, G.L.; Ress, M.; Pigozzi, R.; Boner, A.L.; Peroni, D.G. Transforming growth factor-beta and interleukin-10 in breast milk and development of atopic diseases in infants. *Clin. Exp. Allergy* **2006**, *36*, 614–618. [CrossRef] [PubMed]
116. Munblit, D.; Treneva, M.; Peroni, D.G.; Colicino, S.; Chow, L.; Dissanayeke, S.; Abrol, P.; Sheth, S.; Pampura, A.; Boner, A.L.; et al. Colostrum and mature human milk of women from london, moscow, and verona: Determinants of immune composition. *Nutrients* **2016**, *8*, 695. [CrossRef] [PubMed]
117. Minniti, F.; Comberiati, P.; Munblit, D.; Piacentini, G.L.; Antoniazzi, E.; Zanoni, L.; Boner, A.L.; Peroni, D.G. Breast-milk characteristics protecting against allergy. *Endocr. Metab. Immune Disord. Drug Targets* **2014**, *14*, 9–15. [CrossRef] [PubMed]

118. Munblit, D.; Boyle, R.J.; Warner, J.O. Factors affecting breast milk composition and potential consequences for development of the allergic phenotype. *Clin. Exp. Allergy* **2015**, *45*, 583–601. [CrossRef] [PubMed]
119. Hawkes, J.S.; Bryan, D.L.; Neumann, M.A.; Makrides, M.; Gibson, R.A. Transforming growth factor beta in human milk does not change in response to modest intakes of docosahexaenoic acid. *Lipids* **2001**, *36*, 1179–1181. [CrossRef] [PubMed]
120. Dunstan, J.A.; Roper, J.; Mitoulas, L.; Hartmann, P.E.; Simmer, K.; Prescott, S.L. The effect of supplementation with fish oil during pregnancy on breast milk immunoglobulin a, soluble cd14, cytokine levels and fatty acid composition. *Clin. Exp. Allergy* **2004**, *34*, 1237–1242. [CrossRef] [PubMed]
121. Urwin, H.J.; Miles, E.A.; Noakes, P.S.; Kremmyda, L.S.; Vlachava, M.; Diaper, N.D.; Perez-Cano, F.J.; Godfrey, K.M.; Calder, P.C.; Yaqoob, P. Salmon consumption during pregnancy alters fatty acid composition and secretory iga concentration in human breast milk. *J. Nutr.* **2012**, *142*, 1603–1610. [CrossRef] [PubMed]
122. Bottcher, M.F.; Abrahamsson, T.R.; Fredriksson, M.; Jakobsson, T.; Bjorksten, B. Low breast milk tgf-beta2 is induced by lactobacillus reuteri supplementation and associates with reduced risk of sensitization during infancy. *Pediatr. Allergy Immunol.* **2008**, *19*, 497–504. [CrossRef] [PubMed]
123. Prescott, S.L.; Wickens, K.; Westcott, L.; Jung, W.; Currie, H.; Black, P.N.; Stanley, T.V.; Mitchell, E.A.; Fitzharris, P.; Siebers, R.; et al. Supplementation with lactobacillus rhamnosus or bifidobacterium lactis probiotics in pregnancy increases cord blood interferon-gamma and breast milk transforming growth factor-beta and immunoglobin a detection. *Clin. Exp. Allergy* **2008**, *38*, 1606–1614. [CrossRef] [PubMed]
124. Boyle, R.J.; Ismail, I.H.; Kivivuori, S.; Licciardi, P.V.; Robins-Browne, R.M.; Mah, L.J.; Axelrad, C.; Moore, S.; Donath, S.; Carlin, J.B.; et al. Lactobacillus gg treatment during pregnancy for the prevention of eczema: A randomized controlled trial. *Allergy* **2011**, *66*, 509–516. [CrossRef] [PubMed]
125. Hoppu, U.; Isolauri, E.; Laakso, P.; Matomaki, J.; Laitinen, K. Probiotics and dietary counselling targeting maternal dietary fat intake modifies breast milk fatty acids and cytokines. *Eur. J. Nutr.* **2012**, *51*, 211–219. [CrossRef] [PubMed]
126. Kuitunen, M.; Kukkonen, A.K.; Savilahti, E. Impact of maternal allergy and use of probiotics during pregnancy on breast milk cytokines and food antibodies and development of allergy in children until 5 years. *Int. Arch. Allergy Immunol.* **2012**, *159*, 162–170. [CrossRef] [PubMed]
127. Savilahti, E.M.; Kukkonen, A.K.; Kuitunen, M.; Savilahti, E. Soluble cd14, alpha-and beta-defensins in breast milk: Association with the emergence of allergy in a high-risk population. *Innate Immun.* **2015**, *21*, 332–337. [CrossRef] [PubMed]
128. Linnamaa, P.; Nieminen, K.; Koulu, L.; Tuomasjukka, S.; Kallio, H.; Yang, B.; Tahvonen, R.; Savolainen, J. Black currant seed oil supplementation of mothers enhances ifn-gamma and suppresses il-4 production in breast milk. *Pediatr. Allergy Immunol.* **2013**, *24*, 562–566. [CrossRef] [PubMed]
129. Nikniaz, L.; Ostadrahimi, A.; Mahdavi, R.; Hejazi, M.A.; Salekdeh, G.H. Effects of synbiotic supplementation on breast milk levels of iga, tgf-beta1, and tgf-beta2. *J. Hum. Lact.* **2013**, *29*, 591–596. [CrossRef] [PubMed]
130. Kalliomaki, M.; Ouwehand, A.; Arvilommi, H.; Kero, P.; Isolauri, E. Transforming growth factor-beta in breast milk: A potential regulator of atopic disease at an early age. *J. Allergy Clin. Immunol.* **1999**, *104*, 1251–1257. [CrossRef]
131. Jones, C.A.; Holloway, J.A.; Popplewell, E.J.; Diaper, N.D.; Holloway, J.W.; Vance, G.H.; Warner, J.A.; Warner, J.O. Reduced soluble cd14 levels in amniotic fluid and breast milk are associated with the subsequent development of atopy, eczema, or both. *J. Allergy Clin. Immunol.* **2002**, *109*, 858–866. [CrossRef] [PubMed]
132. Bottcher, M.F.; Jenmalm, M.C.; Bjorksten, B. Cytokine, chemokine and secretory iga levels in human milk in relation to atopic disease and iga production in infants. *Pediatr. Allergy Immunol.* **2003**, *14*, 35–41. [CrossRef] [PubMed]
133. Oddy, W.H.; Halonen, M.; Martinez, F.D.; Lohman, I.C.; Stern, D.A.; Kurzius-Spencer, M.; Guerra, S.; Wright, A.L. Tgf-beta in human milk is associated with wheeze in infancy. *J. Allergy Clin. Immunol.* **2003**, *112*, 723–728. [CrossRef]
134. Savilahti, E.; Siltanen, M.; Kajosaari, M.; Vaarala, O.; Saarinen, K.M. Iga antibodies, tgf-beta1 and -beta2, and soluble cd14 in the colostrum and development of atopy by age 4. *Pediatr. Res.* **2005**, *58*, 1300–1305. [CrossRef] [PubMed]
135. Snijders, B.E.; Damoiseaux, J.G.; Penders, J.; Kummeling, I.; Stelma, F.F.; van Ree, R.; van den Brandt, P.A.; Thijs, C. Cytokines and soluble cd14 in breast milk in relation with atopic manifestations in mother and infant (koala study). *Clin. Exp. Allergy* **2006**, *36*, 1609–1615. [CrossRef] [PubMed]

136. Soto-Ramirez, N.; Karmaus, W.; Yousefi, M.; Zhang, H.; Liu, J.; Gangur, V. Maternal immune markers in serum during gestation and in breast milk and the risk of asthma-like symptoms at ages 6 and 12 months: A longitudinal study. *Allergy Asthma Clin. Immunol.* **2012**, *8*, 11. [CrossRef] [PubMed]
137. Ismail, I.H.; Licciardi, P.V.; Oppedisano, F.; Boyle, R.J.; Tang, M.L. Relationship between breast milk scd14, tgf-beta1 and total iga in the first month and development of eczema during infancy. *Pediatr. Allergy Immunol.* **2013**, *24*, 352–360. [CrossRef] [PubMed]
138. Orivuori, L.; Loss, G.; Roduit, C.; Dalphin, J.C.; Depner, M.; Genuneit, J.; Lauener, R.; Pekkanen, J.; Pfefferle, P.; Riedler, J.; et al. Soluble immunoglobulin a in breast milk is inversely associated with atopic dermatitis at early age: The pasture cohort study. *Clin. Exp. Allergy* **2014**, *44*, 102–112. [CrossRef] [PubMed]
139. Munblit, D.; Treneva, M.; Peroni, D.G.; Colicino, S.; Chow, L.Y.; Dissanayeke, S.; Pampura, A.; Boner, A.L.; Geddes, D.T.; Boyle, R.J.; et al. Immune components in human milk are associated with early infant immunological health outcomes: A prospective three-country analysis. *Nutrients* **2017**, *9*, 532. [CrossRef] [PubMed]
140. Oddy, W.H.; Rosales, F. A systematic review of the importance of milk tgf-beta on immunological outcomes in the infant and young child. *Pediatr. Allergy Immunol.* **2010**, *21*, 47–59. [CrossRef] [PubMed]
141. Ogawa, J.; Sasahara, A.; Yoshida, T.; Sira, M.M.; Futatani, T.; Kanegane, H.; Miyawaki, T. Role of transforming growth factor-beta in breast milk for initiation of iga production in newborn infants. *Early Hum. Dev.* **2004**, *77*, 67–75. [CrossRef] [PubMed]
142. Ulevitch, R.J.; Tobias, P.S. Receptor-dependent mechanisms of cell stimulation by bacterial endotoxin. *Annu. Rev. Immunol.* **1995**, *13*, 437–457. [CrossRef] [PubMed]
143. Pugin, J.; Heumann, I.D.; Tomasz, A.; Kravchenko, V.V.; Akamatsu, Y.; Nishijima, M.; Glauser, M.P.; Tobias, P.S.; Ulevitch, R.J. Cd14 is a pattern recognition receptor. *Immunity* **1994**, *1*, 509–516. [CrossRef]
144. Holt, P.G.; Sly, P.D.; Bjorksten, B. Atopic versus infectious diseases in childhood: A question of balance? *Pediatr. Allergy Immunol.* **1997**, *8*, 53–58. [CrossRef] [PubMed]
145. Labeta, M.O.; Vidal, K.; Nores, J.E.; Arias, M.; Vita, N.; Morgan, B.P.; Guillemot, J.C.; Loyaux, D.; Ferrara, P.; Schmid, D.; et al. Innate recognition of bacteria in human milk is mediated by a milk-derived highly expressed pattern recognition receptor, soluble cd14. *J. Exp. Med.* **2000**, *191*, 1807–1812. [CrossRef] [PubMed]
146. Vidal, K.; Labeta, M.O.; Schiffrin, E.J.; Donnet-Hughes, A. Soluble cd14 in human breast milk and its role in innate immune responses. *Acta Odontol. Scand.* **2001**, *59*, 330–334. [CrossRef] [PubMed]
147. Jarvinen, K.M.; Suarez-Farinas, M.; Savilahti, E.; Sampson, H.A.; Berin, M.C. Immune factors in breast milk related to infant milk allergy are independent of maternal atopy. *J. Allergy Clin. Immunol.* **2015**, *135*, 1390–1393. [CrossRef] [PubMed]
148. Walter, J.; Kuhn, L.; Ghosh, M.K.; Kankasa, C.; Semrau, K.; Sinkala, M.; Mwiya, M.; Thea, D.M.; Aldrovandi, G.M. Low and undetectable breast milk interleukin-7 concentrations are associated with reduced risk of postnatal hiv transmission. *J. Acquir. Immune Defic. Syndr.* **2007**, *46*, 200–207. [CrossRef] [PubMed]
149. Castellote, C.; Casillas, R.; Ramirez-Santana, C.; Perez-Cano, F.J.; Castell, M.; Moretones, M.G.; Lopez-Sabater, M.C.; Franch, A. Premature delivery influences the immunological composition of colostrum and transitional and mature human milk. *J. Nutr.* **2011**, *141*, 1181–1187. [CrossRef] [PubMed]
150. Zuccotti, G.; Meneghin, F.; Aceti, A.; Barone, G.; Callegari, M.L.; Di Mauro, A.; Fantini, M.P.; Gori, D.; Indrio, F.; Maggio, L.; et al. Probiotics for prevention of atopic diseases in infants: Systematic review and meta-analysis. *Allergy* **2015**, *70*, 1356–1371. [CrossRef] [PubMed]
151. Kondo, N.; Suda, Y.; Nakao, A.; Oh-Oka, K.; Suzuki, K.; Ishimaru, K.; Sato, M.; Tanaka, T.; Nagai, A.; Yamagata, Z. Maternal psychosocial factors determining the concentrations of transforming growth factor-beta in breast milk. *Pediatr. Allergy Immunol.* **2011**, *22*, 853–861. [CrossRef] [PubMed]
152. Rautava, S.; Kalliomaki, M.; Isolauri, E. Probiotics during pregnancy and breast-feeding might confer immunomodulatory protection against atopic disease in the infant. *J. Allergy Clin. Immunol.* **2002**, *109*, 119–121. [CrossRef] [PubMed]
153. Osborn, D.A.; Sinn, J.K. Prebiotics in infants for prevention of allergy. *Cochrane Database Syst. Rev.* **2013**, CD006474. [CrossRef]
154. Dotterud, C.K.; Storro, O.; Johnsen, R.; Oien, T. Probiotics in pregnant women to prevent allergic disease: A randomized, double-blind trial. *Br. J. Dermatol.* **2010**, *163*, 616–623. [CrossRef] [PubMed]
155. Xiao, L.; Stahl, B.; Folkerts, G.; Garssen, J.; van't-Land, B. The immunological benefits for complex

oligosaccharides in human milk. In *Nutrition, Immunity & Infection*; CRC Press: Boca Raton, FL, USA, 2017; in press.

156. Thurl, S.; Munzert, M.; Henker, J.; Boehm, G.; Muller-Werner, B.; Jelinek, J.; Stahl, B. Variation of human milk oligosaccharides in relation to milk groups and lactational periods. *Br. J. Nutr.* **2010**, *104*, 1261–1271. [CrossRef] [PubMed]
157. Erney, R.M.; Malone, W.T.; Skelding, M.B.; Marcon, A.A.; Kleman-Leyer, K.M.; O'Ryan, M.L.; Ruiz-Palacios, G.; Hilty, M.D.; Pickering, L.K.; Prieto, P.A. Variability of human milk neutral oligosaccharides in a diverse population. *J. Pediatr. Gastroenterol. Nutr.* **2000**, *30*, 181–192. [CrossRef] [PubMed]
158. Chaturvedi, P.; Warren, C.D.; Altaye, M.; Morrow, A.L.; Ruiz-Palacios, G.; Pickering, L.K.; Newburg, D.S. Fucosylated human milk oligosaccharides vary between individuals and over the course of lactation. *Glycobiology* **2001**, *11*, 365–372. [CrossRef] [PubMed]
159. Morrow, A.L.; Meinzen-Derr, J.; Huang, P.; Schibler, K.R.; Cahill, T.; Keddache, M.; Kallapur, S.G.; Newburg, D.S.; Tabangin, M.; Warner, B.B.; et al. Fucosyltransferase 2 non-secretor and low secretor status predicts severe outcomes in premature infants. *J. Pediatr.* **2011**, *158*, 745–751. [CrossRef] [PubMed]
160. Smilowitz, J.T.; O'Sullivan, A.; Barile, D.; German, J.B.; Lonnerdal, B.; Slupsky, C.M. The human milk metabolome reveals diverse oligosaccharide profiles. *J. Nutr.* **2013**, *143*, 1709–1718. [CrossRef] [PubMed]
161. Spevacek, A.R.; Smilowitz, J.T.; Chin, E.L.; Underwood, M.A.; German, J.B.; Slupsky, C.M. Infant maturity at birth reveals minor differences in the maternal milk metabolome in the first month of lactation. *J. Nutr.* **2015**, *145*, 1698–1708. [CrossRef] [PubMed]
162. Verhasselt, V.; Milcent, V.; Cazareth, J.; Kanda, A.; Fleury, S.; Dombrowicz, D.; Glaichenhaus, N.; Julia, V. Breast milk-mediated transfer of an antigen induces tolerance and protection from allergic asthma. *Nat. Med.* **2008**, *14*, 170–175. [CrossRef] [PubMed]
163. Walker, W.A.; Iyengar, R.S. Breast milk, microbiota, and intestinal immune homeostasis. *Pediatr. Res.* **2015**, *77*, 220–228. [PubMed]
164. Atarashi, K.; Tanoue, T.; Oshima, K.; Suda, W.; Nagano, Y.; Nishikawa, H.; Fukuda, S.; Saito, T.; Narushima, S.; Hase, K.; et al. Treg induction by a rationally selected mixture of clostridia strains from the human microbiota. *Nature* **2013**, *500*, 232–236. [CrossRef] [PubMed]
165. Round, J.L.; Mazmanian, S.K. Inducible foxp3+ regulatory t-cell development by a commensal bacterium of the intestinal microbiota. *Proc. Natl. Acad Sci. USA* **2010**, *107*, 12204–12209. [CrossRef] [PubMed]
166. Schijf, M.A.; Kruijsen, D.; Bastiaans, J.; Coenjaerts, F.E.; Garssen, J.; van Bleek, G.M.; van't Land, B. Specific dietary oligosaccharides increase th1 responses in a mouse respiratory syncytial virus infection model. *J. Virol.* **2012**, *86*, 11472–11482. [CrossRef] [PubMed]
167. Diesner, S.C.; Bergmayr, C.; Pfitzner, B.; Assmann, V.; Krishnamurthy, D.; Starkl, P.; Endesfelder, D.; Rothballer, M.; Welzl, G.; Rattei, T.; et al. A distinct microbiota composition is associated with protection from food allergy in an oral mouse immunization model. *Clin. Immunol.* **2016**, *173*, 10–18. [CrossRef] [PubMed]
168. Hua, X.; Goedert, J.J.; Pu, A.; Yu, G.; Shi, J. Allergy associations with the adult fecal microbiota: Analysis of the american gut project. *EBioMedicine* **2016**, *3*, 172–179. [CrossRef] [PubMed]
169. Noval Rivas, M.; Burton, O.T.; Wise, P.; Zhang, Y.-Q.; Hobson, S.A.; Garcia Lloret, M.; Chehoud, C.; Kuczynski, J.; DeSantis, T.; Warrington, J.; et al. A microbiota signature associated with experimental food allergy promotes allergic sensitization and anaphylaxis. *J. Allergy Clin. Immunol.* **2013**, *131*, 201–212. [CrossRef] [PubMed]
170. Ruokolainen, L.; Paalanen, L.; Karkman, A.; Laatikainen, T.; von Hertzen, L.; Vlasoff, T.; Markelova, O.; Masyuk, V.; Auvinen, P.; Paulin, L.; et al. Significant disparities in allergy prevalence and microbiota between the young people in finnish and russian karelia. *Clin. Exp. Allergy* **2017**, *47*, 665–674. [CrossRef] [PubMed]
171. Zhang, L.-L.; Chen, X.; Zheng, P.-Y.; Luo, Y.; Lu, G.-F.; Liu, Z.-Q.; Huang, H.; Yang, P.-C. Oral bifidobacterium modulates intestinal immune inflammation in mice with food allergy. *J. Gastroenterol. Hepatol.* **2010**, *25*, 928–934. [CrossRef] [PubMed]
172. Gensollen, T.; Iyer, S.S.; Kasper, D.L.; Blumberg, R.S. How colonization by microbiota in early life shapes the immune system. *Science* **2016**, *352*, 539–544. [CrossRef] [PubMed]
173. An, D.; Oh, S.F.; Olszak, T.; Neves, J.F.; Avci, F.Y. Sphingolipids from a symbiotic microbe regulate homeostasis of host intestinal natural killer t cells. *Cell* **2014**, *156*, 123–133. [CrossRef] [PubMed]
174. El Aidy, S.; Hooiveld, G.; Tremaroli, V.; Backhed, F.; Kleerebezem, M. The gut microbiota and mucosal homeostasis. *Gut Microbes* **2014**, *4*, 118–124. [CrossRef] [PubMed]

175. Olszak, T.; An, D.; Zeissig, S.; Vera, M.P.; Richter, J.; Franke, A.; Glickman, J.N.; Siebert, R.; Baron, R.M.; Kasper, D.L.; et al. Microbial exposure during early life has persistent effects on natural killer t cell function. *Science* **2012**, *336*, 489–493. [CrossRef] [PubMed]
176. Marcobal, A.; Barboza, M.; Froehlich, J.W.; Block, D.E.; German, J.B.; Lebrilla, C.B.; Mills, D.A. Consumption of human milk oligosaccharides by gut-related microbes. *J. Agric. Food Chem.* **2010**, *58*, 5334–5340. [CrossRef] [PubMed]
177. De Leoz, M.L.A.; Kalanetra, K.M.; Bokulich, N.A.; Strum, J.S.; Underwood, M.A.; German, J.B.; Mills, D.A.; Lebrilla, C.B. Human milk glycomics and gut microbial genomics in infant feces show a correlation between human milk oligosaccharides and gut microbiota: A proof-of-concept study. *J. Proteome Res.* **2015**, *14*, 491–502. [CrossRef] [PubMed]
178. Garrido, D.; Barile, D.; Mills, D.A. A molecular basis for bifidobacterial enrichment in the infant gastrointestinal tract. *Adv. Nutr.* **2012**, *3*, 415S–421S. [CrossRef] [PubMed]
179. LoCascio, R.G.; Ninonuevo, M.R.; Freeman, S.L.; Sela, D.A.; Grimm, R.; Lebrilla, C.B.; Mills, D.A.; German, J.B. Glycoprofiling of bifidobacterial consumption of human milk oligosaccharides demonstrates strain specific, preferential consumption of small chain glycans secreted in early human lactation. *J. Agric. Food Chem.* **2007**, *55*, 8914–8919. [CrossRef] [PubMed]
180. Marcobal, A.; Sonnenburg, J.L. Human milk oligosaccharide consumption by intestinal microbiota. *Clin. Microbiol. Infect.* **2012**, *18*, 12–15. [CrossRef] [PubMed]
181. Ward, R.E.; Ni onuevo, M.; Mills, D.A.; Lebrilla, C.B.; German, J.B. In vitro fermentability of human milk oligosaccharides by several strains of bifidobacteria. *Mol. Nutr. Food Res.* **2007**, *51*, 1398–1405. [CrossRef] [PubMed]
182. Boudry, G.; Hamilton, M.K.; Chichlowski, M.; Wickramasinghe, S.; Barile, D.; Kalanetra, K.M.; Mills, D.A.; Raybould, H.E. Bovine milk oligosaccharides decrease gut permeability and improve inflammation and microbial dysbiosis in diet-induced obese mice. *J. Dairy Sci.* **2017**, *100*, 2471–2481. [CrossRef] [PubMed]
183. Liu, M.-Y.; Yang, Z.-Y.; Dai, W.-K.; Huang, J.-Q.; Li, Y.-H.; Zhang, J.; Qiu, C.-Z.; Wei, C.; Zhou, Q.; Sun, X.; et al. Protective effect of *Bifidobacterium infantis* cgmcc313-2 on ovalbumin-induced airway asthma and β-lactoglobulin-induced intestinal food allergy mouse models. *World J. Gastroenterol.* **2017**, *23*, 2149–2158. [CrossRef] [PubMed]
184. Schouten, B.; van Esch, B.C.; Hofman, G.A.; van Doorn, S.A.; Knol, J.; Nauta, A.J.; Garssen, J.; Willemsen, L.E.; Knippels, L.M. Cow milk allergy symptoms are reduced in mice fed dietary synbiotics during oral sensitization with whey. *J. Nutr.* **2009**, *139*, 1398–1403. [CrossRef] [PubMed]
185. Lewis, Z.T.; Totten, S.M.; Smilowitz, J.T.; Popovic, M.; Parker, E.; Lemay, D.G.; Van Tassell, M.L.; Miller, M.J.; Jin, Y.-S.; German, J.B.; et al. Maternal fucosyltransferase 2 status affects the gut bifidobacterial communities of breastfed infants. *Microbiome* **2015**, *3*, 13. [CrossRef] [PubMed]
186. Ackerman, D.L.; Doster, R.S.; Weitkamp, J.-H.; Aronoff, D.; Gaddy, J.A.; Townsend, S.D. Human milk oligosaccharides exhibit antimicrobial and anti-biofilm properties against group b streptococcus. *ACS Infect. Dis.* **2017**, *3*, 595–605. [CrossRef] [PubMed]
187. Bode, L. The functional biology of human milk oligosaccharides. *Early Hum. Dev.* **2015**, *91*, 619–622. [CrossRef] [PubMed]
188. Lin, A.E.; Autran, C.A.; Szyszka, A.; Escajadillo, T.; Huang, M.; Godula, K.; Prudden, A.R.; Boons, G.-J.; Lewis, A.L.; Doran, K.S.; et al. Human milk oligosaccharides inhibit growth of group *B streptococcus*. *J. Biol. Chem.* **2017**. [CrossRef] [PubMed]
189. Goldsmith, A.J.; Koplin, J.J.; Lowe, A.J.; Tang, M.L.; Matheson, M.C.; Robinson, M.; Peters, R.; Dharmage, S.C.; Allen, K.J. Formula and breast feeding in infant food allergy: A population-based study. *J. Paediatr. Child Health* **2016**, *52*, 377–384. [CrossRef] [PubMed]
190. Hoyt, A.E.W.; Medico, T.; Commins, S.P. Breast milk and food allergy: Connections and current recommendations. *Pediatr. Clin. N. Am.* **2015**, *62*, 1493–1507. [CrossRef] [PubMed]
191. Chua, M.C.; Ben-Amor, K.; Lay, C.; Neo, A.G.E.; Chiang, W.C.; Rao, R.; Chew, C.; Chaithongwongwatthana, S.; Khemapech, N.; Knol, J.; et al. Effect of synbiotic on the gut microbiota of caesarean delivered infants: A randomized, double-blind, multicenter study. *J. Pediatr. Gastroenterol. Nutr.* **2017**. [CrossRef] [PubMed]
192. Ley, D.; Desseyn, J.L.; Mischke, M.; Knol, J.; Turck, D.; Gottrand, F. Early-life origin of intestinal inflammatory disorders. *Nutr. Rev.* **2017**, *75*, 175–187. [CrossRef] [PubMed]

193. Naarding, M.A.; Ludwig, I.S.; Groot, F.; Berkhout, B.; Geijtenbeek, T.B.; Pollakis, G.; Paxton, W.A. Lewis x component in human milk binds dc-sign and inhibits hiv-1 transfer to cd4+ t lymphocytes. *J. Clin. Investig.* **2005**, *115*, 3256–3264. [CrossRef] [PubMed]
194. Lehmann, S.; Hiller, J.; van Bergenhenegouwen, J.; Knippels, L.M.; Garssen, J.; Traidl-Hoffmann, C. In vitro evidence for immune-modulatory properties of non-digestible oligosaccharides: Direct effect on human monocyte derived dendritic cells. *PLoS ONE* **2015**, *10*, e0132304. [CrossRef] [PubMed]
195. He, Y.; Lawlor, N.T.; Newburg, D.S. Human milk components modulate toll-like receptor-mediated inflammation. *Adv. Nutr.* **2016**, *7*, 102–111. [CrossRef] [PubMed]
196. Gringhuis, S.I.; Kaptein, T.M.; Wevers, B.A.; Mesman, A.W.; Geijtenbeek, T.B. Fucose-specific dc-sign signalling directs t helper cell type-2 responses via ikkepsilon- and cyld-dependent bcl3 activation. *Nat. Commun.* **2014**, *5*, 3898. [CrossRef] [PubMed]
197. Noll, A.J.; Yu, Y.; Lasanajak, Y.; Duska-McEwen, G.; Buck, R.H.; Smith, D.F.; Cummings, R.D. Human dc-sign binds specific human milk glycans. *Biochem. J.* **2016**, *473*, 1343–1353. [CrossRef] [PubMed]
198. De Kivit, S.; Kostadinova, A.I.; Kerperien, J.; Morgan, M.E.; Muruzabal, V.A.; Hofman, G.A.; Knippels, L.M.J.; Kraneveld, A.D.; Garssen, J.; Willemsen, L.E.M. Dietary, nondigestible oligosaccharides and bifidobacterium breve m-16v suppress allergic inflammation in intestine via targeting dendritic cell maturation. *J. Leukoc. Biol.* **2017**, *102*, 105–115. [CrossRef] [PubMed]
199. Marriage, B.J.; Buck, R.H.; Goehring, K.C.; Oliver, J.S.; Williams, J.A. Infants fed a lower calorie formula with 2′fl show growth and 2′fl uptake like breast-fed infants. *J. Pediatr. Gastroenterol. Nutr.* **2015**, *61*, 649–658. [CrossRef] [PubMed]
200. Arslanoglu, S.; Moro, G.E.; Boehm, G.; Wienz, F.; Stahl, B.; Bertino, E. Early neutral prebiotic oligosaccharide supplementation reduces the incidence of some allergic manifestations in the first 5 years of life. *J. Biol. Regul. Homeost. Agents* **2012**, *26*, 49–59. [PubMed]
201. Moro, G.; Arslanoglu, S.; Stahl, B.; Jelinek, J.; Wahn, U.; Boehm, G. A mixture of prebiotic oligosaccharides reduces the incidence of atopic dermatitis during the first six months of age. *Arch. Dis. Child.* **2006**, *91*, 814–819. [CrossRef] [PubMed]
202. Bollrath, J.; Powrie, F. Immunology. Feed your tregs more fiber. *Science* **2013**, *341*, 463–464. [CrossRef] [PubMed]
203. Bendiks, M.; Kopp, M.V. The relationship between advances in understanding the microbiome and the maturing hygiene hypothesis. *Curr. Allergy Asthma Rep.* **2013**, *13*, 487–494. [CrossRef] [PubMed]
204. Rodriguez, J.M.; Murphy, K.; Stanton, C.; Ross, R.P.; Kober, O.I.; Juge, N.; Avershina, E.; Rudi, K.; Narbad, A.; Jenmalm, M.C.; et al. The composition of the gut microbiota throughout life, with an emphasis on early life. *Microb. Ecol. Health Dis.* **2015**, *26*, 26050. [CrossRef] [PubMed]
205. Bridgman, S.L.; Kozyrskyj, A.L.; Scott, J.A.; Becker, A.B.; Azad, M.B. Gut microbiota and allergic disease in children. *Ann. Allergy Asthma Immunol.* **2016**, *116*, 99–105. [CrossRef] [PubMed]
206. Guaraldi, F.; Salvatori, G. Effect of breast and formula feeding on gut microbiota shaping in newborns. *Front. Cell. Infect. Microbiol.* **2012**, *2*, 94. [CrossRef] [PubMed]
207. Perez, P.F.; Dore, J.; Leclerc, M.; Levenez, F.; Benyacoub, J.; Serrant, P.; Segura-Roggero, I.; Schiffrin, E.J.; Donnet-Hughes, A. Bacterial imprinting of the neonatal immune system: Lessons from maternal cells? *Pediatrics* **2007**, *119*, e724–e732. [CrossRef] [PubMed]
208. Martín, R.; Langa, S.; Reviriego, C.; Jiménez, E.; Marín, M.L.; Olivares, M.; Boza, J.; Jiménez, J.; Fernández, L.; Xaus, J.; et al. The commensal microflora of human milk: New perspectives for food bacteriotherapy and probiotics. *Trends Food Sci. Technol.* **2004**, *15*, 121–127. [CrossRef]
209. McGuire, M.K.; McGuire, M.A. Human milk: Mother nature's prototypical probiotic food? *Adv. Nutr.* **2015**, *6*, 112–123. [CrossRef] [PubMed]
210. Abrahamsson, T.R.; Sinkiewicz, G.; Jakobsson, T.; Fredrikson, M.; Bjorksten, B. Probiotic lactobacilli in breast milk and infant stool in relation to oral intake during the first year of life. *J. Pediatr. Gastroenterol. Nutr.* **2009**, *49*, 349–354. [CrossRef] [PubMed]
211. Cabrera-Rubio, R.; Collado, M.C.; Laitinen, K.; Salminen, S.; Isolauri, E.; Mira, A. The human milk microbiome changes over lactation and is shaped by maternal weight and mode of delivery. *Am. J. Clin. Nutr.* **2012**, *96*, 544–551. [CrossRef] [PubMed]
212. Boix-Amoros, A.; Collado, M.C.; Mira, A. Relationship between milk microbiota, bacterial load, macronutrients, and human cells during lactation. *Front. Microbiol.* **2016** *7*, 492. [CrossRef] [PubMed]

213. Fitzstevens, J.L.; Smith, K.C.; Hagadorn, J.I.; Caimano, M.J.; Matson, A.P.; Brownell, E.A. Systematic review of the human milk microbiota. *Nutr. Clin. Pract.* **2017**, *32*, 354–364. [CrossRef] [PubMed]
214. Gomez-Gallego, C.; Garcia-Mantrana, I.; Salminen, S.; Collado, M.C. The human milk microbiome and factors influencing its composition and activity. *Semin. Fetal Neonatal Med.* **2016**, *21*, 400–405. [CrossRef] [PubMed]
215. Drago, L.; Toscano, M.; De Grandi, R.; Grossi, E.; Padovani, E.M.; Peroni, D.G. Microbiota network and mathematic microbe mutualism in colostrum and mature milk collected in two different geographic areas: Italy versus burundi. *ISME J.* **2017**, *11*, 875–884. [CrossRef] [PubMed]
216. Dave, V.; Street, K.; Francis, S.; Bradman, A.; Riley, L.; Eskenazi, B.; Holland, N. Bacterial microbiome of breast milk and child saliva from low-income mexican-american women and children. *Pediatr. Res.* **2016**, *79*, 846–854. [CrossRef] [PubMed]
217. Soto, A.; Martin, V.; Jimenez, E.; Mader, I.; Rodriguez, J.M.; Fernandez, L. Lactobacilli and bifidobacteria in human breast milk: Influence of antibiotherapy and other host and clinical factors. *J. Pediatr. Gastroenterol. Nutr.* **2014**, *59*, 78–88. [CrossRef] [PubMed]
218. Urbaniak, C.; Angelini, M.; Gloor, G.B.; Reid, G. Human milk microbiota profiles in relation to birthing method, gestation and infant gender. *Microbiome* **2016**, *4*, 1. [CrossRef] [PubMed]
219. Contreras, G.A.; Rodriguez, J.M. Mastitis: Comparative etiology and epidemiology. *J. Mammary Gland Biol. Neoplasia* **2011**, *16*, 339–356. [CrossRef] [PubMed]
220. Jimenez, E.; de Andres, J.; Manrique, M.; Pareja-Tobes, P.; Tobes, R.; Martinez-Blanch, J.F.; Codoner, F.M.; Ramon, D.; Fernandez, L.; Rodriguez, J.M. Metagenomic analysis of milk of healthy and mastitis-suffering women. *J. Human Lact.* **2015**, *31*, 406–415. [CrossRef] [PubMed]
221. Rodriguez, J.M. The origin of human milk bacteria: Is there a bacterial entero-mammary pathway during late pregnancy and lactation? *Adv. Nutr.* **2014**, *5*, 779–784. [CrossRef] [PubMed]
222. Xuan, C.; Shamonki, J.M.; Chung, A.; Dinome, M.L.; Chung, M.; Sieling, P.A.; Lee, D.J. Microbial dysbiosis is associated with human breast cancer. *PLoS ONE* **2014**, *9*, e83744. [CrossRef] [PubMed]
223. Urbaniak, C.; Cummins, J.; Brackstone, M.; Macklaim, J.M.; Gloor, G.B.; Baban, C.K.; Scott, L.; O'Hanlon, D.M.; Burton, J.P.; Francis, K.P.; et al. Microbiota of human breast tissue. *Appl. Environ. Microbiol.* **2014**, *80*, 3007–3014. [CrossRef] [PubMed]
224. Martin, V.; Maldonado-Barragan, A.; Moles, L.; Rodriguez-Banos, M.; Campo, R.D.; Fernandez, L.; Rodriguez, J.M.; Jimenez, E. Sharing of bacterial strains between breast milk and infant feces. *J. Hum. Lact.* **2012**, *28*, 36–44. [CrossRef] [PubMed]
225. Diaz-Ropero, M.P.; Martin, R.; Sierra, S.; Lara-Villoslada, F.; Rodriguez, J.M.; Xaus, J.; Olivares, M. Two lactobacillus strains, isolated from breast milk, differently modulate the immune response. *J. Appl. Microbiol.* **2007**, *102*, 337–343. [CrossRef] [PubMed]
226. Gronlund, M.M.; Gueimonde, M.; Laitinen, K.; Kociubinski, G.; Gronroos, T.; Salminen, S.; Isolauri, E. Maternal breast-milk and intestinal bifidobacteria guide the compositional development of the bifidobacterium microbiota in infants at risk of allergic disease. *Clin. Exp. Allergy* **2007**, *37*, 1764–1772. [CrossRef] [PubMed]
227. Dzidic, M.; Abrahamsson, T.R.; Artacho, A.; Bjorksten, B.; Collado, M.C.; Mira, A.; Jenmalm, M.C. Aberrant iga responses to the gut microbiota during infancy precede asthma and allergy development. *J. Allergy Clin. Immunol.* **2017**, *139*, 1017–1025. [CrossRef] [PubMed]
228. Waidyatillake, N.T.; Stoney, R.; Thien, F.; Lodge, C.J.; Simpson, J.A.; Allen, K.J.; Abramson, M.J.; Erbas, B.; Svanes, C.; Dharmage, S.C.; et al. Breast milk polyunsaturated fatty acids: Associations with adolescent allergic disease and lung function. *Allergy* **2017**, *72*, 1193–1201. [CrossRef] [PubMed]
229. Seppo, A.E.; Autran, C.A.; Bode, L.; Jarvinen, K.M. Human milk oligosaccharides and development of cow's milk allergy in infants. *J. Allergy Clin. Immunol.* **2017**, *139*, 708–711. [CrossRef] [PubMed]
230. Baiz, N.; Macchiaverni, P.; Tulic, M.K.; Rekima, A.; Annesi-Maesano, I.; Verhasselt, V.; EDEN Mother-Child Cohort Study Group. Early oral exposure to house dust mite allergen through breast milk: A potential risk factor for allergic sensitization and respiratory allergies in children. *J. Allergy Clin. Immunol.* **2017**, *139*, 369–372. [CrossRef] [PubMed]
231. Braun-Fahrlander, C.; von Mutius, E. Can farm milk consumption prevent allergic diseases? *Clin. Exp. Allergy* **2011**, *41*, 29–35. [CrossRef] [PubMed]

232. Barthow, C.; Wickens, K.; Stanley, T.; Mitchell, E.A.; Maude, R.; Abels, P.; Purdie, G.; Murphy, R.; Stone, P.; Kang, J.; et al. The probiotics in pregnancy study (pip study): Rationale and design of a double-blind randomised controlled trial to improve maternal health during pregnancy and prevent infant eczema and allergy. *BMC Pregnancy Childbirth* **2016**, *16*, 133. [CrossRef] [PubMed]
233. Gueimonde, M.; Sakata, S.; Kalliomaki, M.; Isolauri, E.; Benno, Y.; Salminen, S. Effect of maternal consumption of lactobacillus gg on transfer and establishment of fecal bifidobacterial microbiota in neonates. *J. Pediatr. Gastroenterol. Nutr.* **2006**, *42*, 166–170. [CrossRef] [PubMed]
234. Mastromarino, P.; Capobianco, D.; Miccheli, A.; Pratico, G.; Campagna, G.; Laforgia, N.; Capursi, T.; Baldassarre, M.E. Administration of a multistrain probiotic product (vsl#3) to women in the perinatal period differentially affects breast milk beneficial microbiota in relation to mode of delivery. *Pharmacol. Res.* **2015**, *95–96*, 63–70. [PubMed]
235. Niers, L.; Martin, R.; Rijkers, G.; Sengers, F.; Timmerman, H.; van Uden, N.; Smidt, H.; Kimpen, J.; Hoekstra, M. The effects of selected probiotic strains on the development of eczema (the panda study). *Allergy* **2009**, *64*, 1349–1358. [CrossRef] [PubMed]
236. Rautava, S.; Kainonen, E.; Salminen, S.; Isolauri, E. Maternal probiotic supplementation during pregnancy and breast-feeding reduces the risk of eczema in the infant. *J. Allergy Clin. Immunol.* **2012**, *130*, 1355–1360. [CrossRef] [PubMed]
237. Kramer, M.S.; Kakuma, R. The optimal duration of exclusive breastfeeding: A systematic review. *Adv. Exp. Med. Biol.* **2004**, *554*, 63–77. [PubMed]
238. Allen, L.H. Current information gaps in micronutrient research, programs and policy: How can we fill them? *World Rev. Nutr. Diet.* **2016**, *115*, 109–117. [PubMed]
239. Hampel, D.; Allen, L.H. Analyzing b-vitamins in human milk: Methodological approaches. *Crit. Rev. Food Sci. Nutr.* **2016**, *56*, 494–511. [CrossRef] [PubMed]
240. Barker, D.J. The developmental origins of chronic adult disease. *Acta Paediatr.* **2004**, *93*, 26–33. [CrossRef]
241. Jensen, R.G. *Handbook of Milk Composition*; Academic Press Inc.: San Deigo, CA, USA, 1995.
242. Kamao, M.; Tsugawa, N.; Suhara, Y.; Wada, A.; Mori, T.; Murata, K.; Nishino, R.; Ukita, T.; Uenishi, K.; Tanaka, K.; et al. Quantification of fat-soluble vitamins in human breast milk by liquid chromatography-tandem mass spectrometry. *J. Chromatogr. B Anal. Technol. Biomed. Life Sci.* **2007**, *859*, 192–200. [CrossRef] [PubMed]
243. Bolisetty, S.; Gupta, J.M.; Graham, G.G.; Salonikas, C.; Naidoo, D. Vitamin k in preterm breastmilk with maternal supplementation. *Acta Paediatr.* **1998**, *87*, 960–962. [CrossRef] [PubMed]
244. Lima, M.S.; Dimenstein, R.; Ribeiro, K.D. Vitamin e concentration in human milk and associated factors: A literature review. *J. Pediatr.* **2014**, *90*, 440–448. [CrossRef] [PubMed]
245. Kim, H.; Jung, B.M.; Lee, B.N.; Kim, Y.J.; Jung, J.A.; Chang, N. Retinol, alpha-tocopherol, and selected minerals in breast milk of lactating women with full-term infants in south korea. *Nutr. Res. Pract.* **2017**, *11*, 64–69. [CrossRef] [PubMed]
246. Sakurai, T.; Furukawa, M.; Asoh, M.; Kanno, T.; Kojima, T.; Yonekubo, A. Fat-soluble and water-soluble vitamin contents of breast milk from japanese women. *J. Nutr. Sci. Vitaminol.* **2005**, *51*, 239–247. [CrossRef] [PubMed]
247. Picciano, M.F. *Clinical Nutrition of the Essential Trace Elements and Minerals*; Springer Science and Business Media: New York, NY, USA, 2000.
248. Dawodu, A.; Tsang, R.C. Maternal vitamin d status: Effect on milk vitamin d content and vitamin d status of breastfeeding infants. *Adv. Nutr.* **2012**, *3*, 353–361. [CrossRef] [PubMed]
249. Allen, L.H. Multiple micronutrients in pregnancy and lactation: An overview. *Am. J. Clin. Nutr.* **2005**, *81*, 1206S–1212S. [PubMed]
250. Hampel, D.; Shahab-Ferdows, S.; Adair, L.S.; Bentley, M.E.; Flax, V.L.; Jamieson, D.J.; Ellington, S.R.; Tegha, G.; Chasela, C.S.; Kamwendo, D.; et al. Thiamin and riboflavin in human milk: Effects of lipid-based nutrient supplementation and stage of lactation on vitamer secretion and contributions to total vitamin content. *PLoS ONE* **2016**, *11*, e0149479. [CrossRef] [PubMed]
251. Treneva, M.; Munblit, D.; Pampura, A. Moscow infants: Atopic dermatitis, skin reactions to the dietary intake at 1-year of age followed to 2-years of age and sensitization at the age of 1 year. *Allergy* **2015**, *70*, 306.
252. Page, R.; Robichaud, A.; Arbuckle, T.E.; Fraser, W.D.; MacFarlane, A.J. Total folate and unmetabolized folic acid in the breast milk of a cross-section of canadian women. *Am. J. Clin. Nutr.* **2017**, *105*, 1101–1109. [CrossRef] [PubMed]

253. Houghton, L.A.; Yang, J.; O'Connor, D.L. Unmetabolized folic acid and total folate concentrations in breast milk are unaffected by low-dose folate supplements. *Am. J. Clin. Nutr.* **2009**, *89*, 216–220. [CrossRef] [PubMed]
254. Hampel, D.; Shahab-Ferdows, S.; Islam, M.M.; Peerson, J.M.; Allen, L.H. Vitamin concentrations in human milk vary with time within feed, circadian rhythm, and single-dose supplementation. *J. Nutr.* **2017**, *147*, 603–611. [CrossRef] [PubMed]
255. Williams, A.M.; Chantry, C.J.; Young, S.L.; Achando, B.S.; Allen, L.H.; Arnold, B.F.; Colford, J.M., Jr.; Dentz, H.N.; Hampel, D.; Kiprotich, M.C.; et al. Vitamin b-12 concentrations in breast milk are low and are not associated with reported household hunger, recent animal-source food, or vitamin b-12 intake in women in rural kenya. *J. Nutr.* **2016**, *146*, 1125–1131. [CrossRef] [PubMed]
256. Deegan, K.L.; Jones, K.M.; Zuleta, C.; Ramirez-Zea, M.; Lildballe, D.L.; Nexo, E.; Allen, L.H. Breast milk vitamin b-12 concentrations in guatemalan women are correlated with maternal but not infant vitamin b-12 status at 12 months postpartum. *J. Nutr.* **2012**, *142*, 112–116. [CrossRef] [PubMed]
257. Maas, C.; Franz, A.R.; Shunova, A.; Mathes, M.; Bleeker, C.; Poets, C.F.; Schleicher, E.; Bernhard, W. Choline and polyunsaturated fatty acids in preterm infants' maternal milk. *Eur. J. Nutr.* **2017**, *56*, 1733–1742. [CrossRef] [PubMed]
258. Gaxiola-Robles, R.; Labrada-Martagon, V.; Celis de la Rosa Ade, J.; Acosta-Vargas, B.; Mendez-Rodriguez, L.C.; Zenteno-Savin, T. Interaction between mercury (hg), arsenic (as) and selenium (se) affects the activity of glutathione s-transferase in breast milk; possible relationship with fish and sellfish intake. *Nutr. Hosp.* **2014**, *30*, 436–446. [PubMed]
259. Shearer, T.R.; Hadjimarkos, D.M. Geographic distribution of selenium in human milk. *Arch. Environ. Health* **1975**, *30*, 230–233. [CrossRef] [PubMed]
260. Kim, S.Y.; Park, J.H.; Kim, E.A.; Lee-Kim, Y.C. Longitudinal study on trace mineral compositions (selenium, zinc, copper, manganese) in korean human preterm milk. *J. Korean Med. Sci.* **2012**, *27*, 532–536. [CrossRef] [PubMed]
261. Djurovic, D.; Milisavljevic, B.; Mugosa, B.; Lugonja, N.; Miletic, S.; Spasic, S.; Vrvic, M. Zinc concentrations in human milk and infant serum during the first six months of lactation. *J. Trace Elem. Med. Biol.* **2017**, *41*, 75–78. [CrossRef] [PubMed]
262. Qian, J.; Chen, T.; Lu, W.; Wu, S.; Zhu, J. Breast milk macro- and micronutrient composition in lactating mothers from suburban and urban shanghai. *J. Paediatr. Child Health* **2010**, *46*, 115–120. [CrossRef] [PubMed]
263. Jorgensen, A.; O'Leary, P.; James, I.; Skeaff, S.; Sherriff, J. Assessment of breast milk iodine concentrations in lactating women in western australia. *Nutrients* **2016**, *8*, 699. [CrossRef] [PubMed]
264. Henjum, S.; Kjellevold, M.; Ulak, M.; Chandyo, R.K.; Shrestha, P.S.; Froyland, L.; Strydom, E.E.; Dhansay, M.A.; Strand, T.A. Iodine concentration in breastmilk and urine among lactating women of bhaktapur, nepal. *Nutrients* **2016**, *8*, 255. [CrossRef] [PubMed]
265. Osei, J.; Andersson, M.; Reijden, O.V.; Dold, S.; Smuts, C.M.; Baumgartner, J. Breast-milk iodine concentrations, iodine status, and thyroid function of breastfed infants aged 2–4 months and their mothers residing in a south african township. *J. Clin. Res. Pediatr. Endocrinol.* **2016**, *8*, 381–391. [CrossRef] [PubMed]
266. Domellof, M.; Braegger, C.; Campoy, C.; Colomb, V.; Decsi, T.; Fewtrell, M.; Hojsak, I.; Mihatsch, W.; Molgaard, C.; Shamir, R.; et al. Iron requirements of infants and toddlers. *J. Pediatr. Gastroenterol. Nutr.* **2014**, *58*, 119–129. [CrossRef] [PubMed]
267. Haskell, M.J.; Brown, K.H. Maternal vitamin a nutriture and the vitamin a content of human milk. *J. Mammary Gland Biol. Neoplasia* **1999**, *4*, 243–257. [CrossRef] [PubMed]
268. Turfkruyer, M.; Rekima, A.; Macchiaverni, P.; Le Bourhis, L.; Muncan, V.; van den Brink, G.R.; Tulic, M.K.; Verhasselt, V. Oral tolerance is inefficient in neonatal mice due to a physiological vitamin a deficiency. *Mucosal Immunol.* **2016**, *9*, 479–491. [CrossRef] [PubMed]
269. Nurmatov, U.; Devereux, G.; Sheikh, A. Nutrients and foods for the primary prevention of asthma and allergy: Systematic review and meta-analysis. *J. Allergy Clin. Immunol.* **2011**, *127*, 724–733. [CrossRef] [PubMed]
270. Aage, S.; Kiraly, N.; Da Costa, K.; Byberg, S.; Bjerregaard-Andersen, M.; Fisker, A.B.; Aaby, P.; Benn, C.S. Neonatal vitamin a supplementation associated with increased atopy in girls. *Allergy* **2015**, *70*, 985–994. [CrossRef] [PubMed]

271. Duggan, C.; Srinivasan, K.; Thomas, T.; Samuel, T.; Rajendran, R.; Muthayya, S.; Finkelstein, J.L.; Lukose, A.; Fawzi, W.; Allen, L.H.; et al. Vitamin b-12 supplementation during pregnancy and early lactation increases maternal, breast milk, and infant measures of vitamin b-12 status. *J. Nutr.* **2014**, *144*, 758–764. [CrossRef] [PubMed]
272. Allen, L.H. B vitamins in breast milk: Relative importance of maternal status and intake, and effects on infant status and function. *Adv. Nutr.* **2012**, *3*, 362–369. [CrossRef] [PubMed]
273. Miyake, Y.; Sasaki, S.; Tanaka, K.; Hirota, Y. Maternal b vitamin intake during pregnancy and wheeze and eczemea in japanese infants aged 16–24 months: The osaka maternal and child health study. *Pediatr. Allergy Immunol.* **2011**, *22*, 67–74.
274. Ala-Houhala, M.; Koskinen, T.; Parviainen, M.T.; Visakorpi, J.K. 25-hydroxyvitamin d and vitamin d in human milk: Effects of supplementation and season. *Am. J. Clin. Nutr.* **1988**, *48*, 1057–1060. [PubMed]
275. Greer, F.R.; Hollis, B.W.; Cripps, D.J.; Tsang, R.C. Effects of maternal ultraviolet b irradiation on vitamin d content of human milk. *J. Pediatr.* **1984**, *105*, 431–433. [CrossRef]
276. Specker, B.L.; Tsang, R.C.; Hollis, B.W. Effect of race and diet on human-milk vitamin d and 25-hydroxyvitamin d. *Am. J. Dis. Child.* **1985**, *139*, 1134–1137. [CrossRef] [PubMed]
277. Pugliese, M.T.; Blumberg, D.L.; Hludzinski, J.; Kay, S. Nutritional rickets in suburbia. *J. Am. Coll. Nutr.* **1998**, *17*, 637–641. [CrossRef] [PubMed]
278. Thiele, D.K.; Senti, J.L.; Anderson, C.M. Maternal vitamin d supplementation to meet the needs of the breastfed infant: A systematic review. *J. Hum. Lact.* **2013**, *29*, 163–170. [CrossRef] [PubMed]
279. Wagner, C.L.; Greer, F.R. Prevention of rickets and vitamin d deficiency in infants, children, and adolescents. *Pediatrics* **2008**, *122*, 1142–1152. [CrossRef] [PubMed]
280. Weisse, K.; Winkler, S.; Hirche, F.; Herberth, G.; Hinz, D.; Bauer, M.; Roder, S.; Rolle-Kampczyk, U.; von Bergen, M.; Olek, S.; et al. Maternal and newborn vitamin d status and its impact on food allergy development in the german lina cohort study. *Allergy* **2013**, *68*, 220–228. [CrossRef] [PubMed]
281. Gale, C.R.; Robinson, S.M.; Harvey, N.C.; Javaid, M.K.; Jiang, B.; Martyn, C.N.; Godfrey, K.M.; Cooper, C.; Princess Anne Hospital Study Group. Maternal vitamin d status during pregnancy and child outcomes. *Eur. J. Clin. Nutr.* **2008**, *62*, 68–77. [CrossRef] [PubMed]
282. Erkkola, M.; Kaila, M.; Nwaru, B.I.; Kronberg-Kippila, C.; Ahonen, S.; Nevalainen, J.; Veijola, R.; Pekkanen, J.; Ilonen, J.; Simell, O.; et al. Maternal vitamin d intake during pregnancy is inversely associated with asthma and allergic rhinitis in 5-year-old children. *Clin. Exp. Allergy* **2009**, *39*, 875–882. [CrossRef] [PubMed]
283. Allen, K.J.; Ponsonby, A.; Gurrin, L.C.; Wake, M.; Vuillermin, P.; Martin, P.; Matheson, M.L.A.; Robinson, M.; Tey, D.; Osborne, N.J.; et al. Vitamin d insufficiency is associated with challenge-proven food allergy in infants. *J. Allergy Clin. Immunol.* **2013**, *131*, 1109–1116. [CrossRef] [PubMed]
284. Wang, S.S.; Hon, K.L.; Kong, A.P.; Pong, H.N.; Wong, G.W.; Leung, T.F. Vitamin d deficiency is associated with diagnosis and severity of childhood atopic dermatitis. *Pediatr. Allergy Immunol.* **2014**, *25*, 30–35. [CrossRef] [PubMed]
285. Samochocki, Z.; Bogaczewicz, J.; Jeziorkowska, R.; Sysa-Jedrzejowska, A.; Glinska, O.; Karczmarewicz, E.; McCauliffe, D.P.; Wozniacka, A. Vitamin d effects in atopic dermatitis. *J. Am. Acad. Dermatol.* **2013**, *69*, 238–244. [CrossRef] [PubMed]
286. Litonjua, A.A.; Carey, V.J.; Laranjo, N.; Harshfield, B.J.; McElrath, T.F.; O'Connor, G.T.; Sandel, M.; Iverson, R.E., Jr.; Lee-Paritz, A.; Strunk, R.C.; et al. Effect of prenatal supplementation with vitamin d on asthma or recurrent wheezing in offspring by age 3 years: The vdaart randomized clinical trial. *J. Am. Med. Assoc.* **2016**, *315*, 362–370. [CrossRef] [PubMed]
287. Goldring, S.T.; Griffiths, C.J.; Martineau, A.R.; Robinson, S.; Yu, C.; Poulton, S.; Kirkby, J.C.; Stocks, J.; Hooper, R.; Shaheen, S.O.; et al. Prenatal vitamin d supplementation and child respiratory health: A randomised controlled trial. *PLoS ONE* **2013**, *8*, e66627. [CrossRef] [PubMed]
288. Chawes, B.L.; Bonnelykke, K.; Stokholm, J.; Vissing, N.H.; Bjarnadottir, E.; Schoos, A.M.; Wolsk, H.M.; Pedersen, T.M.; Vinding, R.K.; Thorsteinsdottir, S.; et al. Effect of vitamin d3 supplementation during pregnancy on risk of persistent wheeze in the offspring: A randomized clinical trial. *J. Am. Med. Assoc.* **2016**, *315*, 353–361. [CrossRef] [PubMed]
289. Tuokkola, J.; Luukkainen, P.; Kaila, M.; Takkinen, H.M.; Niinisto, S.; Veijola, R.; Virta, L.J.; Knip, M.; Simell, O.; Ilonen, J.; et al. Maternal dietary folate, folic acid and vitamin d intakes during pregnancy and lactation and the risk of cows' milk allergy in the offspring. *Br. J. Nutr.* **2016**, *116*, 710–718. [CrossRef] [PubMed]

290. Cuello-Garcia, C.A.; Fiocchi, A.; Pawankar, R.; Yepes-Nuñez, J.J.; Morgano, G.P.; Zhang, Y.; Ahn, K.; Al-Hammadi, S.; Agarwal, A.; Gandhi, S.; et al. World allergy organization-mcmaster university guidelines for allergic disease prevention (glad-p): Vitamin d. *World Allergy Organ. J.* **2016**, *9*, 17. [CrossRef] [PubMed]
291. Hernell, O.; Fewtrell, M.S.; Georgieff, M.K.; Krebs, N.F.; Lonnerdal, B. Summary of current recommendations on iron provision and monitoring of iron status for breastfed and formula-fed infants in resource-rich and resource-constrained countries. *J. Pediatr.* **2015**, *167*, S40–S47. [CrossRef] [PubMed]
292. Georgieff, M.K.; Wewerka, S.W.; Nelson, C.A.; Deregnier, R.A. Iron status at 9 months of infants with low iron stores at birth. *J. Pediatr.* **2002**, *141*, 405–409. [CrossRef] [PubMed]
293. Fewtrell, M.; Bronsky, J.; Campoy, C.; Domellof, M.; Embleton, N.; Fidler Mis, N.; Hojsak, I.; Hulst, J.M.; Indrio, F.; Lapillonne, A.; et al. Complementary feeding: A position paper by the european society for paediatric gastroenterology, hepatology, and nutrition (espghan) committee on nutrition. *J. Pediatr. Gastroenterol. Nutr.* **2017**, *64*, 119–132. [CrossRef] [PubMed]
294. Krebs, N.F.; Sherlock, L.G.; Westcott, J.; Culbertson, D.; Hambidge, K.M.; Feazel, L.M.; Robertson, C.E.; Frank, D.N. Effects of different complementary feeding regimens on iron status and enteric microbiota in breastfed infants. *J. Pediatr.* **2013**, *163*, 416–423. [CrossRef] [PubMed]
295. Friel, J.K.; Aziz, K.; Andrews, W.L.; Harding, S.V.; Courage, M.L.; Adams, R.J. A double-masked, randomized control trial of iron supplementation in early infancy in healthy term breast-fed infants. *J. Pediatr.* **2003**, *143*, 582–586. [CrossRef]
296. Baker, R.D.; Greer, F.R. Diagnosis and prevention of iron deficiency and iron-deficiency anemia in infants and young children (0–3 years of age). *Pediatrics* **2010**, *126*, 1040–1050. [CrossRef] [PubMed]
297. WHO. *The Global Prevalence of Anaemia in 2011*; WHO: Geneva, Switzerland, 2015.
298. Toyran, M.; Kaymak, M.; Vezir, E.; Harmanci, K.; Kaya, A.; Ginis, T.; Kose, G.; Kocabas, C.N. Trace element levels in children with atopic dermatitis. *J. Investig. Allergol. Clin. Immunol.* **2012**, *22*, 341–344. [PubMed]
299. Gibson, R.S. A historical review of progress in the assessment of dietary zinc intake as an indicator of population zinc status. *Adv. Nutr.* **2012**, *3*, 772–782. [CrossRef] [PubMed]
300. Brown, K.H.; Rivera, J.A.; Bhutta, Z.; Gibson, R.S.; King, J.C.; Lonnerdal, B.; Ruel, M.T.; Sandtrom, B.; Wasantwisut, E.; Hotz, C. International zinc nutrition consultative group (izincg) technical document #1. Assessment of the risk of zinc deficiency in populations and options for its control. *Food Nutr. Bull.* **2004**, *25*, S99–S203. [PubMed]
301. Krebs, N.F.; Miller, L.V.; Michael Hambidge, K. Zinc deficiency in infants and children: A review of its complex and synergistic interactions. *Paediatr. Int. Child. Health* **2014**, *34*, 279–288. [CrossRef] [PubMed]
302. Kent, J.C.; Mitoulas, L.R.; Cregan, M.D.; Ramsay, D.T.; Doherty, D.A.; Hartmann, P.E. Volume and frequency of breastfeedings and fat content of breast milk throughout the day. *Pediatrics* **2006**, *117*, e387–e395. [CrossRef] [PubMed]
303. Moco, S.; Collino, S.; Rezzi, S.; Martin, F.P. Metabolomics perspectives in pediatric research. *Pediatr. Res.* **2013**, *73*, 570–576. [CrossRef] [PubMed]
304. Sundekilde, U.K.; Downey, E.; O'Mahony, J.A.; O'Shea, C.A.; Ryan, C.A.; Kelly, A.L.; Bertram, H.C. The effect of gestational and lactational age on the human milk metabolome. *Nutrients* **2016**, *8*. [CrossRef] [PubMed]
305. Andreas, N.J.; Hyde, M.J.; Gomez-Romero, M.; Lopez-Gonzalvez, M.A.; Villasenor, A.; Wijeyesekera, A.; Barbas, C.; Modi, N.; Holmes, E.; Garcia-Perez, I. Multiplatform characterization of dynamic changes in breast milk during lactation. *Electrophoresis* **2015**. [CrossRef] [PubMed]
306. Villasenor, A.; Garcia-Perez, I.; Garcia, A.; Posma, J.M.; Fernandez-Lopez, M.; Nicholas, A.J.; Modi, N.; Holmes, E.; Barbas, C. Breast milk metabolome characterization in a single-phase extraction, multiplatform analytical approach. *Anal. Chem.* **2014**, *86*, 8245–8252. [CrossRef] [PubMed]
307. Wu, J.; Domellof, M.; Zivkovic, A.M.; Larsson, G.; Ohman, A.; Nording, M.L. Nmr-based metabolite profiling of human milk: A pilot study of methods for investigating compositional changes during lactation. *Biochem. Biophys. Res. Commun.* **2016**, *469*, 626–632. [CrossRef] [PubMed]
308. Palmas, F.; Fattuoni, C.; Noto, A.; Barberini, L.; Dessi, A.; Fanos, V. The choice of amniotic fluid in metabolomics for the monitoring of fetus health. *Expert Rev. Mol. Diagn.* **2016**, *16*, 473–486. [CrossRef] [PubMed]
309. Jantscher-Krenn, E.; Zherebtsov, M.; Nissan, C.; Goth, K.; Guner, Y.S.; Naidu, N.; Choudhury, B.; Grishin, A.V.; Ford, H.R.; Bode, L. The human milk oligosaccharide disialyllacto-n-tetraose prevents necrotising enterocolitis in neonatal rats. *Gut* **2012** *61*, 1417–1425. [CrossRef] [PubMed]

310. Autran, C.A.; Kellman, B.P.; Kim, J.H.; Asztalos, E.; Blood, A.B.; Spence, E.C.; Patel, A.L.; Hou, J.; Lewis, N.E.; Bode, L. Human milk oligosaccharide composition predicts risk of necrotising enterocolitis in preterm infants. *Gut* **2017**. [CrossRef] [PubMed]
311. Wang, M.; Li, M.; Wu, S.; Lebrilla, C.B.; Chapkin, R.S.; Ivanov, I.; Donovan, S.M. Fecal microbiota composition of breast-fed infants is correlated with human milk oligosaccharides consumed. *J. Pediatr. Gastroenterol. Nutr.* **2015**, *60*, 825–833. [CrossRef] [PubMed]
312. Mosconi, E.; Rekima, A.; Seitz-Polski, B.; Kanda, A.; Fleury, S.; Tissandie, E.; Monteiro, R.; Dombrowicz, D.D.; Julia, V.; Glaichenhaus, N.; et al. Breast milk immune complexes are potent inducers of oral tolerance in neonates and prevent asthma development. *Mucosal Immunol.* **2010**, *3*, 461–474. [CrossRef] [PubMed]
313. Verhasselt, V. Neonatal tolerance under breastfeeding influence: The presence of allergen and transforming growth factor-beta in breast milk protects the progeny from allergic asthma. *J. Pediatr.* **2010**, *156*, S16–S20. [CrossRef] [PubMed]
314. Kumari, M.; Kozyrskyj, A.L. Gut microbial metabolism defines host metabolism: An emerging perspective in obesity and allergic inflammation. *Obes. Rev.* **2017**, *18*, 18–31. [CrossRef] [PubMed]
315. Julia, V.; Macia, L.; Dombrowicz, D. The impact of diet on asthma and allergic diseases. *Nat. Rev. Immunol.* **2015**, *15*, 308–322. [CrossRef] [PubMed]
316. Corthesy, B. Multi-faceted functions of secretory iga at mucosal surfaces. *Front. Immunol.* **2013**, *4*, 185. [CrossRef] [PubMed]
317. Hennet, T.; Borsig, L. Breastfed at tiffany's. *Trends Biochem. Sci.* **2016**, *41*, 508–518. [CrossRef] [PubMed]
318. Brandtzaeg, P. The mucosal immune system and its integration with the mammary glands. *J. Pediatr.* **2010**, *156*, S8–S15. [CrossRef] [PubMed]
319. Maruyama, K.; Hida, M.; Kohgo, T.; Fukunaga, Y. Changes in salivary and fecal secretory iga in infants under different feeding regimens. *Pediatr. Int.* **2009**, *51*, 342–345. [CrossRef] [PubMed]
320. Urwin, H.J.; Miles, E.A.; Noakes, P.S.; Kremmyda, L.S.; Vlachava, M.; Diaper, N.D.; Godfrey, K.M.; Calder, P.C.; Vulevic, J.; Yaqoob, P. Effect of salmon consumption during pregnancy on maternal and infant faecal microbiota, secretory iga and calprotectin. *Br. J. Nutr.* **2014**, *111*, 773–784. [CrossRef] [PubMed]
321. Kukkonen, K.; Kuitunen, M.; Haahtela, T.; Korpela, R.; Poussa, T.; Savilahti, E. High intestinal iga associates with reduced risk of ige-associated allergic diseases. *Pediatr. Allergy Immunol.* **2010**, *21*, 67–73. [CrossRef] [PubMed]
322. Koutras, A.K.; Vigorita, V.J. Fecal secretory immunoglobulin a in breast milk versus formula feeding in early infancy. *J. Pediatr. Gastroenterol. Nutr.* **1989**, *9*, 58–61. [CrossRef] [PubMed]
323. Munblit, D.; Sheth, S.; Abrol, P.; Treneva, M.; Peroni, D.G.; Chow, L.Y.; Boner, A.L.; Pampura, A.; Warner, J.O.; Boyle, R.J. Exposures influencing total iga level in colostrum. *J. Dev. Orig. Health Dis.* **2016**, *7*, 61–67. [CrossRef] [PubMed]
324. Breakey, A.A.; Hinde, K.; Valeggia, C.R.; Sinofsky, A.; Ellison, P.T. Illness in breastfeeding infants relates to concentration of lactoferrin and secretory immunoglobulin a in mother's milk. *Evol. Med. Public Health* **2015**, *2015*, 21–31. [CrossRef] [PubMed]
325. Bridgman, S.L.; Konya, T.; Azad, M.B.; Sears, M.R.; Becker, A.B.; Turvey, S.E.; Mandhane, P.J.; Subbarao, P.; Investigators, C.S.; Scott, J.A.; et al. Infant gut immunity: A preliminary study of iga associations with breastfeeding. *J. Dev. Orig. Health Dis.* **2016**, *7*, 68–72. [CrossRef] [PubMed]
326. Bridgman, S.L.; Konya, T.; Azad, M.B.; Guttman, D.S.; Sears, M.R.; Becker, A.B.; Turvey, S.E.; Mandhane, P.J.; Subbarao, P.; Investigators, C.S.; et al. High fecal iga is associated with reduced clostridium difficile colonization in infants. *Microbes Infect. Inst. Pasteur* **2016**, *18*, 543–549. [CrossRef] [PubMed]
327. Adlerberth, I.; Wold, A.E. Establishment of the gut microbiota in western infants. *Acta Paediatr.* **2009**, *98*, 229–238. [CrossRef] [PubMed]
328. Penders, J.; Thijs, C.; van den Brandt, P.A.; Kummeling, I.; Snijders, B.; Stelma, F.; Adams, H.; van Ree, R.; Stobberingh, E.E. Gut microbiota composition and development of atopic manifestations in infancy: The koala birth cohort study. *Gut* **2007**, *56*, 661–667. [CrossRef] [PubMed]
329. Mastromarino, P.; Capobianco, D.; Campagna, G.; Laforgia, N.; Drimaco, P.; Dileone, A.; Baldassarre, M.E. Correlation between lactoferrin and beneficial microbiota in breast milk and infant's feces. *Biometals* **2014**, *27*, 1077–1086. [CrossRef] [PubMed]

330. Cacho, N.T.; Lawrence, R.M. Innate immunity and breast milk. *Front. Immunol.* **2017**, *8*, 584. [CrossRef] [PubMed]
331. Johansson, M.A.; Sjogren, Y.M.; Persson, J.O.; Nilsson, C.; Sverremark-Ekstrom, E. Early colonization with a group of lactobacilli decreases the risk for allergy at five years of age despite allergic heredity. *PLoS ONE* **2011**, *6*, e23031. [CrossRef] [PubMed]
332. Zhang, G.; Lai, C.T.; Hartmann, P.; Oddy, W.H.; Kusel, M.M.; Sly, P.D.; Holt, P.G. Anti-infective proteins in breast milk and asthma-associated phenotypes during early childhood. *Pediatr. Allergy Immunol.* **2014**, *25*, 544–551. [CrossRef] [PubMed]
333. Yates, C.M.; Calder, P.C.; Ed Rainger, G. Pharmacology and therapeutics of omega-3 polyunsaturated fatty acids in chronic inflammatory disease. *Pharmacol. Ther.* **2014**, *141*, 272–282. [CrossRef] [PubMed]
334. Serhan, C.N.; Chiang, N.; Van Dyke, T.E. Resolving inflammation: Dual anti-inflammatory and pro-resolution lipid mediators. *Nat. Rev. Immunol.* **2008**, *8*, 349–361. [CrossRef] [PubMed]
335. Miyata, J.; Arita, M. Role of omega-3 fatty acids and their metabolites in asthma and allergic diseases. *Allergol. Int.* **2015**, *64*, 27–34. [CrossRef] [PubMed]
336. Koltsida, O.; Karamnov, S.; Pyrillou, K.; Vickery, T.; Chairakaki, A.D.; Tamvakopoulos, C.; Sideras, P.; Serhan, C.N.; Andreakos, E. Toll-like receptor 7 stimulates production of specialized pro-resolving lipid mediators and promotes resolution of airway inflammation. *EMBO Mol. Med.* **2013**, *5*, 762–775. [CrossRef] [PubMed]
337. Thorburn, A.N.; McKenzie, C.I.; Shen, S.; Stanley, D.; Macia, L.; Mason, L.J.; Roberts, L.K.; Wong, C.H.; Shim, R.; Robert, R.; et al. Evidence that asthma is a developmental origin disease influenced by maternal diet and bacterial metabolites. *Nat. Commun.* **2015**, *6*, 7320. [CrossRef] [PubMed]
338. Rasmussen, H.S.; Holtug, K.; Ynggard, C.; Mortensen, P.B. Faecal concentrations and production rates of short chain fatty acids in normal neonates. *Acta Paediatr. Scand.* **1988**, *77*, 365–368. [CrossRef] [PubMed]
339. Bridgman, S.L.; Azad, M.B.; Field, C.J.; Haqq, A.M.; Becker, A.B.; Mandhane, P.J.; Subbarao, P.; Turvey, S.E.; Sears, M.R.; Scott, J.A.; et al. Fecal short-chain fatty acid variations by breastfeeding status in infants at 4 months: Differences in relative versus absolute concentrations. *Front. Nutr.* **2017**, *4*, 11. [CrossRef] [PubMed]
340. Tan, J.; McKenzie, C.; Vuillermin, P.J.; Goverse, G.; Vinuesa, C.G.; Mebius, R.E.; Macia, L.; Mackay, C.R. Dietary fiber and bacterial scfa enhance oral tolerance and protect against food allergy through diverse cellular pathways. *Cell Rep.* **2016**, *15*, 2809–2824. [CrossRef] [PubMed]
341. Stefka, A.T.; Feehley, T.; Tripathi, P.; Qiu, J.; McCoy, K.; Mazmanian, S.K.; Tjota, M.Y.; Seo, G.Y.; Cao, S.; Theriault, B.R.; et al. Commensal bacteria protect against food allergen sensitization. *Proc. Natl. Acad. Sci. USA* **2014**, *111*, 13145–13150. [CrossRef] [PubMed]
342. Albright, C.D.; Tsai, A.Y.; Friedrich, C.B.; Mar, M.H.; Zeisel, S.H. Choline availability alters embryonic development of the hippocampus and septum in the rat. *Brain Res. Dev. Brain Res.* **1999**, *113*, 13–20. [CrossRef]
343. Ilcol, Y.O.; Ozbek, R.; Hamurtekin, E.; Ulus, I.H. Choline status in newborns, infants, children, breast-feeding women, breast-fed infants and human breast milk. *J. Nutr. Biochem.* **2005**, *16*, 489–499. [CrossRef] [PubMed]
344. Ozarda, Y.; Cansev, M.; Ulus, I.H. Breast milk choline contents are associated with inflammatory status of breastfeeding women. *J. Hum. Lact.* **2014**, *30*, 161–166. [CrossRef] [PubMed]
345. Marnell, L.; Mold, C.; Du Clos, T.W. C-reactive protein: Ligands, receptors and role in inflammation. *Clin. Immunol.* **2005**, *117*, 104–111. [CrossRef] [PubMed]
346. Kushner, I.; Rzewnicki, D.; Samols, D. What does minor elevation of c-reactive protein signify? *Am. J. Med.* **2006**, *119*, 166. [CrossRef] [PubMed]
347. Detopoulou, P.; Panagiotakos, D.B.; Antonopoulou, S.; Pitsavos, C.; Stefanadis, C. Dietary choline and betaine intakes in relation to concentrations of inflammatory markers in healthy adults: The attica study. *Am. J. Clin. Nutr.* **2008**, *87*, 424–430. [PubMed]
348. Bager, P.; Wohlfahrt, J.; Westergaard, T. Caesarean delivery and risk of atopy and allergic disease: Meta-analyses. *Clin. Exp. Allergy* **2008**, *38*, 634–642. [CrossRef] [PubMed]
349. Cederlund, A.; Kai-Larsen, Y.; Printz, G.; Yoshio, H.; Alvelius, G.; Lagercrantz, H.; Stromberg, R.; Jornvall, H.; Gudmundsson, G.H.; Agerberth, B. Lactose in human breast milk an inducer of innate immunity with implications for a role in intestinal homeostasis. *PLoS ONE* **2013**, *8*, e53876. [CrossRef] [PubMed]

350. Marincola, F.C.; Noto, A.; Caboni, P.; Reali, A.; Barberini, L.; Lussu, M.; Murgia, F.; Santoru, M.L.; Atzori, L.; Fanos, V. A metabolomic study of preterm human and formula milk by high resolution nmr and gc/ms analysis: Preliminary results. *J. Matern. Fetal Neonatal Med.* **2012**, *25*, 62–67. [CrossRef] [PubMed]
351. Skovbjerg, H.; Sjostrom, H.; Noren, O. Purification and characterisation of amphiphilic lactase/phlorizin hydrolase from human small intestine. *Eur. J. Biochem.* **1981**, *114*, 653–661. [CrossRef] [PubMed]
352. Hove, H.; Norgaard, H.; Mortensen, P.B. Lactic acid bacteria and the human gastrointestinal tract. *Eur. J. Clin. Nutr.* **1999**, *53*, 339–350. [CrossRef] [PubMed]
353. Levin, A.M.; Sitarik, A.R.; Havstad, S.L.; Fujimura, K.E.; Wegienka, G.; Cassidy-Bushrow, A.E.; Kim, H.; Zoratti, E.M.; Lukacs, N.W.; Boushey, H.A.; et al. Joint effects of pregnancy, sociocultural, and environmental factors on early life gut microbiome structure and diversity. *Sci. Rep.* **2016**, *6*, 31775. [CrossRef] [PubMed]
354. Madan, J.C.; Hoen, A.G.; Lundgren, S.N.; Farzan, S.F.; Cottingham, K.L.; Morrison, H.G.; Sogin, M.L.; Li, H.; Moore, J.H.; Karagas, M.R. Association of cesarean delivery and formula supplementation with the intestinal microbiome of 6-week-old infants. *JAMA Pediatr.* **2016**, *170*, 212–219. [CrossRef] [PubMed]
355. Azad, M.B.; Konya, T.; Persaud, R.R.; Guttman, D.S.; Chari, R.S.; Field, C.J.; Sears, M.R.; Mandhane, P.J.; Turvey, S.E.; Subbarao, P.; et al. Impact of maternal intrapartum antibiotics, method of birth and breastfeeding on gut microbiota during the first year of life: A prospective cohort study. *Int. J. Obstet. Gynaecol.* **2016**, *123*, 983–993. [CrossRef] [PubMed]
356. Kramer, M.S. Does breast feeding help protect against atopic disease? Biology, methodology, and a golden jubilee of controversy. *J. Pediatr.* **1988**, *112*, 181–190. [CrossRef]

5

Prevention and Management of Cow's Milk Allergy in Non-Exclusively Breastfed Infants

Yvan Vandenplas

Kidz Health Castle, UZ Brussel, Vrije Universiteit Brussel, Laarbeeklaan 101, 1090 Brussels, Belgium; yvan.vandenplas@uzbrussel.be

Abstract: **Introduction:** The prevention and management of cow milk allergy (CMA) is still debated. Since CMA is much less frequent in breastfed infants, breastfeeding should be stimulated. **Method:** Literature was searched using databases to find original papers and reviews on this topic. **Results:** Hydrolysates with a clinical proof of efficacy are recommended in the prevention and treatment of CMA. However, not all meta-analyses conclude that hydrolysates do prevent CMA or other atopic manifestations such as atopic dermatitis. There are pros and cons to consider partially hydrolysed protein as an option for starter infant formula for each non-exclusively breastfed infant. A challenge test is still recommended as the most specific and sensitive diagnostic test, although a positive challenge test does not proof that the immune system is involved. The Cow Milk Symptom Score (CoMiSS™) is an awareness tool that enables healthcare professionals to better recognize symptoms related to the ingestion of cow milk, but it still needs validation as diagnostic tool. The current recommended elimination diet is a cow milk based extensive hydrolysate, although rice hydrolysates or soy infant formula can be considered in some cases. About 10 to 15% of infants allergic to cow milk will also react to soy. Mainly because of the higher cost, amino acid based formula is reserved for severe cases. There is no place for infant formula with intact protein from other animals as cross-over allergenicity is high. During recent years, attention focused also on the bifidogenic effect of prebiotics and more recently also on human milk oligosaccharides. A bifidogenic gastrointestinal microbiome may decrease the risk to develop allergic disease. The addition of probiotics and prebiotics to the elimination diet in treatment may enhance the development of tolerance development. **Conclusion:** Breastfeeding is the best way to feed infants. Cow milk based extensive hydrolysates remain the first option for the treatment of CMA for the majority of patients, while amino acid formulas are reserved for the most severe cases. Rice hydrolysates and soy infant formula are second choice options. Partial hydrolysates with clinical proof of efficacy are recommended in some guidelines in the prevention of CMA and allergic disease in at risk infants, and may be considered as an option as protein source in starter infant formula.

Keywords: cow milk allergy; hydrolysate; infant formula; functional gastrointestinal disorder; prevention; treatment

---

1. Introduction

This manuscript discusses the prevention and management of cow's milk allergy (CMA) in non-exclusively breastfed infants. CMA is an adverse health effect arising from a specific immune response that occurs reproducibly on exposure to a protein present in cow milk. Breastfeeding is the first choice feeding for infants, and allergic and functional gastrointestinal disorders occur more often in non-exclusively breastfed than in breastfed infants. The prevalence of allergic diseases involving the gastrointestinal (GI) tract, respiratory tract and the skin is likely to be rising worldwide [1]. Food allergy is a growing health concern in the westernized world with approximately 6% of children suffering from it [2]. CMA is one of the most frequent causes of food allergies in young children with an estimated prevalence between 1.9% and 4.9% in the first year of life [3,4]. Whether there has also been an increase in CMA has not been thoroughly studied [5]. According to a report from Denmark, CMA is up to half of the allergic children immunoglobulin E (IgE) mediated [6]. The risk to develop allergic disease is multifactorial. Recent evidence suggests that low blood vitamin D level is a risk factor for food allergy; vitamin D deficiency predisposes to GI infections, which may promote the development of food allergy. Several data suggest that serum 25-hydroxyvitamin D levels are often insufficient in children with asthma, atopic dermatitis, and food allergy [7]. There is no evidence that supplementation of poly-unsaturated fatty acids in infancy has an effect on infant or childhood allergy, asthma, dermatitis/eczema or food allergy [8]. Many infants present with symptoms related to milk ingestion. The most frequent symptoms and signs related to CMA are listed in Table 1. Both IgE and non-IgE mediated CMA exist. Allergic symptoms must be reproducible. The involvement of the immune system in non-IgE mediated allergy is difficult to demonstrate. Non-IgE mediated allergy is the cause of symptoms in a subset of patients with "hypersensitivity". Sometimes the symptoms caused by ingestion of milk are very likely to be immune mediated, as in the case of atopic dermatitis improving during a cow milk elimination diet. However, in the case of GI symptoms, such as regurgitation, constipation or general symptoms such as crying or distress, the involvement of the immune system cannot (easily) be demonstrated. . It is likely that there is overlap between the latter and functional GI symptoms. Experts agreed that the likely prevalence for colic, regurgitation, and functional constipation is 20%, 30% and 15%, respectively [9]. The perception of parents that an infant may have cow milk related symptoms is much greater than the reported incidence of CMA since parents report an incidence of up to 17% [10]. The relationship between some of these common symptoms of infancy and CMA is not clear. The best example may be upper respiratory tract symptoms which can seldom be related to CMA, but most frequently are caused by viral infections. It is only in a minority of infants that functional GI symptoms such as regurgitation, constipation and colic are of allergic origin. Intolerance is the consequence of lactase deficiency, the brush border enzyme that digests lactose, the predominant sugar in milk, and is almost always secondary to another condition in young infants. The meaning and definition of a "hypo-allergenic formula" varies in different parts of the world. While in Europe a "hypo-allergenic formula" means a formula that contains hydrolyzed protein and thus a reduced allergenicity, the American Academy of Pediatrics defined it as a formula that is effective in the treatment of at least 90% of the children with CMA, with a 95% confidence interval. It has to be recognized that an extensive hydrolysate is "tolerated" by the vast majority of CMA-patients but that such an elimination diet is not really "treatment" as the elimination diet does not change the immune response. Oral immunotherapy or anti-IgE actually modify the individual propensity to react to cow's milk and are therefore therapeutic. However, since most literature, including guidelines, recommend the use of extensive hydrolysates as first choice in the management, "treatment" is used in this context.

Tolerance of cow milk will have developed in 85% to 90% of the infants with CMA by the age of three years. High IgE levels predict a longer persistence of allergic reactions to cow milk. In particular, GI symptoms show a good prognosis, suggesting again an overlap between functional GI symptoms and CMA [3,6]. However, most of the information on the natural evolution of CMA comes from tertiary care or specialized centers and only the most severe cases are seen in these centers. This means that data on the natural evolution of CMA at the primary healthcare level are missing.

Table 1. Symptoms and signs related to CMA.

General
• Anaphylaxis • Food protein induced enterocolitis syndrome (FPIES; shock-like symptoms with severe metabolic acidosis, vomiting and diarrhea)
Gastro-Intestinal
• Failure to thrive, anorexia, refusal to feed, early satiety • Dysphagia, dyspepsia • Abdominal pain, colic • Nausea, regurgitation, emesis • Diarrhea with or without protein loss or bleeding • Constipation with or without perianal rash • Iron-defeiciency anemia due to occult blood loss
Respiratory
• Respiratory distress • Runny nose, chronic coughing • Wheezing/stridor
Dermatological
• Urticaria, atopic eczema, angioedema.

2. Methods

The PubMed and Cochrane Library databases were searched up to July 2016. The searches were limited to human studies and to studies published in English. Only published data were considered.

3. Prevention

The allergic march describes the order in which atopic disease develops, starting with atopic dermatitis followed by asthma to end with rhinoconjunctivitis [11]. The development of atopic disease is influenced by environmental and genetic, thus epi-genetic, confounders.

Two meta-analyses including selected papers on one partial hydrolysate conclude that selected partially and extensive hydrolyzed infant formula may prevent the development of atopic dermatitis and possibly that of CMA [12,13]. Boyle et al concluded in a meta-analysis including much more trials (37 compared to 11 and 15 [14]) that overall there was no consistent evidence that partially or extensively hydrolysed formulas reduce risk of allergic or autoimmune outcomes in infants at high pre-existing risk of these outcomes [14]. Odds ratios for eczema at age 0–4, compared with standard cows' milk formula, were 0.84 (95% confidence interval 0.67 to 1.07) for partially hydrolysed formula; 0.55 (0.28 to 1.09) for extensively hydrolysed casein based formula; and 1.12 (0.88 to 1.42) for extensively hydrolysed whey based formula [14]. A large study with a negative outcome with a different partial whey hydrolysate than the one included in the above mentioned two meta-analyses contributes largely to these findings [15]. These findings also suggest that outcomes obtained with one hydrolysate may not be extrapolated to another hydrolysate, and that findings are hydrolysate-specific. According to Boyle et al, there is no evidence to support the health claim approved by the US Food and Drug Administration that a partially hydrolysed formula could reduce the risk of eczema nor the conclusion of the Cochrane review that hydrolysed formula could allergy to cows' milk [14]. This is only partially confirmed by the recent Cochrane review reported that in infants at high risk of allergy not exclusively breast fed, very low-quality evidence suggests that prolonged hydrolysed formula feeding compared with CMF feeding reduces infant allergy and infant CMA ([16] -Cochrane review withdrawn). Studies have found no difference in childhood allergy and no difference in specific allergy, including infant and childhood asthma, eczema and rhinitis and infant food allergy [16]. Although extensively hydrolyzed formulas (eHF) can be used in prevention, they are not considered as first option as they are much more expensive that partially HF (pHF). Because of their bitter taste, eHF have a poor palatability. In theory, the allergenic epitopes are destroyed in the manufacturing process of eHF. pHF has been developed to decrease the amount of epitopes that possibly induce sensitization, while still having peptides of sufficient immunogenicity to induce oral tolerance. Only these pHF can be recommended for prevention for which there are sufficient clinical data to support their efficacy, which are missing for the majority of the commercialized pHFs. Some guidelines recommend the use of pHFs in "at risk" infants, which are defined as infants born in a family in which at least one of the family members (parents, brother, sister) has atopic disease. There is no consensus if this diagnosis of atopic disease should be "doctor confirmed" or not. As a consequence of the ongoing debate some countries (e.g., Japan, UK, Finland, Australia) do not recommend the use of pHF to prevent allergy. There is no place for infant formula with intact protein from different origin in the prevention of allergic disease. Soy protein infant formula has no place in the prevention of atopic disease.

Epidemiological data show that about half of the infants that will develop allergy are not part of this "at risk" group [17]. This is due to the fact that although the risk is lower in the non-at risk group, the number of infants in the non-at risk group is much larger. In other words: guidelines recommend today prevention only for half of the infants that will develop atopic disease, and not for the other half. A recent analysis from the 15 year follow-up of the two German birth cohorts GINI-plus and LISA-plus reported for the first time that parental allergic diseases increase the risk of childhood allergic diseases, especially for asthma, independent on whether the first onsets was before or after the birth of a child [18]. Knowledge on the long-term effects of pHF on growth and body composition outcomes in healthy infants later in life is still limited [19]. There are some indications that hydrolysed protein results in metabolic responses more distinctly different from those of human milk and different metabolic organ development compared to intact protein [19,20]. However, FDA and EFSA regulatory authorities consider a partially hydrolysed protein source as a protein source that can be used in starter infant formula, irrespective of the fact if there would be some prevention of allergy or not. All studies with pHF show no or some benefit, but never an increased risk for adverse effects. So the question should be asked is pHF should not be considered as the best second choice infant feeding for every infant, at least for those pHFs with clinical data supporting their efficacy (Figure 1), irrespective of the fact if there is a preventive effect on allergy or not. Opponents to this viewpoint state that breast milk contains intact protein, and a pHF does not. This is true. But: breast milk contains also proteases, digesting protein. The role of these proteases is yet unknown. And breast milk does not contain intact cow milk protein, but contains cow milk peptides. The digestion of partially hydrolysed protein may result in different metabolites than intact protein. Whether this is clinically relevant or not, is yet unknown. Overall, it is the opinion of the author that a partially hydrolysed protein may be considered as an option as protein source of a starter formula for every non-exclusively breastfed infants. It then becomes a cost/benefit discussion, which is difficult because cost of formula does vary substantially from country to country [19].

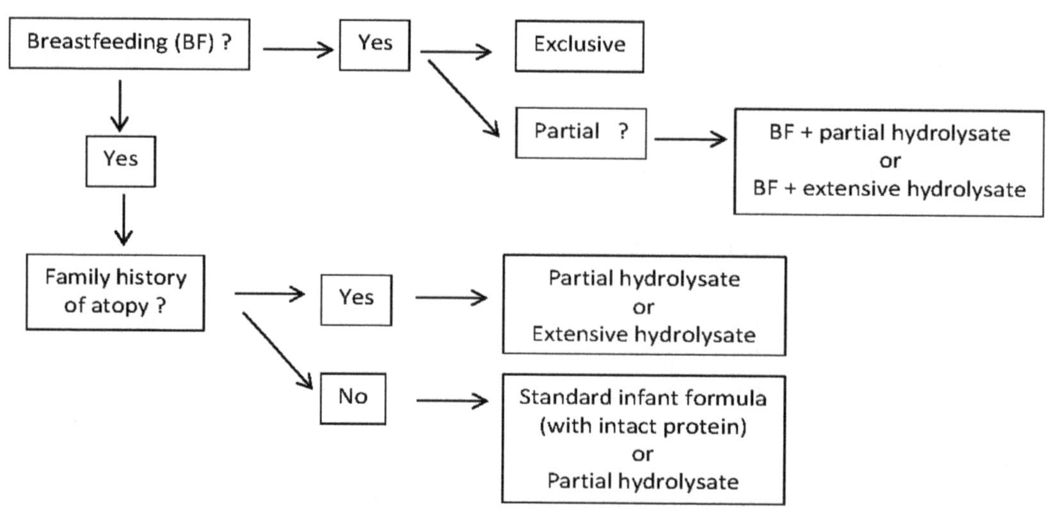

Figure 1. Proposed dietary options according to breastfeeding and/or family history of atopic disease.

4. Symptoms and Diagnosis

Symptoms related to cow milk intake develop usually within the first two months after its introduction and it is unusual for CMA to develop in a child older than one year of age [21]. Symptoms can be separated in IgE and non-IgE mediated, and according to literature the distribution can be estimated fifty-fifty [21]. Many infants develop symptoms in two or more organ systems. Typical IgE mediated symptoms include urticaria, angioedema, vomiting, diarrhea and anaphylaxis. Dermatitis and rhinitis can be IgE and non-IgE mediated. Vomiting, constipation, hemosiderosis, malabsorption, villous atrophy, eosinophilic proctocolitis, enterocolitis and eosinophilic esophagitis are non-IgE mediated reactions. In addition, respiratory symptoms such as chronic rhinitis and asthma may be caused by CMA [22]. Irritability, fuzziness and colic are sometimes the only symptoms of CMA [3,23]. Whether diagnostic investigations such as IgE, specific RAST and skin prick tests should be performed depends on local facilities and routines, but they are not routinely recommended in the guidelines [3,21]. Total IgE is not helpful in the diagnosis of CMA, but the IgE level is related to the development of tolerance: the lower the total IgE, the more rapidly tolerance develops [21]. Specific IgE and skin prick tests may contribute to confirm the suspected diagnosis, although false positive results do exist. The atopy patch test, which is popular in France, has not been considered as a recommended diagnostic test in guidelines [3,21]. Negative test results do not exclude allergy [3]. Other diagnostic tests are only possible in specialized laboratories or indicated in very distinct clinical conditions, such as mucosal biopsies in infants presenting with blood in their stools. There is no place for the (expensive) determination of IgG4-antibody levels as these are considered to demonstrate contact of the immune system with the antigens but do not suggest an allergic reaction [3,21,23].

A symptom-based score, the Cow Milk Related Symptom Score (CoMiSS™) has recently been developed to raise awareness of symptoms related to the ingestion of cow milk [24]. A challenge test is likely to be positive in 80% of patients if an initial score of more than 12 decreases to less than half with an eHF [25]. Therefore, it is hoped that, when it is validated, the CoMiSS™ may become a valuable diagnostic tool [24].

The majority of the guidelines accept an open challenge in infants suspected of CMA, although a double-blind challenge test is considered to be the gold standard for diagnosing CMA [3,21,23]. Standardized procedures on how to perform a challenge test have been published (Table 2) [3,21,23]. A challenge test should always be performed under medical supervision, but it does not have to be systematically performed in a hospital environment. Hospitalization is recommended if it is suspected that acute, severe or unpredictable symptoms could occur [3]. Parents are often reluctant to perform a challenge test, because it will make the allergic child sick again. In addition, the results of a challenge are often difficult to interpret. While immediate reactions are relatively easy to pick up, delayed reactions are more difficult to detect. A group of experts published a standardized double-blind placebo-controlled food challenge [24]. This certainly has the merit to be scientifically sound but has the disadvantage to be difficult to apply in daily practice in not experienced centers or at primary health care level. Specifically for a cow's milk challenge, European experts have proposed an open prolonged challenge: after a half day challenge under medical supervision, the patient returns home and parents need to continue the challenge by providing a sufficient daily intake of at least 200 mL of milk per day [3,21]. Indeed, about half of the children will develop a delayed reaction, which will only be picked up if the parents are collaborating and the follow up is adequate. Double-blind challenge tests cover only the first part of the challenge test, which is under medical supervision.

Table 2. Example of standardized protocol for open challenge test.

- Drop of formula on the lips
- If there is no reaction after 15 min, the formula is given orally and the dose is increased stepwise (0.5, 1, 3, 10, 30, 50 to 100 mL) every 30 min
- Additional observation for at least 2 h

If negative, the infant should drink at least 200 m of cows' milk-based infant formula each day for the next 2 weeks and the parents should be contacted daily by a healthcare professional or should contact a healthcare professional if symptoms occur so that a late reaction can be documented.

5. Treatment

The vast majority of infants with suspected CMA will be formula-fed and present with a combination of the symptoms listed in the CoMiSS™ [24]. Guidelines recommend an elimination diet with a whey or casein-based eHF with clinical proof of efficacy for two to four weeks as the first option [3,23] (Table 3). The CoMiSS™ score can contribute to quantify clinical improvement. Hydrolysates strengthen the epithelial barrier, modulate T-cell differentiation and decrease inflammation [26]. Some studies suggest a role for hydrolysates in manipulating pathogen recognition receptors signaling as underlying mechanism. Peptides from hydrolysates have been shown to bind to TLR2 and TLR4 and influence cytokine production in epithelial cells and macrophages. Current insight suggests that hydrolysates may actively participate in modulating the immune responses in subjects with and those at risk to develop CMA [26]. If the symptoms do not improve, then CMA is unlikely. The percentage of patients tolerating the eHF will depend on the selection of patients. In eHFs, most of the nitrogen is present as free amino acids and peptides <1500 kDa [27]. During CMA treatment, allergenic peptides may be potentially harmful. Therefore, peptides that have reduced allergenicity but are capable to induce tolerance are recommended. The World Allergy Organization Diagnosis and Rationale for Action against Cow's Milk Allergy (WAO-DRACMA) guidelines recommend cow milk based eHF over soy infant formula in IgE-mediated CMA [10]. Amino acid based formula (AAF) is recommended if formula-fed infants present with the rare condition of anaphylaxis and in eosinophilic esophagitis, or when the child does not tolerate to the eHF and CMA is a likely diagnosis (because failure of eHF has been reported) or when the cost/benefit analysis is in favor of the AAF [3,21]. However, eHFs have been reported to be effective in adults with eosinophilic esophagitis caused by cow milk [28]. If a strict AAF diet does not result in an improvement of the symptoms, the patient does not suffer CMA. In case of anaphylaxis, the long-term management of such infants should include a challenge with an eHF before cow milk is (re-)introduced. This should be carried out after 6 to 9 months or when the infant is one year old and always in a hospital environment [3,23].

Table 3. Recommended therapeutic options according to different guidelines for different symptoms and signs of cow's milk allergy.

	Australia [29]		Dracma [10]		Espghan [3]	
	1st choice	2nd choice	1st choice	2nd choice	1st choice	2nd choice
GI syndromes	eHF soy (if >6 months)	AAF eHF	eHF	AAF	eHF	AAF
proctocolitis	eHF	AAF			eHF	AAF
Eos Eso	AAF		AAF		AAF	
Immediate FA	eHF soy (if >6 months)	AAF eHF	eHF	AAF/Soy	eHF	AAF
FPIES	eHF	AAF	eHF	AAF	eHF	AAF
Atopic eczema	eHF soy	AAF eHF	eHF	AAF/Soy	eHF	AAF
urticaria			eHF	AAF/Soy	eHF	AAF
Constipation			eHF	AAF		
Heiner syndrome			AAF	eHF		

If an eHF is not available, if the infant refuses to drink it or if it is too expensive, a rice hydrolysate or a soy infant formula are considered as second choices. Since pHF has longer peptides than eHF, pHF may trigger symptoms in sensitized infants (3,10,23). Therefore, a cow milk based pHF is not suitable for treating CMA. While eHF needs to be tolerated by >90% of patients, pHF will be tolerated by less than half of infants with CMA [3].

Thickened eHF and AAF are commercially available [30,31] to treat simultaneously CMA and infant regurgitation. Whether an eHF is thickened or not seems not to be relevant in CMA; however, when the challenge test is negative, the thickened eHF is more effective in reducing regurgitation than the non-thickened [30]. Up to now allergic reactions to the thickening agent in these formulas have not been reported.

Partial and extensively rice hydrolyzed formula are commercialized and, in some parts of the world, soy (hydrolyzed) infant formula also exists. Since rice hydrolysates are relatively new, they are not (yet) considered in published guidelines. The clinical efficacy of rice hydrolysates, partial and extensive, seems excellent [32,33]. Rice hydrolysates are free of CMP allergens. Rice hydrolysates are less expensive than cow milk based eHF. The content of arsenic in rice may be a safety issue limiting the use of rice. There is an FDA warning against the use of rice in infants and young children regarding rice feed thickeners and rice cereals. Therefore the arsenic content in rice based infant formula should be determined and declared on the label [34]. The arsenic content in infant formula is reported to be within the safety limits. Other mammalian milks such as sheep milk and goat milk are not indicated in the treatment of CMA [3]. Infant formulas based on goat milk are on the market in a substantial number of countries, but the high incidence of cross-reactivity in CMA patients results in the fact that they cannot be recommended for infants with CMA [35]. Significant cross-sensitization to milk proteins derived from kosher animals exist in patients allergic to CMP, but far less so than the milk proteins tested from non-kosher animals [35,36]. Camel and mare milk have not been evaluated as possible options [37–39], but ass milk in particular has been shown to be effective in treating CMA [40,41]. The DRACMA guidelines even recommend donkeys milk as third option in constipation due to CMA. However, none of these alternative options fulfill the nutritional and compositional requirements for infant formula and as a result they cannot be recommended in the treatment of CMA. Consumption of unprocessed cow milk in young infants protects against respiratory infections [42]. However, unprocessed cow milk can as well not be recommended in infants for nutritional reasons. The epitopes in raw, cooked or baked milk differ [43] as baked milk was reported to be tolerated in patients with eosinophilic esophagitis as presentation of CMA [43]. Although use of hypoallergenic baked milk in oral immune therapy is a promising therapy, care must be taken before its administration in baked milk-reactive patients because of the risk for anaphylaxis and only limited increase in challenge threshold attained [44].

Soy infant formula has existed for longer than one century, but its popularity varies greatly [23]. The Agence Française de Sécurité Sanitaire des Aliments drew attention to the presence of isoflavones and their unknown impact on infant health. Isoflavones have been shown to induce estradiol-like effects in animal models [45]. The American Academy of Pediatrics reviewed the literature and summarized that 10% to 14% of infants with CMA will become soy-sensitized, with a higher incidence in non-IgE mediated CMA than in IgE mediated CMA [46]. According to a recent meta-analysis, the prevalence of soy allergy was 0.5% in the general population, but the prevalence of sensitization after the use of soy infant formula was 8.7% [47]. Therefore, it seems logic today to recommend a clinically tested eHF as first option in the management of CMA, and to recommend rice hydrolysates as a second option and soy as third option.

A lack of effective and approved treatment has led to strict avoidance of the culprit food proteins being the only standard of care [2]. Several food immunotherapies are being developed; these involve oral, sublingual, epicutaneous, or subcutaneous administration of small amounts of native or modified allergens to induce immune tolerance [2,48]. Oral immunotherapy is a promising but still experimental method to treat children with cow's milk allergy [49]. The approach generally follows the same principles as immunotherapy of other allergic disorders and involves the administration of small increasing doses of food during an induction phase followed by a maintenance phase with regular intake of a maximum tolerated amount of food [50]. Most research has been conducted with oral immunotherapy due to its efficacious and relatively safe profile but remains an investigational treatment to be further studied before advancing into clinical practice [2,48]. Determination of IgE and IgG4 epitope binding may contribute to select candidates for oral immune therapy [51]. Oral immune therapy carries significant risk of allergic reactions [51]. The ability of oral immune therapy to desensitize patients to particular foods is well-documented, although the ability to induce tolerance has not been established [51]. Recent data suggest that oral immune therapy may induce long term tolerance in half of the children [52]. Markers of allergy such as blood eosinophils and serum IgE decreased and milk-specific IgG and IgG4 increased during oral immune therapy [49]. Adipokines, leptin and resistin, which functionally are cytokines linked to Th1-type response, increase during oral immune therapy [49]. The high frequency of allergic adverse reactions of the various approaches highlighted the need of refinements in the strategies. A careful review of the patients who received food oral immune therapy in controlled trials confirmed that adverse events were not rare but that ~90% of children could achieve an effective desensitization [53]. A promising strategy for preventing IgE cross-linking and thus enhancing safety of immune therapy, while still activating T cells, is the use of tolerogenic peptides [2]. Additional bigger, multicentric and randomized-controlled studies must answer multiple questions including optimal dose, ideal duration of immunotherapy, degree of protection, efficacy for different ages, severity and type of food allergy responsive to treatment [48]. The procedure remains investigational and should be performed only by trained physicians, especially in the pediatric setting [53]. Immunotherapy for food allergy is still not ready for the clinic, but current and upcoming studies are dedicated to collect enough evidence for the possible implementation of allergen-SIT as a standard treatment for food allergy [2].

6. Gut Microbiota

The role of the GI microbiota in food allergy has been a topic of major interest since many years. Oral tolerance is the consequence of a systemic absence of a response to dietary antigens. Early infancy is a window during which gut microbiota may shape food allergy outcomes in childhood [54]. Dietary antigens and intestinal microbiota are known to make up the majority of the antigen load in the intestine. The GI microbiome plays a strong role in the orientation of the immune response [55].

Food allergy is associated with alterations in the gut microbiota or dysbiosis early in life that may be predictive of disease persistence versus tolerance acquisition [56]. Qualitative and quantitative differences in the composition of the gut microbiota between infants who will and infants who will not develop allergy are demonstrable before the development of any clinical manifestations of atopy [57,58]. Gut microbiome composition at age 3 to 6 months was associated with acquisition of tolerance to milk proteins by age 8 years, with enrichment of Clostridia and Firmicutes in the infant gut microbiome of subjects with resolved CMA [54]. Metagenome functional prediction supported decreased fatty acid metabolism in the gut microbiome of subjects whose CMA resolved [54]. As a consequence, bacterial taxa within Clostridia and Firmicutes could be studied as probiotic candidates for milk allergy therapy [54]. Data obtained in murine models of food allergy suggest that microbial therapy with protolerogenic bacteria such as certain Clostridial species holds promise in future applications for prevention or therapy of food allergy [59]. Extrapolation from in vitro data suggests that supplementing infant formulas such as eHF with prebiotics or probiotics (*Lactobacillus* (L.) *rhamnosus* GG, *Bifidobacteria* (B.) breve) may offer an additional benefit [60].

6.1. Prebiotics

Dietary supplementation with short chain galacto-oligosaccharides (scGOS), long chain fructo-olgosaccharides (lcFOS) and/or pectin-derived acidic oligosaccharides during sensitization effectively reduce allergic symptoms but differentially affect mucosal immune activation in whey-sensitized mice [61]. A beneficial effect of prebiotics on the development of atopic dermatitis in a high risk population of infants was shown for the first time in this paper [62]. Although the mechanism of this effect requires further investigation, it appears likely that oligosaccharides modulate postnatal immune development by altering bowel flora and have a potential role in primary allergy prevention during infancy [63]. These findings were confirmed by demonstrating that early dietary intervention with oligosaccharide prebiotics has a protective effect against both allergic manifestations and infections [64]. Later, this effect was also shown in non-at-risk infants [63]. The observed dual protection lasting beyond the intervention period, up to the age of five years, suggests that an immune modulating effect through the intestinal flora modification may be the principal mechanism of action [60,63]. This mechanism has now been demonstrated [64].

The addition of lactose to an eHF is able to positively modulate the composition of gut microbiota by increasing the total fecal counts of L/B and decreasing that of Bacteroides/Clostridia [65]. The positive effect is completed by the increase of median concentration of short chain fatty acids, especially for acetic and butyric acids demonstrated by the metabolomic analysis [66]. However, the ESPGHAN Committee on Nutrition concluded in 2011 that there was insufficient evidence to recommend the use of prebiotics in infant formula to prevent atopic disease [67]. But, based on GRADE evidence to decision frameworks, the WAO guideline panel suggests using prebiotic supplementation in not-exclusively breastfed infants and not using prebiotic supplementation in exclusively breastfed infants [68]. Both recommendations are conditional and based on very low certainty of the evidence [68].

Human milk oligosaccharides (HMOs) are a group of complex sugars that are highly abundant in human milk, but currently not present in infant formula. Literature indicating that HMOs play a major beneficial and facilitating role in the development of the infant's microbiome and thus immune development is abundant and unequivocal. However, there are over 100 different HMOs, with specific properties and functions. HMOs are not digested by the infant and serve as metabolic substrates for select microbes, contributing to shape the infant gut microbiome. HMOs provide a main substrate to help shape the infant's gut microbiota and affect the maturation of the intestinal mucosal immune system [69]. Higher HMO diversity at the age of one month was associated with lower total and percentage fat mass [69]. At the age of 6 months, each 1-μg/mL increase in lacto-N-fucopentaose was associated with a 1.11-kg lower weight and a 0.85-g lower lean mass [69]. These findings support the hypothesis that differences in HMO composition in mother's milk are associated with infant growth and body composition [69].

HMOs act as soluble decoy receptors that block the attachment of viral, bacterial or protozoan parasite pathogens to epithelial cell surface sugars, which may help prevent infectious diseases in the gut and also the respiratory and urinary tracts. HMOs alter host epithelial and immune cell responses. Secretor milk contains higher concentrations of total and fucosylated HMOs than does nonsecretor milk. These HMO concentrations can be correlated to the health of breastfed infants in order to investigate the protective effects of milk components [70]. HMOs have the potential to selectively enrich the beneficial intestinal microbiota in breast-fed infants. Infants that received human milk with low Lacto-N-fucopentaose III concentrations were more likely to become affected with cow's milk allergy when compared to high LNFP III-containing milk (odds ratio 6.7, 95% CI 2.0–22) [71].

Up to now, only a limited number of HMOs have been synthetized and studied in infant formula, showing beneficial results. It is however unclear if a single HMO is more beneficial for the infant's immune system development than the artificial prebiotic oligosaccharides such as galacto- and fructo-oligosaccharides.

6.2. Probiotics

The administration of probiotics may contribute to the restoration of the healthy equilibrium of the GI microbiota and contribute to the efficacy of an elimination diet in CMA. Probiotics are known to cross-talk with the intestinal immune cells. Probiotic bacteria have different modes of action in the intestinal lumen: they hydrolyze peptides that are potentially antigenic to non-antigenic peptides; they decrease the intestinal permeability and, as a consequence reduce the penetration of antigens from the gut lumen to the systemic circulation; they stimulate the local production of IgA and they regulate local inflammatory responses and stimulate the differentiation and growth of the GI mucosa [41]. Administration of L GG to children under the age of 2 years suffering from eczema and with a challenge-proven food allergy has been shown to result in a significant decrease in the eczema score [72]. A formula supplemented with L GG also decreased GI symptoms in infants with eczema [73]. A cow milk challenge in allergic infants resulted in an increase of fecal IgA levels and a decrease of the TNF-α level compared to a placebo [74]. L. GG has been shown to substantially increase the memory B cells and stimulate interferon-γ secretion in infants with CMA and with IgE-associated dermatitis, but not in healthy infants [75]. These findings support the hypothesis that infants with an atopic predisposition may have an aberrant pattern of intestinal microbiota and this explains why the beneficial effects of probiotics are only seen in this group [76]. In infants with colitis, supplementing a casein eHF with L. GG significantly enhanced the recovery of the inflammation in the colonic mucosa in comparison to the same hydrolysate without the probiotics [76]. In the group that received the probiotic, fecal calprotectin and the number of infants with ongoing occult blood in stools after one month were significantly smaller [77]. The primary goal in the treatment of CMA is, of course, for the symptoms to disappear. However, the second, and almost equally important objective, is to acquire oral tolerance. As an eHF supplemented with L casei CRL431 and B lactis BB-12 failed to accelerate tolerance, this effect may be strain specific [78]. In a trial that compared an eHF without and with L GG, a double-blind placebo-controlled food challenge (at least 1.4×10^7 CFU/100 mL) was negative in 15/28 (53.6%) infants without L. GG and in 22/27 (81.5%, $p = 0.027$) with L. GG. These findings may prove innovative in the therapeutic approach to treating infants with CMA by accelerating the acquisition of tolerance [79].

Consumption of probiotic milk products was related to a reduced incidence of atopic eczema and rhinoconjunctivitis, but not associated to the incidence of asthma by 36 months of age [80].

Most tolerant infants showed a significant increase in fecal butyrate levels, and those taxa that were significantly enriched in these samples [81], exhibited specific strain-level demarcations between tolerant and allergic infants. Data suggest that a casein eHF with L. GG promotes tolerance in infants with CMA, in part, by influencing the strain-level bacterial community structure of the infant gut [81].

Perinatal probiotic administration is safe in long-term follow-up [82]. Children receiving L. rhamnosus GG perinatally tended to have decreased allergy prevalence [82]. The subgroup analysis based on the type of treatment suggested that both L. alone and L. with B. are protective against atopic dermatitis (OR = 0.70, $p = 0.004$; OR = 0.62, $p < 0.001$). Probiotics seem to have a protective role in atopic dermatitis prevention if these are administered during the pre- and postnatal period in both general and allergic risk populations [82]. However, the ESPGHAN Committee on Nutrition concluded in 2011 that there was insufficient evidence to recommend probiotics to prevent atopic disease [67]. However, considering all critical outcomes in this context, the WAO guideline panel determined that there is a likely net benefit from using probiotics resulting primarily from prevention of eczema. The WAO guideline panel suggests: (i) using probiotics in pregnant women at high risk for having an allergic child; (ii) using probiotics in women who breastfeed infants at high risk of developing allergy; and (iii) using probiotics in infants at high risk of developing allergy [83]. Probiotic compounds may contain hidden allergens of food and may not be safe for subjects with allergy to cow milk or hen's egg [84,85].

Post-sensitization administration of non-digestible oligosaccharides and *Bifidobacterium breve* M-16 V were shown to reduce allergic symptoms in mice [86]. Studies demonstrate that an AAF with synbiotics is safe and well tolerated and promotes normal growth when fed to healthy full-term infants as the sole source of nutrition and is hypoallergenic in subjects with CMA [87].

7. Conclusions

The diagnosis of CMA is still a challenge. Cow milk based eHF remains the recommended and preferred therapeutic choice, while AAF is reserved for the most severe cases. Rice hydrolysates and soy informant formulas are second choice options. Manipulation of the gut microbiotica may enhance the development of oral tolerance. Hydrolysates, in particular pHF with proven efficacy, may become a protein source in starter infant formula. Since the efficacy of hydrolysates in the prevention of allergic disease is debated, some guidelines recommend these formulas in infants at risk for atopic disease, while other meta-analyses and some countries do not recommend the use of these formulas in prevention. However, it is obvious that these formulas do not harm. Similar, although the clinical evidence for a benefit of additional prebiotics or HMOs and/or probiotics is limited, supplementation of hydrolysates should be considered as adverse effects have not been reported.

References

1. Sicherer, S.H. Epidemiology of food allergy. *J. Allergy Clin. Immunol.* **2011**, *127*, 594–602. [CrossRef] [PubMed]
2. Kostadinova, A.I.; Willemsen, L.E.; Knippels, L.M.; Garssen, J. Immunotherapy-risk/benefit in food allergy. *Pediatr. Allergy Immunol.* **2013**, *24*, 633–644. [CrossRef] [PubMed]
3. Koletzko, S.; Niggemann, B.; Arato, A.; Dias, J.A.; Heuschkel, R.; Husby, S.; Mearin, M.L.; Papadopoulou, A.; Ruemmele, F.M.; Staiano, A.; et al. European Society of Pediatric Gastroenterology, Hepatology, and, Nutrition. Diagnostic approach and management of cow's-milk protein allergy in infants and children: ESPGHAN GI Committee practical guidelines. *J. Pediatr. Gastroenterol. Nutr.* **2012**, *55*, 221–229. [CrossRef] [PubMed]
4. Host, A. Frequency of cow's milk allergy in childhood. *Ann. Allergy Asthma Immunol.* **2002**, *89*, 33–37. [CrossRef]
5. Sackesen, C. Epidemiology of cow's milk allergy: Has it changed? *Clin. Trans. Allergy* **2011**, *1*, S50. [CrossRef]
6. Host, A.; Halken, S. A prospective study of cow milk allergy in Danish infants during the first 3 years of life. Clinical course in relation to clinical and immunological type of hypersensitivity reaction. *Allergy* **1990**, *45*, 587–596. [CrossRef] [PubMed]
7. Miraglia Del Giudice, M.; Allegorico, A. The role of vitamin D in allergic diseases in children. *J. Clin. Gastroenterol.* **2016**, *50*, S133–S135. [CrossRef] [PubMed]
8. Schindler, T.; Sinn, J.K.; Osborn, D.A. Polyunsaturated fatty acid supplementation in infancy for the prevention of allergy. *Cochrane Database Syst. Rev.* **2016**, *10*. [CrossRef]
9. Vandenplas, Y.; Abkari, A.; Bellaiche, M.; Benninga, M.; Chouraqui, J.P.; Çokura, F.; Harb, T.; Hegar, B.; Lifschitz, C.; Ludwig, T.; et al. Prevalence and health outcomes of functional gastrointestinal symptoms in infants from birth to 12 months of age. *J. Pediatr. Gastroenterol. Nutr.* **2015**, *61*, 531–537. [CrossRef] [PubMed]
10. Fiocchi, A.; Brozek, J.; Schünemann, H. World Allergy Organization (WAO) Diagnosis and Rationale for Action against Cow's Milk Allergy (DRACMA) Guidelines. *World Allergy Organ. J.* **2010**, *3*, 157–161. [CrossRef] [PubMed]
11. Gordon, B.R. The allergic march: Can we prevent allergies and asthma? *Otolaryngol. Clin. N. Am.* **2011**, *44*, 765–777. [CrossRef] [PubMed]
12. Alexander, D.D.; Cabana, M.D. Partially hydrolyzed 100% whey protein infant formula and reduced risk of atopic dermatitis: a meta-analysis. *J. Pediatr. Gastroenterol. Nutr.* **2010**, *50*, 422–430. [CrossRef] [PubMed]
13. Szajewska, H.; Horvath, A. Meta-analysis of the evidence for a partially hydrolyzed 100% whey formula for the prevention of allergic diseases. *Curr. Med. Res. Opin.* **2010**, *26*, 423–437. [CrossRef] [PubMed]
14. Boyle, R.J.; Ierodiakonou, D.; Khan, T.; Chivinge, J.; Robinson, Z.; Geoghegan, N.; Jarrold, K.; Afxentiou, T.; Reeves, T.; Cunhalibrarian, S.; et al. Hydrolysed formula and risk of allergic or autoimmune disease: Systematic review and meta-analysis. *BMJ* **2016**, *352*, i974. [CrossRef] [PubMed]
15. Boyle, R.J.; Tang, M.L.; Chiang, W.C.; Chua, M.C.; Ismail, I.; Nauta, A.; Hourihane, J.O.; Smith, P.; Gold, M.; Ziegler, J.; et al. PATCH study investigators. Prebiotic-supplemented partially hydrolysed cow's milk formula for the prevention of eczema in high-risk infants: A randomized controlled trial. *Allergy* **2016**, *71*, 701–710. [CrossRef] [PubMed]
16. Osborn, D.A.; Sinn, J.K.; Jones, L.J. Infant formulas containing hydrolysed protein for prevention of allergic disease and food allergy. *Cochrane Database Syst. Rev.* **2017**, *3*, CD003664. [PubMed]
17. Halken, S. Prevention of allergic disease in childhood: Clinical and epidemiological aspects of primary and secondary allergy prevention. *Pediatr. Allergy Immunol.* **2004**, *15*, 9–32. [CrossRef] [PubMed]
18. Fuertes, E.; Standl, M.; von Berg, A.; Lehmann, I.; Hoffmann, B.; Bauer, C.P.; Koletzko, S.; Berdel, D.; Heinrich, J. Parental allergic disease before and after child birth poses similar risk for childhood allergies. *Allergy* **2015** *70*, 873–876. [CrossRef] [PubMed]

19. Vandenplas, Y.; Alarcon, P.; Fleischer, D.; Hernell, O.; Kolacek, S.; Laignelet, H.; Lönnerdal, B.; Raman, R.; Rigo, J.; Salvatore, S.; et al. Should Partial Hydrolysates Be Used as Starter Infant Formula? A Working Group Consensus. *J. Pediatr. Gastroenterol. Nutr.* **2016**, *62*, 22–35. [CrossRef] [PubMed]
20. Vandenplas, Y.; Cruchet, S.; Faure, C.; Lee, H.; Di Lorenzo, C.; Staiano, A.; Chundi, X.; Aw, M.; Gutiérrez-Castrellón, P.; Asery, A.; et al. When should we use partially hydrolysed formulae for frequent gastrointestinal symptoms and allergy prevention? *Acta Paediatr.* **2014**, *103*, 689–695. [CrossRef] [PubMed]
21. Vandenplas, Y.; Koletzko, S.; Isolauri, E.; Brueton, M.; Dupont, C.; Hill, D.; Koletzko, S.; Oranje, A.P.; Staiano, A. Guidelines for the diagnosis and management of cow's milk protein allergy in infants. *Arch. Dis. Child.* **2007**, *92*, 902–908. [CrossRef] [PubMed]
22. Papadopoulou, A.; Tsoukala, D.; Tsoumakas, K. Rhinitis and asthma in children: Comorbitity or united airway disease? *Curr. Pediatr. Rev.* **2014**, *10*, 275–281. [CrossRef] [PubMed]
23. Vandenplas, Y.; Alarcon, P.; Alliet, P.; De Greef, E.; De Ronne, N.; Hoffman, I.; Van Winckel, M.; Hauser, B. Algorithms for managing infant constipation, colic, regurgitation and cow's milk allergy in formula-fed infants. *Acta Paediatr.* **2015**, *104*, 449–457. [CrossRef] [PubMed]
24. Vandenplas, Y.; Dupont, C.; Eigenmann, P.; Host, A.; Kuitunen, M.; Ribes-Koninckx, C.; Shah, N.; Shamir, R.; Staiano, A.; Szajewska, H.; et al. A workshop report on the development of the Cow's Milk-related Symptom Score awareness tool for young children. *Acta Paediatr.* **2015**, *104*, 334–339. [CrossRef] [PubMed]
25. Vandenplas, Y.; Steenhout, P.; Järvi, A.; Garreau, A.-S.; Mukherjee, R. Pooled analysis of the cow's milk-related-symptom-score (CoMiSS™) as a predictor for cow's milk related symptoms. *Pediatr. Gastroenterol. Hepatol. Nutr.* **2017**, *20*, 22–26. [CrossRef] [PubMed]
26. Kiewiet, M.B.; Gros, M.; van Neerven, R.J.; Faas, M.M.; de Vos, P. Immunomodulating properties of protein hydrolysates for application in cow's milk allergy. *Pediatr. Allergy Immunol.* **2015**, *26*, 206–217. [CrossRef] [PubMed]
27. Lowe, A.J.; Dharmage, S.C.; Allen, K.J.; Tang, M.L.; Hill, D.J. The role of partially hydrolyzed whey formula for the prevention of allergic disease: Evidence and gaps. *Expert Rev. Clin. Immunol.* **2013**, *9*, 31–41. [CrossRef] [PubMed]
28. Lucendo, A.J.; Arias, Á.; González-Cervera, J.; Mota-Huertas, T.; Yagüe-Compadre, J.L. Tolerance of a cow's milk-based hydrolyzed formula in patients with eosinophilic esophagitis triggered by milk. *Allergy* **2013**, *68*, 1065–1072. [CrossRef] [PubMed]
29. Kemp, A.S.; Hill, D.J.; Allen, K.J.; Anderson, K.; Davidson, G.P.; Day, A.S.; Heine, R.G.; Peake, J.E.; Prescott, S.L.; Shugg, A.W. Guidelines for the use of infant formulas to treat cows milk protein allergy: an Australian consensus panel opinion. *Med. J. Aust.* **2008**, *188*, 109–112. [PubMed]
30. Vandenplas, Y.; De Greef, E.; Xinias, I.; Vrani, O.; Mavroudi, A.; Hammoud, M.; Al Refai, F.; Khalife, M.C.; Sayad, A.; Noun, P.; et al. Safety of a thickened extensive casein hydrolysate formula. *Nutrition* **2016**, *32*, 206–212. [CrossRef] [PubMed]
31. Dupont, C.; Kalach, N.; Soulaines, P.; Bradatan, E.; Lachaux, A.; Payot, F.; De Blay, F.; Guénard-Bilbault, L.; Hatahet, R.; Mulier, S.; et al. Safety of a new amino acid formula in infants allergic to cow's milk and intolerant to hydrolysates. *J. Pediatr. Gastroenterol. Nutr.* **2015**, *61*, 456–463. [CrossRef] [PubMed]
32. Vandenplas, Y.; De Greef, E.; Hauser, B.; Paradice Study Group. Safety and tolerance of a new extensively hydrolyzed rice protein-based formula in the management of infants with cow's milk protein allergy. *Eur. J. Pediatr.* **2014**, *173*, 1209–1216.
33. Vandenplas, Y.; De Greef, E.; Hauser, B.; Paradice Study Group. An extensively hydrolysed rice protein-based formula in the management of infants with cow's milk protein allergy: Preliminary results after 1 month. *Arch. Dis. Child.* **2014**, *99*, 933–936. [CrossRef] [PubMed]
34. Hojsak, I.; Braegger, C.; Bronsky, J.; Campoy, C.; Colomb, V.; Decsi, T.; Domellöf, M.; Fewtrell, M.; Mis, N.F.; Mihatsch, W.; et al. Arsenic in rice: A cause for concern. *J. Pediatr. Gastroenterol. Nutr.* **2015**, *60*, 142–145. [CrossRef] [PubMed]
35. Ah-Leung, S.; Bernard, H.; Bidat, E.; Paty, E.; Rancé, F.; Scheinmann, P.; Wal, J.M. Allergy to goat and sheep milk without allergy to cow's milk. *Allergy* **2006**, *61*, 1358–1365. [CrossRef] [PubMed]
36. Katz, Y.; Goldberg, M.R.; Zadik-Mnuhin, G.; Leshno, M.; Heyman, E. Cross-sensitization between milk proteins: Reactivity to a "kosher" epitope? *Isr. Med. Assoc. J.* **2008**, *10*, 85–88. [PubMed]
37. Ehlayel, M.S.; Hazeima, K.A.; Al-Mesaifri, F.; Bener, A. Camel milk: An alternative for cow's milk allergy in children. *Allergy Asthma Proc.* **2011**, *32*, 255–258. [CrossRef] [PubMed]

38. Businco, L.; Giampietro, P.G.; Lucenti, P.; Lucaroni, F.; Pini, C.; Di Felice, G.; Iacovacci, P.; Curadi, C.; Orlandi, M. Allergenicity of mare's milk in children with cow's milk allergy. *J. Allergy Clin. Immunol.* **2000**, *105*, 1031–1034. [CrossRef] [PubMed]
39. Vincenzetti, S.; Foghini, L.; Pucciarelli, S.; Polzonetti, V.; Cammertoni, N.; Beghelli, D.; Polidori, P. Hypoallergenic properties of donkey's milk: A preliminary study. *Vet. Ital.* **2014**, *50*, 99–107. [PubMed]
40. Iacono, G.; Carroccio, A.; Cavataio, F.; Montalto, G.; Soresi, M.; Balsamo, V. Use of ass's milk in multiple food allergy. *J. Pediatr. Gastr. Nutr.* **1992**, *14*, 177–181. [CrossRef]
41. Monti, G.; Bertino, E.; Muratore, M.C.; Coscia, A.; Cresi, F.; Silvestro, L.; Fabris, C.; Fortunato, D.; Giuffrida, M.G.; Conti, A. Efficacy of donkey's milk in treating highly problematic cow's milk allergic children: An in vivo and in vitro study. *Pediatr. Allergy Immunol.* **2007**, *18*, 258–264. [CrossRef] [PubMed]
42. Loss, G.; Depner, M.; Ulfman, L.H.; van Neerven, R.J.; Hose, A.J.; Genuneit, J.; Karvonen, A.M.; Hyvärinen, A.; Kaulek, V.; Roduit, C.; et al. Consumption of unprocessed cow's milk protects infants from common respiratory infections. *Allergy Clin. Immunol.* **2015**, *135*, 56–62. [CrossRef] [PubMed]
43. Leung, J.; Hundal, N.V.; Katz, A.J.; Shreffler, W.G.; Yuan, Q.; Butterworth, C.A.; Hesterberg, P.E. Tolerance of baked milk in patients with cow's milk-mediated eosinophilic esophagitis. *J. Allergy Clin. Immunol.* **2013**, *132*, 1215–1216. [CrossRef] [PubMed]
44. Goldberg, M.R.; Nachshon, L.; Appel, M.Y.; Elizur, A.; Levy, M.B.; Eisenberg, E.; Sampson, H.A.; Katz, Y. Efficacy of baked milk oral immunotherapy in baked milk-reactive allergic patients. *J. Allergy Clin. Immunol.* **2015**, *136*, 1601–1606. [CrossRef] [PubMed]
45. Mars. Available online: www.afssa.fr (accessed on 16 June 2017).
46. American Academy of Pediatrics; Committee on Nutrition. Hypoallergenic infant formulas. *Pediatrics* **2000**, *106*, 346–349.
47. Katz, Y.; Gutierrez-Castrellon, P.; González, M.G.; Rivas, R.; Lee, B.W.; Alarcon, P. A comprehensive review of sensitization and allergy to soy-based products. *Clin. Rev. Allergy Immunol.* **2014**, *46*, 272–281. [CrossRef] [PubMed]
48. Martinolli, F.; Carraro, S.; Berardi, M.; Ferraro, V.; Baraldi, E.; Zanconato, S. Immunother for food allergies in children. *Curr. Pharm. Des.* **2014**, *20*, 906–923. [CrossRef] [PubMed]
49. Salmivesi, S.; Paassilta, M.; Huhtala, H.; Nieminen, R.; Moilanen, E.; Korppi, M. Changes in biomarkers during a six-month oral immunotherapy intervention for cow's milk allergy. *Acta Paediatr.* **2016**, *105*, 1349–1354. [CrossRef] [PubMed]
50. Burbank, A.J.; Sood, P.; Vickery, B.P.; Wood, R.A. Oral Immunotherapy for Food Allergy. *Immunol. Allergy Clin. N. Am.* **2016**, *36*, 55–69. [CrossRef] [PubMed]
51. Savilahti, E.M.; Kuitunen, M.; Valori, M.; Rantanen, V.; Bardina, L.; Gimenez, G.; Mäkelä, M.J.; Hautaniemi, S.; Savilahti, E.; Sampson, H.A. Use of IgE and IgG4 epitope binding to predict the outcome of oral immunotherapy in cow's milk allergy. *Pediatr. Allergy Immunol.* **2014**, *25*, 227–235. [CrossRef] [PubMed]
52. Kivistö, J.E.; Korppi, M.; Helminen, M.; Mäki, T.; Paassilta, M. Half of the children who received oral immunotherapy for a cows' milk allergy consumed milk freely after 2.5 years. *Acta Paediatr.* **2015**, *104*, 1164–1168.
53. Pajno, G.B.; Caminiti, L.; Chiera, F.; Crisafulli, G.; Salzano, G.; Arasi, S.; Passalacqua, G. Safety profile of oral immunotherapy with cow's milk and hen egg: A 10-year experience in controlled trials. *Allergy Asthma Proc.* **2016**, *37*, 400–403. [CrossRef] [PubMed]
54. Bunyavanich, S.; Shen, N.; Grishin, A.; Wood, R.; Burks, W.; Dawson, P.; Jones, S.M.; Leung, D.Y.; Sampson, H.; Sicherer, S.; et al. Early-life gut microbiome composition and milk allergy resolution. *J. Allergy Clin. Immunol.* **2016**, *138*, 1122–1130. [CrossRef] [PubMed]
55. Mowat, A.M. Anatomical basis of tolerance and immunity to intestinal antigens. *Nat. Rev. Immunol.* **2003**, *3*, 331–341. [CrossRef] [PubMed]
56. Rachid, R.; Chatila, T.A. The role of the gut microbiota in food allergy. *Curr. Opin. Pediatr.* **2016**, *28*, 748–753. [CrossRef] [PubMed]
57. Björkstén, B.; Sepp, E.; Julge, K.; Voor, T.; Mikelsaar, M. Allergy development and the intestinal microflora during the first year of life. *J. Allergy Clin. Immunol.* **2001**, *108*, 516–520. [CrossRef] [PubMed]
58. Canani, R.B.; Di Costanzo, M. Gut microbiota as potential therapeutic target for the treatment of cow's milk allergy. *Nutrients* **2013**, *5*, 651–662. [CrossRef] [PubMed]

59. Lundelin, K.; Poussa, T.; Salminen, S.; Isolauri, E3. Long-term safety and efficacy of perinatal probiotic intervention: Evidence from a follow-up study of four randomized, double-blind, placebo-controlled trials. *Pediatr. Allergy Immunol.* **2016**, *28*, 170–175. [CrossRef] [PubMed]
60. Vandenplas, Y.; Steenhout, P.; Planoudis, Y.; Grathwohl, D.; Althera Study Group. Treating cow's milk protein allergy: A double-blind randomized trial comparing two extensively hydrolysed formulas with probiotics. *Acta Paediatr.* **2013**, *102*, 990–998. [CrossRef] [PubMed]
61. Kerperien, J.; Jeurink, P.V.; Wehkamp, T.; van der Veer, A.; van de Kant, H.J.; Hofman, G.A.; van Esch, E.C.; Garssen, J.; Willemsen, L.E.; Knippels, L.M. Non-digestible oligosaccharides modulate intestinal immune activation and suppress cow's milk allergic symptoms. *Pediatr. Allergy Immunol.* **2014**, *25*, 747–754. [CrossRef] [PubMed]
62. Moro, G.; Arslanoglu, S.; Stahl, B.; Jelinek, J.; Wahn, U.; Boehm, G. A mixture of prebiotic oligosaccharides reduces the incidence of atopic dermatitis during the first six months of age. *Arch. Dis. Child.* **2006**, *91*, 814–819. [CrossRef] [PubMed]
63. Arslanoglu, S.; Moro, G.E.; Schmitt, J.; Tandoi, L.; Rizzardi, S.; Boehm, G. Early dietary intervention with a mixture of prebiotic oligosaccharides reduces the incidence of allergic manifestations and infections during the first two years of life. *J. Nutr.* **2008**, *138*, 1091–1095. [PubMed]
64. Grüber, C.; van Stuijvenberg, M.; Mosca, F.; Moro, G.; Chirico, G.; Braegger, C.P.; Riedler, J.; Boehm, G.; Wahn, U.; MIPS 1 Working Group. Reduced occurrence of early atopic dermatitis because of immunoactive prebiotics among low-atopy-risk infants. *J. Allergy Clin. Immunol.* **2010**, *126*, 791–797.
65. Arslanoglu, S.; Moro, G.E.; Boehm, G.; Wienz, F.; Stahl, B.; Bertino, E. Early neutral prebiotic oligosaccharide supplementation reduces the incidence of some allergic manifestations in the first 5 years of life. *J. Biol. Regul. Homeost. Agents* **2012**, *26*, 49–59. [PubMed]
66. Francavilla, R.; Calasso, M.; Calace, L.; Siragusa, S.; Ndagijimana, M.; Vernocchi, P.; Brunetti, L.; Mancino, G.; Tedeschi, G.; Guerzoni, E.; et al. Effect of lactose on gut microbiota and metabolome of infants with cow's milk allergy. *Pediatr. Allergy Immunol.* **2012**, *23*, 420–427. [CrossRef] [PubMed]
67. Braegger, C.; Chmielewska, A.; Decsi, T.; Kolacek, S.; Mihatsch, W.; Moreno, L.; Pieścik, M.; Puntis, J.; Shamir, R.; Szajewska, H.; et al. Supplementation of infant formula with probiotics and/or prebiotics: A systematic review and comment by the ESPGHAN committee on nutrition. *J. Pediatr. Gastroenterol. Nutr.* **2011**, *52*, 238–250. [CrossRef] [PubMed]
68. Cuello-Garcia, C.A.; Fiocchi, A.; Pawankar, R.; Yepes-Nuñez, J.J.; Morgano, G.P.; Zhang, Y.; Ahn, K.; Al-Hammadi, S.; Agarwal, A.; Gandhi, S.; et al. World Allergy Organization-McMaster University Guidelines for Allergic Disease Prevention (GLAD-P): Prebiotics. *World Allergy Organ. J.* **2016**, *9*, 10. [CrossRef] [PubMed]
69. Alderete, T.L.; Autran, C.; Brekke, B.E.; Knight, R.; Bode, L.; Goran, M.I.; Fields, D.A. Associations between human milk oligosaccharides and infant body composition in the first 6 mo of life. *Am. J. Clin. Nutr.* **2015**, *102*, 1381–1388. [CrossRef] [PubMed]
70. Bode, L.; Contractor, N.; Barile, D.; Pohl, N.; Prudden, A.R.; Boons, G.J.; Jin, Y.S.; Jennewein, S. Overcoming the limited availability of human milk oligosaccharides: Challenges and opportunities for research and application. *Nutr. Rev.* **2016**, *74*, 635–644. [CrossRef] [PubMed]
71. Seppo, A.E.; Autran, C.A.; Bode, L.; Järvinen, K.M. Human milk oligosaccharides and development of cow's milk allergy in infants. *J. Allergy Clin. Immunol.* **2017**, *139*, 708–711. [CrossRef] [PubMed]
72. Majamaa, H.; Isolauri, E. Probiotics: A novel approach in the management of food allergy. *J. Allergy Clin. Immunol.* **1997**, *99*, 179–185. [CrossRef]
73. Isolauri, E.; Arvola, T.; Sutas, Y.; Moilanen, E.; Salminen, S. Probiotics in the management of atopic eczema. *Clin. Exp. Allergy* **2000**, *30*, 1604–1610. [CrossRef] [PubMed]
74. Isolauri, E. Studies on Lactobacillus GG in food hypersensitivity disorders. *Nutr. Today Suppl.* **1996**, *31*, 285–315. [CrossRef]
75. Nermes, M.; Kantele, J.M.; Atosuo, T.J.; Salminen, S.; Isolauri, E. Interaction of orally administered Lactobacillus rhamnosus GG with skin and gut microbiota and humoral immunity in infants with atopic dermatitis. *Clin. Exp. Allergy* **2010**, *41*, 370–377. [CrossRef] [PubMed]
76. Pohjavuori, E.; Viljanen, M.; Korpela, R.; Kuitunen, M.; Tiittanen, M.; Vaarala, O.; Savilahti, E. Lactobacillus GG effect in increasing IFN-γ production in infants with cow's milk allergy. *J. Allergy Clin. Immunol.* **2004**, *114*, 131–136. [CrossRef] [PubMed]

77. Baldassarre, M.E.; Laforgia, N.; Fanelli, M.; Laneve, A.; Grosso, R.; Lifschitz, C. Lactobacillus, G.G improves recovery in infants with blood in the stools and presumptive allergic colitis compared with extensively hydrolyzed formula alone. *J. Pediatr.* **2010**, *156*, 397–401. [CrossRef] [PubMed]
78. Hol, J.; van Leer, E.H.; Elink Schuurman, B.E.; de Ruiter, L.F.; Samsom, J.N.; Hop, W.; Neijens, H.J.; de Jongste, J.C.; Nieuwenhuis, E.E.; Cow's Milk Allergy Modified by Elimination and Lactobacilli Study Group. The acquisition of tolerance toward cow's milk through probiotic supplementation: A randomized, controlled trial. *J. Allergy Clin. Immunol.* **2008**, *121*, 1448–1454. [CrossRef] [PubMed]
79. Berni Canani, R.; Nocerino, R.; Terrin, G.; Coruzzo, A.; Cosenza, L.; Leone, L.; Troncone, R. Effect of extensively hydrolyzed casein formula supplemented with Lactobacillus GG on tolerance acquisition in infants with cow's milk allergy: A randomized trial. *J. Allergy Clin. Immunol.* **2012**, *129*, 580–582. [CrossRef] [PubMed]
80. Bertelsen, R.J.; Brantsæter, A.L.; Magnus, M.C.; Haugen, M.; Myhre, R.; Jacobsson, B.; Longnecker, M.P.; Meltzer, H.M.; London, S.J. Probiotic milk consumption in pregnancy and infancy and subsequent childhood allergic diseases. *J. Allergy Clin. Immunol.* **2014**, *133*, 165–171. [CrossRef] [PubMed]
81. Berni Canani, R.; Sangwan, N.; Stefka, A.T.; Nocerino, R.; Paparo, L.; Aitoro, R.; Calignano, A.; Khan, A.A.; Gilbert, J.A.; Nagler, C.R. Lactobacillus rhamnosus GG-supplemented formula expands butyrate-producing bacterial strains in food allergic infants. *ISME J.* **2016**, *10*, 742–750. [CrossRef] [PubMed]
82. Panduru, M.; Panduru, N.M.; Sălăvăstru, C.M.; Tiplica, G.S. Probiotics and primary prevention of atopic dermatitis: A meta-analysis of randomized controlled trials. *J. Eur. Acad. Dermatol. Venereol.* **2015**, *29*, 232–242. [CrossRef] [PubMed]
83. Fiocchi, A.; Pawankar, R.; Cuello-Garcia, C.; Ahn, K.; Al-Hammadi, S.; Agarwal, A.; Beyer, K.; Burks, W.; Canonica, G.W.; Ebisawa, M.; et al. World Allergy Organization-McMaster University Guidelines for Allergic Disease Prevention (GLAD-P): Probiotics. *World Allergy Organ. J.* **2015**, *8*, 4. [CrossRef] [PubMed]
84. Martín-Muñoz, M.F.; Fortuni, M.; Caminoa, M.; Belver, T.; Quirce, S.; Caballero, T. Anaphylactic reaction to probiotics. Cow's milk and hen's egg allergens in probiotic compounds. *Pediatr. Allergy Immunol.* **2012**, *23*, 778–784. [CrossRef] [PubMed]
85. Lee, T.T.; Morisset, M.; Astier, C.; Moneret-Vautrin, D.A.; Cordebar, V.; Beaudouin, E.; Codreanu, F.; Bihain, B.E.; Kanny, G. Contamination of probiotic preparations with milk allergens can cause anaphylaxis in children with cow's milk allergy. *J. Allergy Clin. Immunol.* **2007**, *119*, 746–747. [PubMed]
86. Van Esch, B.C.; Abbring, S.; Diks, M.A.; Dingjan, G.M.; Harthoorn, L.F.; Vos, A.P.; Garssen, J. Post-sensitization administration of non-digestible oligosaccharides and Bifidobacterium breve M-16V reduces allergic symptoms in mice. *Immun. Inflamm. Dis.* **2016**, *4*, 155–165. [CrossRef] [PubMed]
87. Harvey, B.M.; Langford, J.E.; Harthoorn, L.F.; Gillman, S.A.; Green, T.D.; Schwartz, R.H.; Burks, A.W. Effects on growth and tolerance and hypoallergenicity of an amino acid-based formula with synbiotics. *Pediatr. Res.* **2014**, *75*, 343–351. [CrossRef] [PubMed]

6

Diet Hypotheses in Light of the Microbiota Revolution

Tomasz P. Wypych * and Benjamin J. Marsland

Faculty of Biology and Medicine, University of Lausanne, Service de Pneumologie, CHUV, Epalinges 1066, Switzerland; benjamin.marsland@chuv.ch
* Correspondence: tomasz.wypych@chuv.ch

Abstract: From an evolutionary standpoint, allergy has only recently emerged as a significant health problem. Various hypotheses were proposed to explain this, but they all indicated the importance of rapid lifestyle changes, which occurred in industrialized countries in the last few decades. In this review, we discuss evidence from epidemiological and experimental studies that indicate changes in dietary habits may have played an important role in this phenomenon. Based on the example of dietary fiber, we discuss molecular mechanisms behind this and point towards the importance of diet-induced changes in the microbiota. Finally, we reason that future studies unraveling mechanisms governing these changes, along with the development of better tools to manipulate microbiota composition in individuals will be crucial for the design of novel strategies to combat numerous inflammatory disorders, including atopic diseases.

Keywords: Western diet; nutrients; allergy; microbiota

---

1. Introduction

Allergy is one of the leading health problems in industrialized countries, affecting around 50 million people in the United States alone, and the number of atopic individuals continues to grow. The hallmark of this disorder is a strong Th2 response with upregulated levels of the interleukin-4 (IL-4), IL-5, and IL-13, which leads to enhanced immunoglobulin E (IgE) and IgG1 production, cell recruitment to the site of allergen exposure, and exaggerated immune responses leading to tissue damage.

From an evolutionary perspective, allergies have only recently appeared as a significant health problem. Therefore, researchers have long linked their emergence with rapid lifestyle changes, which occurred in the course of hominine evolution. The "hygiene hypothesis" and its derivatives (the "old friend" and the "biodiversity" hypotheses) pointed to the reduced exposure to environmental microorganisms and helminths in industrialized countries nowadays [1–3]. The "toxin hypothesis" underlined the presence of plant-derived toxins in contemporary foods and skin-care products [4]. Dietary habits are another example of these rapid lifestyle changes and hence, different forms of "diet hypotheses" have emerged [5–7]. The introduction of animal husbandry and agriculture in the Neolithic period slowly initiated these shifts. The Industrial Revolution and development of better tools for food processing further escalated them. As a result, new food items were introduced, such as refined grains, sugars, and vegetable oils, or manufactured salt. In addition to this, development of a mechanical reaper in 19th century allowed for increased harvest of grains, which coincided with the development of steam engine and railroads—prerequisites for grain and cattle transportation. This created a habit of feeding cattle with grain [8], leading to increased saturated fatty acids (SFA) content and increased ratio of n-6 to n-3 polyunsaturated fatty acids (PUFAs) in their meat [9,10].

The bloom of the aforementioned foods fundamentally influenced nutritional characteristics of industrialized regions, increasing glycemic load (potential of food to increase blood glucose and, in turn, insulin levels), and altering various parameters, including fatty acid composition (elevating levels of n-6 PUFAs while reducing that of n-3 PUFAs), macro- and micronutrient intake (decreasing protein and vitamin/mineral density content, respectively), sodium-potassium ratio (increasing Na^+ while reducing K^+ levels), and finally, the fiber content (leading to its severe reduction) [8]. As an outcome, food in the 20th century substantially differed from what our ancestors consumed. Since these changes occurred so rapidly on an evolutionary scale, our genome could not have adapted to them. This notion stands behind the hypotheses that contemporary diet may contribute to development of so-called "lifestyle diseases".

Unfortunately, developed countries did very little in the last few decades to spread awareness of this phenomenon and counteract it. The ubiquitous presence of highly processed, high fat, and high sugar food and drinks has been a major driver in the development of a so-called "Western diet", in which the trends mentioned above are amplified to their extremes. For example, consumption of refined sugars in the United States increased by 24.5% between 2000 and 1970 while that of refined vegetable oil increased by 170% between the 1990s and the 1940s [8].

In this review, we will look at the epidemiological and experimental evidence that these changes may predispose individuals to develop allergies and reason why current trends in dietary habits of Western civilization might constitute a health threat.

2. Nutrients and Epidemiology of Allergy

One of the earliest notions that nutrients might influence allergic diseases was introduced in the late 1980s when an association between sodium intake and asthma was reported [11,12]. These data were backed-up by several other groups studying asthma in both adults and children [13–15], and although their conclusions were not consistently supported [16–18], they pioneered the notion that diet may influence development of allergy. Soon after the "sodium hypothesis", other diet hypotheses emerged. In 1990, Schwartz and Weiss analyzed data from the Second National Health and Nutrition Examination Survey, taking into account various antioxidants, including vitamin C. This study revealed a negative association between vitamin C intake and bronchitis/wheezing [13], a conclusion that was supported by some, but not all, subsequent studies [19–22]. However, trials to control asthma progression via dietary vitamin C supplementation brought disappointing results, questioning the significance of vitamin C in allergy prevention [23,24]. Similar discrepancies were found for other antioxidants, such as vitamin E, β-caroten, or selenium [19,22,25,26].

Soon after the antioxidant hypothesis, the link between increased intake of n-6 and reduced consumption of n-3 PUFAs with atopy and asthma was suggested [27–29]. However, as in the case of the antioxidant hypothesis, observational studies brought inconsistent results, with some of them supporting it [30–33], some disputing it [34–36], and some even indicating the opposite correlation [37,38]. Similar to the antioxidant hypothesis, interventional studies aiming to improve asthma severity via modification of fatty acid intake have been disappointing [5–7].

One factor which might play a significant role is whether the nutrient is assimilated via diet modification or supplement administration. Observational studies cited in this manuscript relied on food questionnaires and blood or urine analysis and did not provide information regarding this issue [13,15,16,18,19,21,26,30,31,33–35,37,38]. Its potential importance is exemplified in the interventional study by Troisi et al., who dissected the influence of nutrients rich in vitamin C and E from vitamin C or E supplementation [25]. Interestingly, diet-derived vitamin E was inversely associated with asthma, while in the case of supplement-derived vitamin E, a positive association was found. Comparatively, there was no significant influence of diet-derived vitamin C on asthma, while supplement-derived vitamin C correlated positively with this condition [25]. Comparison of the impact of diet and supplement-derived nutrients on allergic conditions will be important for future studies.

3. Milk and Epidemiology of Allergy

Milk is not solely a source of nutrients but contains various other components, such as immunoglobulin A, cytokines, bacterial metabolites, and, in the case of unpasteurized milk, live bacteria. Considering this, we are describing the relationship between milk consumption and allergy in a separate paragraph, starting with the intake of milk from breastfeeding mothers in infancy, followed by consumption of unpasteurized milk.

3.1. Breastfeeding

Breastfeeding is one of the few features linking dietary habits of people today with that of our evolutionary ancestors. The sole fact that it is so highly conserved among mammals highlights its important physiological role. For this reason, it has long been speculated that breastfeeding may protect against development of atopic diseases. One of the first studies to support this idea was published in 1936 when an inverse relation between breastfeeding and infantile eczema was reported [39]. Since then, a number of studies supported the protective role of breastfeeding against atopy in infancy [40–44]. Importantly, Saarinen and colleagues followed up on individuals for 17 years, showing that the protective effect of breastfeeding was maintained during childhood and adolescence [45]. Also, additional studies focusing on children reached similarconclusions [33,46–48].

However, not all studies confirmed this. In the study by Hide and Gruyer initiated in 1981, breast-fed children had the same (in the case of asthma) or even increased (in the case of eczema) risk of developing atopic disease [49]. Also, Wright and colleagues reported that beginning at the age of 6 years, breastfeeding was no longer associated with protection from recurrent wheeze and, in fact, carried an increased risk in the case of atopic children with asthmatic mothers [50]. No protection against asthma or even elevated risk for its occurrence was also reported by other studies [51–53]. The reasons for these discrepancies are not clear, although they might have been caused by variation in milk composition between individuals. Of note, infant formulas have greatly changed over past decades, which constitutes another variable to consider. However, many studies cited above were performed in different decades but reached similar conclusions while others were performed in the same decade but reached conflicting results. These examples suggest that decade-dependent differences in infant formula composition may not be a major confounding factor.

In order to clarify the inconsistencies between the studies, meta-analyses of published reports were undertaken. An analysis of 12 studies concerning bronchial asthma pointed towards an inverse association between breastfeeding and occurrence of this disease during childhood [54]. Also, an analysis of 18 studies regarding atopic dermatitis reached similar conclusions, but the effect was restricted to children with a family history of atopy [55]. Another meta-analysis of six studies underlined a protective role of breastfeeding in the development of allergic rhinitis [56]. Finally, the most comprehensive meta-analysis regarding asthma to date, taking into account 117 studies, found that breastfeeding was a factor reducing the risk of childhood asthma, with the strongest association in infants (0–2 years) [57].

Collectively, although there is still controversy in the field, most studies conclude that breastfeeding protects infants and children from developing allergic diseases [58,59]. The underlying mechanisms are not clear at present but may be associated with immunological components of breast milk (e.g., immunoglobulin A and its immune complexes, cytokines), antigens (e.g., allergens), prebiotics (e.g., human milk oligosaccharides), bacteria and bacterial metabolites, and/or others. Interestingly, many of these components (e.g., IgA [60], human milkoligosaccharides [61], human milk microbiota [62]) have the potential to influence the microbiota and the homeostasis of infant's intestines, which may be of importance for the development of immune tolerance later in life. Detailed description of these putative mechanisms is beyond the scope of this review. Instead, the reader is referred to other recent publications in this field [61–66].

3.2. *Unpasteurized Cow's Milk*

It has been well documented that growing up on a farm protects against development of allergies [67]. One of the proposed factors playing a role in this protection is consumption of raw milk. Indeed, a cross-sectional survey in rural areas of Austria, Germany, and Switzerland inversely associated raw milk consumption with asthma, hay fever, and allergic sensitization [68]. This conclusion has been supported by a cross-sectional multi-center study including almost 15,000 children from five European countries [69]. Also, similar results were obtained by others. For example, Wickens and colleagues found a protective effect of unpasteurized milk consumption against atopic eczema/dermatitis syndrome among farm children from New Zealand [70]. Perkin and Strachan found that consumption of unpasteurized milk protected against development of eczema and atopy in rural England [67]. Finally, the GABRIELA study reported an inverse association between raw milk consumption and asthma, atopy, and hay fever in children from rural areas of Austria, Germany, and Switzerland [71]. Taken together, there is strong evidence that consumption of raw milk early in life protects against development of allergies, perhaps even more convincing than the possible protective effect of breastfeeding. On the other hand, it must be emphasized that raw milk may contain certain human pathogens, such as *Salmonella* spp., *Campylobacter* spp., human pathogenic *Escherichia coli*, and *Listeria monocytogenes*. Therefore, its consumption carries risk for serious infectious diseases and milk processing (pasteurization or ultra heat treatments) effectively minimizes this risk. For this reason, raw milk consumption is not a general solution for allergy prevention. Instead, identification of the mechanisms behind its protective action will be essential for designing novel prophylactic and therapeutic strategies for allergic diseases. Similarly as in the case of breast milk, various mechanisms may play a role, including bovine immunoglobulins, cytokines and oligosaccharides [72], fatty acids [73], miRNA [74], antigens [71], milk microbiota [75], and others. Detailed description of these potential mechanisms is beyond the scope of this review and has been covered elsewhere [72,76].

4. Dietary Fiber and the Lung Function

Western diets are often rich in fat and processed foods, but low in fiber [8]. For this reason, a notion that fiber consumption may reduce symptoms of asthma has been hypothesized [77]. This has been based upon studies using mouse models (discussed in the next chapter) as well observational studies linking fiber intake with improved lung function [78–81]. Kan and colleagues were the first to observe a positive association between fiber intake and better lung function in chronic obstructive pulmonary disease (COPD). Statistically significant trends were found for total fiber intake, cereal fiber, and fruit fiber [78]. Similar conclusions were reached by Varasso et al., who found a negative association between total and cereal fiber intake and the risk of newly diagnosed COPD [79]. An inverse association between dietary fiber and impaired lung function was also found in the case of asthma. Berthon and colleagues compared dietary intake patterns between patients suffering from severe persistent asthma and healthy individuals. Interestingly, a positive association was found for fat (total and monounsaturated fatty acids) and sodium intake while an inverse correlation was observed for fiber and potassium intake [80]. Finally, Root et al. surveyed 15,567 American subjects for their dietary habits and correlated calculated macronutrient intake with their lung function. Total calories as well as saturated fatty acids were inversely associated with the pulmonary function [measured by the ratio of forced expiratory volume in 1 second to forced vital capacity (FEV1/FVC)], while for dietary polyunsaturated fatty acids, long-chain omega-3 fatty acids, dietary fiber, and animal protein, a positive correlation was found [81]. Given the above evidence, Halnes and co-workers hypothesized that high-fiber meal challenge may ameliorate symptoms in asthmatic patients. They recruited 29 individuals with stable asthma and divided them in two groups: 17 patients were challenged with a soluble fiber meal and 12 of them with a control meal. Interestingly, patients receiving a soluble fiber meal had decreased levels of several airway inflammation biomarkers 4 hours post-challenge, including exhaled nitric oxide, sputum total cell, neutrophil, lymphocyte, and macrophage counts as well as sputum IL-8 protein concentration. Intriguingly, these changes correlated with increased expression of GPR41 and GPR43 in the sputum of these patients, suggesting the mechanistic basis for these beneficial changes [77]. The possible importance of GRP41 and GPR43 in triggering anti-inflammatory mechanisms downstream of fiber intake will be discussed in detail in the next chapter.

In conclusion, various nutrients have been proposed in the past to influence risk for allergy development and many epidemiological studies have been launched to investigate their impact. Although "diet hypotheses" are still controversial, it seems that certain nutrients may indeed confer protection, especially in the case of consumption of raw milk. However, epidemiological studies regarding many other nutrients are scarce, including intake of dietary fiber, which has dramatically reduced over the last centuries. In the next section, we will discuss the potential role for dietary fiber intake in protection against diseases, including allergy, based on experimental data using mouse models.

5. Dietary Fiber, Short-Chain Fatty Acids, and Susceptibility to Diseases: Lessons Learned from Animal Studies

Anti-inflammatory properties of butyrate, a short-chain fatty acid produced by fermentation of soluble fibers by commensal bacteria in the gut, have long been recognized. Although initially proposed to exert its function through restoration of energy metabolism in colonocytes [82], later research rather supported its immunomodulatory properties, based on experiments in vitro [83–86]. Apart from the butyrate, in vitro anti-inflammatory properties of other short-chain fatty acids, such as propionate and acetate, have also been proposed [87].

An important step towards unraveling the mechanisms behind short-chain fatty acids (SCFA) action came with identification of G-protein-coupled receptors GPR41 and GPR43 as their extracellular receptors [88,89]. The physiological importance of this finding was first highlighted in a study showing that the protective role of acetate in a mouse model of colitis was dependent on GPR43 [90], although this did not appear to be the case in a mouse model of allergic inflammation, where the effects of acetate did not require GPR43 [91]. Similar discrepancy was observed in the case of propionate. While exerting its anti-inflammatory properties via GPR43 in a mouse model ofcolitis [92], in a mouse model of allergic airway inflammation it was GPR41 but not GPR43 that played a major role [93]. The reasons for these differences are not clear. Finally, GPR109a has been reported as a low-affinity receptor for one of the short chain fatty acids, butyrate [94], and the physiological importance of this finding has been demonstrated in a mouse model of colitis [95,96] and food allergy [97].

Regardless of the surface receptor responsible for the initial recognition of short-chain fatty acids, many studies have focused on downstream mechanisms mediating their anti-inflammatory properties. For example, propionate and butyrate were shown to induce differentiation of regulatory T cells in vitro and in vivo and this process coincided with increased histone H3 acetylation inTregs [92], or more specifically, of *Foxp3* regulatory elements [98,99]. Smith and colleagues proposed that propionate acts directly via GPR43 on colonic Tregs to induce these effects [92]. However, Arpaia et al. pointed out that in the case of butyrate, in addition to imprinting epigenetic effects directly on Tregs, it may also endow dendritic cells with superior capacity to drive differentiation of this subset [99]. Similar conclusions were drawn by Singh and colleagues who demonstrated that colonic dendritic cells (DCs) and macrophages from GPR109a-deficient mice were defective in inducing Treg cell differentiation in vitro [95]. Interestingly, in the mouse model of airway allergic inflammation, anti-inflammatory properties of propionate were not linked to Treg cells but rather to DC function, since propionate treatment in vivo did not affect Treg cell numbers but impaired the ability of dendritic cells to drive Th2 responses [93]. Finally, Macia et al. implicated inflammasome activation as a mechanism through which short chain fatty acids confer protection in a dextran sulfate sodium (DSS)-induced mouse model of colitis [96].

The mechanisms behind anti-inflammatory properties of acetate are also controversial. Furusawa et al. [98] and Arpaia et al. [99] suggested that acetate, unlike propionate and butyrate, lacks HDAC inhibitory properties and fails to induce Treg differentiation in vitro and in vivo. In the study by Fukuda et al., the authors suggest that the protective effects of acetate in their model of enteropathogenic infection may rely on its ability to induce anti-apoptotic and anti-inflammatory gene expression in colonic epithelial cells as well as on its capacity to increase transepithelial electrical resistance [100]. However, Thorburn and colleagues reached different conclusions based on their model of allergic airway inflammation. They observed increased acetylation levels of histones at the *Foxp3* promoter, elevated numbers of Treg cells and their enhanced suppressive activity upon feeding mice with acetate in the drinking water. Importantly, they concluded that the protective effect of acetate in their model of allergic inflammation was dependent on this subset of cells, as Treg depletion abrogated its beneficial role [91].

Since short-chain fatty acids are mostly products of bacterial fermentation of nutrients, the question regarding the interplay between SCFA production, diet, and microbiota composition has been raised. In a study from our group, some light onto these complex interactions was shed. Mice fed on a high fiber diet had increased ratio of *Bacteroidetes/Firmicutes* abundance in the gut and lungs and this coincided with increased cecal and serum levels of SCFA [93]. A similar observation was reported in the study by Thorburn and colleagues [91]. Of note, *Bacteroidetes* are known to be efficient at fermenting fiber into SCFAs, supporting a causative relationship between increased SCFA and the increase of *Bacteroidetes*. Nevertheless, since SCFA may also be produced by other phyla, the importance of *Bacteroidetes* increase in these models should be investigated further. Overall, it is important to note that high fiber diet protected mice against allergic airway inflammation, underlining that protective effects of SCFA are not restricted to the gut, but can influence other peripheral tissues [91,93].

The importance of high fiber diet-induced microbiota changes has also been implicated in a mouse model of colitis [96]. The authors linked the protective role of high fiber diet in this model with inflammasome activation. Interestingly, re-colonization of germ-free mice with microbiota from mice fed on a high fiber diet resulted in increased levels of IL-18 secretion and caspase-1 activity in comparison to the control group [96]. Further insights into the diet-microbiota-SCFA axis were gained by Tan and colleagues [97]. First, they noted that high fiber diet, which protected mice against peanut allergy, changed intestinal microbiota composition and increased levels of SCFA. In order to dissect the impact of these two factors, they re-colonized germ-free mice with fecal matter from mice fed on low-fiber or high fiber diets and showed that the latter were protected against peanut allergy despite having similar levels of SCFA. This indicated that the protective effect of fiber feeding in this model was not due to these metabolites. However, SCFA supplementation was also able to confer similar protection. Therefore, the authors propose that two mechanisms play a role upon feeding mice with a high fiber diet. Importantly, the effects of this diet relied on epithelial GPR43 and immune cell GPR109a, since feeding GPR43 or GPR109a-deficient mice with high fiber diet no longer protected mice against peanut allergy [97].

6. Dietary Fats and Susceptibility to Diseases

As previously mentioned, Western diet contains elevated levels of dietary fats [8]. For this reason, it has long been hypothesized that higher fat intake might be implicated in elevated risk for disease occurrence, including allergy. High fat diet-induced obesity could have a significant contribution to this. Indeed, a positive association between obesity and allergy is well documented in epidemiological studies [101–104] as well as in animal models of allergy [105–108]. Description of the current knowledge regarding this issue is beyond the scope of this review. Instead, the reader is referred to several recent reviews in this field [109–112]. However, it could be hypothesized that high fat diet enhances susceptibility to allergy independently of obesity. Increased free fatty acid release itself could be immunomodulatory and influence disease susceptibility. The effects of high fat meals independently of obesity have been shown in asthmatic patients. In the study by Wood et al., non-obese asthmatic patients receiving a high-fat meal had increased levels of TLR4 mRNA and neutrophils in their sputum cells in comparison to subjects receiving a low-fat meal [113]. In an animal model of allergy, although pups born from mothers fed on a high fat diet did not have increased body weight or blood glucose levels, they displayed a more severe anaphylaxis score after oral sensitization to peanut protein [114]. This study underlined transgenerational effects of high fat diet independently of major confounders, such as obesity or diabetes; however, the exact components of a high fat diet which could imprint these changes were not defined. Saturated fatty acids, which are major components of a high fat diet, could be involved, as their pro-inflammatory potential is well established [115]. Polyunsaturated omega-6 fatty acids could also contribute to this, as they have been described to enhance allergic responses in mouse models of asthma [116–118]. Finally, monounsaturated fatty acids are also candidates, as they constitute a major component of high fat diets, although their immunomodulatory potential in the context of allergy remains unexplored.

Overall, high fat diet may influence susceptibility to allergy through obesity or directly through nutritional composition. Regarding the latter, dietary fatty acids contained within the diet have the potential to induce pro-inflammatory responses. Decreased content of dietary fiber in high fat diets may at the same time lead to downregulation of anti-inflammatory pathways, further escalating the imbalance between pro- and anti-inflammatory responses. Further research is needed to establish the potential of dietary components of high fat diets to influence allergic responses and decipher the molecular mechanisms they trigger.

7. Conclusions and Perspectives

Lifestyle changes, which most rapidly occurred in the last century, have been proposed to increase susceptibility to allergies. The hygiene hypothesis suggested the role of decreased contact with environmental microbes and helminths in this phenomenon, while diet hypotheses pointed towards the importance of changes in dietary habits. The microbiota seems to be a common component of these two views, as it is shaped by various external factors, including environmental microorganisms and diet (Figure 1). Given the vast impact the microbiota exerts on immune responses and susceptibility to diseases, it is crucial to integrate both views and understand how environmental cues influence microbiota composition. Unraveling this may lead to clearer distinctions between pathogenic and beneficial species and indicate ways to manipulate them. This holds promise for the development of novel therapeutic approaches targeting the microbiota for prevention and treatment of inflammatory disorders.

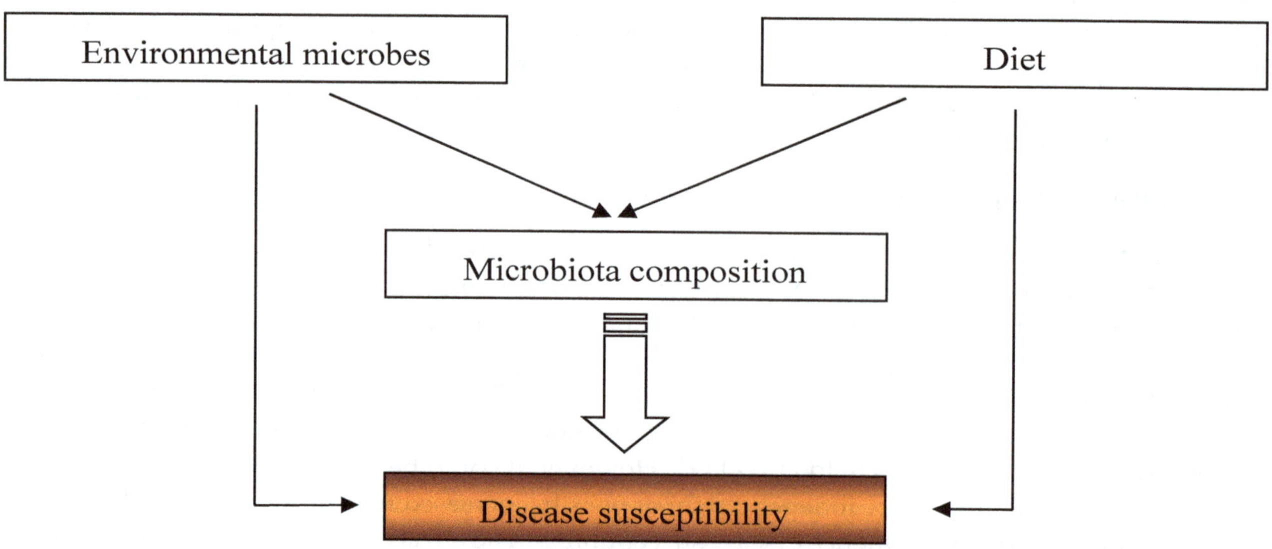

Figure 1. The cross-talk between environmental microorganisms, diet and microbiota composition and its impact of disease susceptibility.

Acknowledgments: This work has been supported by the Swiss National Science Foundation, 310030-166210/1 awarded to B.J.M.

Author Contributions: T.P.W wrote the manuscript, B.J.M edited the manuscript

References

1. Strachan, D.P. Hay fever, hygiene, and household size. *BMJ* **1989**, *299*, 1259–1260. [CrossRef] [PubMed]
2. Rook, G.A.; Martinelli, R.; Brunet, L.R. Innate immune responses to mycobacteria and the downregulation of atopic responses. *Curr. Opin. Allergy Clin. Immunol.* **2003**, *3*, 337–342. [CrossRef] [PubMed]
3. Von Hertzen, L.; Hanski, I.; Haahtela, T. Natural immunity. Biodiversity loss and inflammatory diseases are two global megatrends that might be related. *EMBO Rep.* **2011**, *12*, 1089–1093. [CrossRef] [PubMed]
4. Profet, M. The function of allergy: Immunological defense against toxins. *Q. Rev. Biol.* **1991**, *66*, 23–62. [CrossRef] [PubMed]
5. Devereux, G.; Seaton, A. Diet as a risk factor for atopy and asthma. *J. Allergy Clin. Immunol.* **2005**, *115*, 1109–1117. [CrossRef] [PubMed]
6. Devereux, G. Early life events in asthma—Diet. *Pediatr. Pulmonol.* **2007**, *42*, 663–673. [CrossRef] [PubMed]
7. Kim, J.H.; Ellwood, P.E.; Asher, M.I. Diet and asthma: Looking back, moving forward. *Respir. Res.* **2009**, *10*, 49. [CrossRef] [PubMed]
8. Cordain, L.; Eaton, S.B.; Sebastian, A.; Mann, N.; Lindeberg, S.; Watkins, B.A.; O'Keefe, J.H.; Brand-Miller, J. Origins and evolution of the western diet: Health implications for the 21st century. *Am. J. Clin. Nutr.* **2005**, *81*, 341–354. [PubMed]
9. Cordain, L.; Watkins, B.A.; Florant, G.L.; Kelher, M.; Rogers, L.; Li, Y. Fatty acid analysis of wild ruminant tissues: Evolutionary implications for reducing diet-related chronic disease. *Eur. J. Clin. Nutr.* **2002**, *56*, 181–191. [CrossRef] [PubMed]
10. Rule, D.C.; Broughton, K.S.; Shellito, S.M.; Maiorano, G. Comparison of muscle fatty acid profiles and cholesterol concentrations of bison, beef cattle, elk, and chicken. *J. Anim. Sci.* **2002**, *80*, 1202–1211. [CrossRef] [PubMed]
11. Burney, P. A diet rich in sodium may potentiate asthma. Epidemiologic evidence for a new hypothesis. *Chest* **1987**, *91*, 143S–148S. [CrossRef] [PubMed]
12. Javaid, A.; Cushley, M.J.; Bone, M.F. Effect of dietary salt on bronchial reactivity to histamine in asthma. *BMJ* **1988**, *297*, 454. [CrossRef] [PubMed]
13. Schwartz, J.; Weiss, S.T. Dietary factors and their relation to respiratory symptoms. The second national health and nutrition examination survey. *Am. J. Epidemiol.* **1990**, *132*, 67–76. [CrossRef] [PubMed]
14. Carey, O.J.; Locke, C.; Cookson, J.B. Effect of alterations of dietary sodium on the severity of asthma in men. *Thorax* **1993**, *48*, 714–718. [CrossRef] [PubMed]
15. Pistelli, R.; Forastiere, F.; Corbo, G.M.; Dell'Orco, V.; Brancato, G.; Agabiti, N.; Pizzabiocca, A.; Perucci, C.A. Respiratory symptoms and bronchial responsiveness are related to dietary salt intake and urinary potassium excretion in male children. *Eur. Respir. J.* **1993**, *6*, 517–522. [PubMed]
16. Sparrow, D.; O'Connor, G.T.; Rosner, B.; Weiss, S.T. Methacholine airway responsiveness and 24-hour urine excretion of sodium and potassium. The normative aging study. *Am. Rev. Respir. Dis.* **1991**, *144*, 722–725. [CrossRef] [PubMed]
17. Lieberman, D.; Heimer, D. Effect of dietary sodium on the severity of bronchial asthma. *Thorax* **1992**, *47*, 360–362. [CrossRef] [PubMed]
18. Devereux, G.; Beach, J.R.; Bromly, C.; Avery, A.J.; Ayatollahi, S.M.; Williams, S.M.; Stenton, S.C.; Bourke, S.J.; Hendrick, D.J. Effect of dietary sodium on airways responsiveness and its importance in the epidemiology of asthma: An evaluation in three areas of northern England. *Thorax* **1995**, *50*, 941–947. [CrossRef] [PubMed]
19. Rubin, R.N.; Navon, L.; Cassano, P.A. Relationship of serum antioxidants to asthma prevalence in youth. *Am. J. Respir. Crit. Care Med.* **2004**, *169*, 393–398. [CrossRef] [PubMed]
20. Patel, B.D.; Welch, A.A.; Bingham, S.A.; Luben, R.N.; Day, N.E.; Khaw, K.T.; Lomas, D.A.; Wareham, N.J. Dietary antioxidants and asthma in adults. *Thorax* **2006**, *61*, 388–393. [CrossRef] [PubMed]

21. Picado, C.; Deulofeu, R.; Lleonart, R.; Agusti, M.; Mullol, J.; Quinto, L.; Torra, M. Dietary micronutrients/antioxidants and their relationship with bronchial asthma severity. *Allergy* **2001**, *56*, 43–49. [CrossRef] [PubMed]
22. Gao, J.; Gao, X.; Li, W.; Zhu, Y.; Thompson, P.J. Observational studies on the effect of dietary antioxidants on asthma: A meta-analysis. *Respirology* **2008**, *13*, 528–536. [CrossRef] [PubMed]
23. Kaur, B.; Rowe, B.H.; Ram, F.S. Vitamin C supplementation for asthma. *Cochrane Database Syst. Rev.* **2001**, CD000993.
24. Fogarty, A.; Lewis, S.A.; Scrivener, S.L.; Antoniak, M.; Pacey, S.; Pringle, M.; Britton, J. Oral magnesium and vitamin C supplements in asthma: A parallel group randomized placebo-controlled trial. *Clin. Exp. Allergy* **2003**, *33*, 1355–1359. [CrossRef] [PubMed]
25. Troisi, R.J.; Willett, W.C.; Weiss, S.T.; Trichopoulos, D.; Rosner, B.; Speizer, F.E. A prospective study of diet and adult-onset asthma. *Am. J. Respir. Crit. Care Med.* **1995**, *151*, 1401–1408. [CrossRef] [PubMed]
26. Bodner, C.; Godden, D.; Brown, K.; Little, J.; Ross, S.; Seaton, A. Antioxidant intake and adult-onset wheeze: A case-control study. *Eur. Respir. J.* **1999**, *13*, 22–30. [CrossRef] [PubMed]
27. Chang, C.C.; Phinney, S.D.; Halpern, G.M.; Gershwin, M.E. Asthma mortality: Another opinion—Is it a matter of life and bread? *J. Asthma* **1993**, *30*, 93–103. [CrossRef] [PubMed]
28. Hodge, L.; Peat, J.K.; Salome, C. Increased consumption of polyunsaturated oils may be a cause of increased prevalence of childhood asthma. *Aust. N. Z. J. Med.* **1994**, *24*, 727. [CrossRef] [PubMed]
29. Black, P.N.; Sharpe, S. Dietary fat and asthma: Is there a connection? *Eur. Respir. J.* **1997**, *10*, 6–12. [CrossRef] [PubMed]
30. Dunder, T.; Kuikka, L.; Turtinen, J.; Rasanen, L.; Uhari, M. Diet, serum fatty acids, and atopic diseases in childhood. *Allergy* **2001**, *56*, 425–428. [CrossRef] [PubMed]
31. Bolte, G.; Frye, C.; Hoelscher, B.; Meyer, I.; Wjst, M.; Heinrich, J. Margarine consumption and allergy in children. *Am. J. Respir. Crit. Care Med.* **2001**, *163*, 277–279. [CrossRef] [PubMed]
32. Trak-Fellermeier, M.A.; Brasche, S.; Winkler, G.; Koletzko, B.; Heinrich, J. Food and fatty acid intake and atopic disease in adults. *Eur. Respir. J.* **2004**, *23*, 575–582. [CrossRef] [PubMed]
33. Haby, M.M.; Peat, J.K.; Marks, G.B.; Woolcock, A.J.; Leeder, S.R. Asthma in preschool children: Prevalence and risk factors. *Thorax* **2001**, *56*, 589–595. [CrossRef] [PubMed]
34. Fluge, O.; Omenaas, E.; Eide, G.E.; Gulsvik, A. Fish consumption and respiratory symptoms among young adults in a Norwegian community. *Eur. Respir. J.* **1998**, *12*, 336–340. [CrossRef] [PubMed]
35. Bolte, G.; Kompauer, I.; Fobker, M.; Cullen, P.; Keil, U.; Mutius, E.; Weiland, S.K. Fatty acids in serum cholesteryl esters in relation to asthma and lung function in children. *Clin. Exp. Allergy* **2006**, *36*, 293–302. [CrossRef] [PubMed]
36. Almqvist, C.; Garden, F.; Xuan, W.; Mihrshahi, S.; Leeder, S.R.; Oddy, W.; Webb, K.; Marks, G.B.; Team, C. Omega-3 and omega-6 fatty acid exposure from early life does not affect atopy and asthma at age 5 years. *J. Allergy Clin. Immunol.* **2007**, *119*, 1438–1444. [CrossRef] [PubMed]
37. Takemura, Y.; Sakurai, Y.; Honjo, S.; Tokimatsu, A.; Gibo, M.; Hara, T.; Kusakari, A.; Kugai, N. The relationship between fish intake and the prevalence of asthma: The Tokorozawa childhood asthma and pollinosis study. *Prev. Med.* **2002**, *34*, 221–225. [CrossRef] [PubMed]
38. Broadfield, E.C.; McKeever, T.M.; Whitehurst, A.; Lewis, S.A.; Lawson, N.; Britton, J.; Fogarty, A. A case-control study of dietary and erythrocyte membrane fatty acids in asthma. *Clin. Exp. Allergy* **2004**, *34*, 1232–1236. [CrossRef] [PubMed]
39. Grulee, C.G.; Sanford, H.N. The influence of breast and artificial feeding on infantile eczema. *J. Pediatr.* **1936**, *9*, 223–225. [CrossRef]
40. Saarinen, U.M.; Kajosaari, M.; Backman, A.; Siimes, M.A. Prolonged breast-feeding as prophylaxis for atopic disease. *Lancet* **1979**, *2*, 163–166. [CrossRef]
41. Hide, D.W.; Guyer, B.M. Clinical manifestations of allergy related to breast and cows' milk feeding. *Arch. Dis. Child.* **1981**, *56*, 172–175. [CrossRef] [PubMed]
42. Wright, A.L.; Holberg, C.J.; Martinez, F.D.; Morgan, W.J.; Taussig, L.M. Breast feeding and lower respiratory tract illness in the first year of life. Group health medical associates. *BMJ* **1989**, *299*, 946–949. [CrossRef] [PubMed]
43. Dell, S.; To, T. Breastfeeding and asthma in young children: Findings from a population-based study. *Arch. Pediatr. Adolesc. Med.* **2001**, *155*, 1261–1265. [CrossRef] [PubMed]

44. Kull, I.; Wickman, M.; Lilja, G.; Nordvall, S.L.; Pershagen, G. Breast feeding and allergic diseases in infants-a prospective birth cohort study. *Arch. Dis. Child.* **2002**, *87*, 478–481. [CrossRef] [PubMed]
45. Saarinen, U.M.; Kajosaari, M. Breastfeeding as prophylaxis against atopic disease: Prospective follow-up study until 17 years old. *Lancet* **1995**, *346*, 1065–1069. [CrossRef]
46. Tariq, S.M.; Matthews, S.M.; Hakim, E.A.; Stevens, M.; Arshad, S.H.; Hide, D.W. The prevalence of and risk factors for atopy in early childhood: A whole population birth cohort study. *J. Allergy Clin. Immunol.* **1998**, *101*, 587–593. [CrossRef]
47. Oddy, W.H.; Holt, P.G.; Sly, P.D.; Read, A.W.; Landau, L.I.; Stanley, F.J.; Kendall, G.E.; Burton, P.R. Association between breast feeding and asthma in 6 year old children: Findings of a prospective birth cohort study. *BMJ* **1999**, *319*, 815–819. [CrossRef] [PubMed]
48. Scholtens, S.; Wijga, A.H.; Brunekreef, B.; Kerkhof, M.; Hoekstra, M.O.; Gerritsen, J.; Aalberse, R.; de Jongste, J.C.; Smit, H.A. Breast feeding, parental allergy and asthma in children followed for 8 years. The piama birth cohort study. *Thorax* **2009**, *64*, 604–609. [CrossRef] [PubMed]
49. Hide, D.W.; Guyer, B.M. Clinical manifestations of allergy related to breast- and cow's milk-feeding. *Pediatrics* **1985**, *76*, 973–975. [PubMed]
50. Wright, A.L.; Holberg, C.J.; Taussig, L.M.; Martinez, F.D. Factors influencing the relation of infant feeding to asthma and recurrent wheeze in childhood. *Thorax* **2001**, *56*, 192–197. [CrossRef] [PubMed]
51. Takemura, Y.; Sakurai, Y.; Honjo, S.; Kusakari, A.; Hara, T.; Gibo, M.; Tokimatsu, A.; Kugai, N. Relation between breastfeeding and the prevalence of asthma : The tokorozawa childhood asthma and pollinosis study. *Am. J. Epidemiol.* **2001**, *154*, 115–119. [CrossRef] [PubMed]
52. Sears, M.R.; Greene, J.M.; Willan, A.R.; Taylor, D.R.; Flannery, E.M.; Cowan, J.O.; Herbison, G.P.; Poulton, R. Long-term relation between breastfeeding and development of atopy and asthma in children and young adults: A longitudinal study. *Lancet* **2002**, *360*, 901–907. [CrossRef]
53. Burgess, S.W.; Dakin, C.J.; O'Callaghan, M.J. Breastfeeding does not increase the risk of asthma at 14 years. *Pediatrics* **2006**, *117*, e787–e792. [CrossRef] [PubMed]
54. Gdalevich, M.; Mimouni, D.; Mimouni, M. Breast-feeding and the risk of bronchial asthma in childhood: A systematic review with meta-analysis of prospective studies. *J. Pediatr.* **2001**, *139*, 261–266. [CrossRef] [PubMed]
55. Gdalevich, M.; Mimouni, D.; David, M.; Mimouni, M. Breast-feeding and the onset of atopic dermatitis in childhood: A systematic review and meta-analysis of prospective studies. *J. Am. Acad. Dermatol.* **2001**, *45*, 520–527. [CrossRef] [PubMed]
56. Mimouni Bloch, A.; Mimouni, D.; Mimouni, M.; Gdalevich, M. Does breastfeeding protect against allergic rhinitis during childhood? A meta-analysis of prospective studies. *Acta Paediatr.* **2002**, *91*, 275–279. [CrossRef] [PubMed]
57. Dogaru, C.M.; Nyffenegger, D.; Pescatore, A.M.; Spycher, B.D.; Kuehni, C.E. Breastfeeding and childhood asthma: Systematic review and meta-analysis. *Am. J. Epidemiol.* **2014**, *179*, 1153–1167. [CrossRef] [PubMed]
58. Peat, J.K.; Allen, J.; Oddy, W.; Webb, K. Breastfeeding and asthma: Appraising the controversy. *Pediatr. Pulmonol.* **2003**, *35*, 331–334. [CrossRef] [PubMed]
59. Oddy, W.H.; Peat, J.K. Breastfeeding, asthma, and atopic disease: An epidemiological review of the literature. *J. Hum. Lact.* **2003**, *19*, 250–261. [CrossRef] [PubMed]
60. Rogier, E.W.; Frantz, A.L.; Bruno, M.E.; Wedlund, L.; Cohen, D.A.; Stromberg, A.J.; Kaetzel, C.S. Secretory antibodies in breast milk promote long-term intestinal homeostasis by regulating the gut microbiota and host gene expression. *Proc. Natl. Acad. Sci. USA* **2014**, *111*, 3074–3079. [CrossRef] [PubMed]
61. Chichlowski, M.; German, J.B.; Lebrilla, C.B.; Mills, D.A. The influence of milk oligosaccharides on microbiota of infants: Opportunities for formulas. *Annu. Rev. Food Sci. Technol.* **2011**, *2*, 331–351. [CrossRef] [PubMed]
62. Fernandez, L.; Langa, S.; Martin, V.; Maldonado, A.; Jimenez, E.; Martin, R.; Rodriguez, J.M. The human milk microbiota: Origin and potential roles in health and disease. *Pharmacol. Res.* **2013**, *69*, 1–10. [CrossRef] [PubMed]
63. Kaetzel, C.S. Cooperativity among secretory IgA, the polymeric immunoglobulin receptor, and the gut microbiota promotes host-microbial mutualism. *Immunol. Lett.* **2014**, *162*, 10–21. [CrossRef] [PubMed]
64. Rogier, E.W.; Frantz, A.L.; Bruno, M.E.; Wedlund, L.; Cohen, D.A.; Stromberg, A.J.; Kaetzel, C.S. Lessons from mother: Long-term impact of antibodies in breast milk on the gut microbiota and intestinal immune system of breastfed offspring. *Gut Microbes* **2014**, *5*, 663–668. [CrossRef] [PubMed]

65. Julia, V.; Macia, L.; Dombrowicz, D. The impact of diet on asthma and allergic diseases. *Nat. Rev. Immunol.* **2015**, *15*, 308–322. [CrossRef] [PubMed]
66. Walker, W.A.; Iyengar, R.S. Breast milk, microbiota, and intestinal immune homeostasis. *Pediatr. Res.* **2015**, *77*, 220–228. [PubMed]
67. Perkin, M.R.; Strachan, D.P. Which aspects of the farming lifestyle explain the inverse association with childhood allergy? *J. Allergy Clin. Immunol.* **2006**, *117*, 1374–1381. [CrossRef] [PubMed]
68. Riedler, J.; Braun-Fahrlander, C.; Eder, W.; Schreuer, M.; Waser, M.; Maisch, S.; Carr, D.; Schierl, R.; Nowak, D.; von Mutius, E.; et al. Exposure to farming in early life and development of asthma and allergy: A cross-sectional survey. *Lancet* **2001**, *358*, 1129–1133. [CrossRef]
69. Waser, M.; Michels, K.B.; Bieli, C.; Floistrup, H.; Pershagen, G.; von Mutius, E.; Ege, M.; Riedler, J.; Schram-Bijkerk, D.; Brunekreef, B.; et al. Inverse association of farm milk consumption with asthma and allergy in rural and suburban populations across Europe. *Clin. Exp. Allergy* **2007**, *37*, 661–670. [CrossRef] [PubMed]
70. Wickens, K.; Lane, J.M.; Fitzharris, P.; Siebers, R.; Riley, G.; Douwes, J.; Smith, T.; Crane, J. Farm residence and exposures and the risk of allergic diseases in New Zealand children. *Allergy* **2002**, *57*, 1171–1179. [CrossRef] [PubMed]
71. Loss, G.; Apprich, S.; Waser, M.; Kneifel, W.; Genuneit, J.; Buchele, G.; Weber, J.; Sozanska, B.; Danielewicz, H.; Horak, E.; et al. The protective effect of farm milk consumption on childhood asthma and atopy: The Gabriela study. *J. Allergy Clin. Immunol.* **2011**, *128*, 766–773. [CrossRef] [PubMed]
72. Van Neerven, R.J.; Knol, E.F.; Heck, J.M.; Savelkoul, H.F. Which factors in raw cow's milk contribute to protection against allergies? *J. Allergy Clin. Immunol.* **2012**, *130*, 853–858. [CrossRef] [PubMed]
73. Brick, T.; Schober, Y.; Bocking, C.; Pekkanen, J.; Genuneit, J.; Loss, G.; Dalphin, J.C.; Riedler, J.; Lauener, R.; Nockher, W.A.; et al. Omega-3 fatty acids contribute to the asthma-protective effect of unprocessed cow's milk. *J. Allergy Clin. Immunol.* **2016**, *137*, 1699–1706. [CrossRef] [PubMed]
74. Kirchner, B.; Pfaffl, M.W.; Dumpler, J.; von Mutius, E.; Ege, M.J. MicroRNA in native and processed cow's milk and its implication for the farm milk effect on asthma. *J. Allergy Clin. Immunol.* **2016**, *137*, 1893–1895. [CrossRef] [PubMed]
75. Quigley, L.; O'Sullivan, O.; Stanton, C.; Beresford, T.P.; Ross, R.P.; Fitzgerald, G.F.; Cotter, P.D. The complex microbiota of raw milk. *FEMS Microbiol. Rev.* **2013**, *37*, 664–698. [CrossRef] [PubMed]
76. Braun-Fahrlander, C.; von Mutius, E. Can farm milk consumption prevent allergic diseases? *Clin. Exp. Allergy* **2011**, *41*, 29–35. [CrossRef] [PubMed]
77. Halnes, I.; Baines, K.J.; Berthon, B.S.; MacDonald-Wicks, L.K.; Gibson, P.G.; Wood, L.G. Soluble fibre meal challenge reduces airway inflammation and expression of *gpr43* and *gpr41* in asthma. *Nutrients* **2017**, *9*, 57. [CrossRef] [PubMed]
78. Kan, H.; Stevens, J.; Heiss, G.; Rose, K.M.; London, S.J. Dietary fiber, lung function, and chronic obstructive pulmonary disease in the atherosclerosis risk in communities study. *Am. J. Epidemiol.* **2008**, *167*, 570–578. [CrossRef] [PubMed]
79. Varraso, R.; Willett, W.C.; Camargo, C.A., Jr. Prospective study of dietary fiber and risk of chronic obstructive pulmonary disease among US women and men. *Am. J. Epidemiol.* **2010**, *171*, 776–784. [CrossRef] [PubMed]
80. Berthon, B.S.; Macdonald-Wicks, L.K.; Gibson, P.G.; Wood, L.G. Investigation of the association between dietary intake, disease severity and airway inflammation in asthma. *Respirology* **2013**, *18*, 447–454. [CrossRef] [PubMed]
81. Root, M.M.; Houser, S.M.; Anderson, J.J.; Dawson, H.R. Healthy eating index 2005 and selected macronutrients are correlated with improved lung function in humans. *Nutr. Res.* **2014**, *34*, 277–284. [CrossRef] [PubMed]
82. Roediger, W.E. The colonic epithelium in ulcerative colitis: An energy-deficiency disease? *Lancet* **1980**, *2*, 712–715. [CrossRef]
83. Gilbert, K.M.; Weigle, W.O. Th1 cell anergy and blockade in G1a phase of the cell cycle. *J. Immunol.* **1993**, *151*, 1245–1254. [PubMed]
84. Siavoshian, S.; Blottiere, H.M.; Bentouimou, N.; Cherbut, C.; Galmiche, J.P. Butyrate enhances major histocompatibility complex class I, HLA-DR and ICAM-1 antigen expression on differentiated human intestinal epithelial cells. *Eur. J. Clin. Investig.* **1996**, *26*, 803–810. [CrossRef] [PubMed]

85. Bohmig, G.A.; Krieger, P.M.; Saemann, M.D.; Wenhardt, C.; Pohanka, E.; Zlabinger, G.J. N-butyrate downregulates the stimulatory function of peripheral blood-derived antigen-presenting cells: A potential mechanism for modulating T-cell responses by short-chain fatty acids. *Immunology* **1997**, *92*, 234–243. [CrossRef] [PubMed]
86. Segain, J.P.; Raingeard de la Bletiere, D.; Bourreille, A.; Leray, V.; Gervois, N.; Rosales, C.; Ferrier, L.; Bonnet, C.; Blottiere, H.M.; Galmiche, J.P. Butyrate inhibits inflammatory responses through NF_kB inhibition: Implications for Crohn's disease. *Gut* **2000**, *47*, 397–403. [CrossRef] [PubMed]
87. Tedelind, S.; Westberg, F.; Kjerrulf, M.; Vidal, A. Anti-inflammatory properties of the short-chain fatty acids acetate and propionate: A study with relevance to inflammatory bowel disease. *World J. Gastroenterol.* **2007**, *13*, 2826–2832. [PubMed]
88. Brown, A.J.; Goldsworthy, S.M.; Barnes, A.A.; Eilert, M.M.; Tcheang, L.; Daniels, D.; Muir, A.I.; Wigglesworth, M.J.; Kinghorn, I.; Fraser, N.J.; et al. The Orphan G protein-coupled receptors GPR41 and GPR43 are activated by propionate and other short chain carboxylic acids. *J. Biol. Chem.* **2003**, *278*, 11312–11319. [CrossRef] [PubMed]
89. Le Poul, E.; Loison, C.; Struyf, S.; Springael, J.Y.; Lannoy, V.; Decobecq, M.E.; Brezillon, S.; Dupriez, V.; Vassart, G.; Van Damme, J.; et al. Functional characterization of human receptors for short chain fatty acids and their role in polymorphonuclear cell activation. *J. Biol. Chem.* **2003**, *278*, 25481–25489. [CrossRef] [PubMed]
90. Maslowski, K.M.; Vieira, A.T.; Ng, A.; Kranich, J.; Sierro, F.; Yu, D.; Schilter, H.C.; Rolph, M.S.; Mackay, F.; Artis, D.; et al. Regulation of inflammatory responses by gut microbiota and chemoattractant receptor GPR43. *Nature* **2009**, *461*, 1282–1286. [CrossRef] [PubMed]
91. Thorburn, A.N.; McKenzie, C.I.; Shen, S.; Stanley, D.; Macia, L.; Mason, L.J.; Roberts, L.K.; Wong, C.H.; Shim, R.; Robert, R.; et al. Evidence that asthma is a developmental origin disease influenced by maternal diet and bacterial metabolites. *Nat. Commun.* **2015**, *6*, 7320. [CrossRef] [PubMed]
92. Smith, P.M.; Howitt, M.R.; Panikov, N.; Michaud, M.; Gallini, C.A.; Bohlooly, Y.M.; Glickman, J.N.; Garrett, W.S. The microbial metabolites, short-chain fatty acids, regulate colonic Treg cell homeostasis. *Science* **2013**, *341*, 569–573. [CrossRef] [PubMed]
93. Trompette, A.; Gollwitzer, E.S.; Yadava, K.; Sichelstiel, A.K.; Sprenger, N.; Ngom-Bru, C.; Blanchard, C.; Junt, T.; Nicod, L.P.; Harris, N.L.; et al. Gut microbiota metabolism of dietary fiber influences allergic airway disease and hematopoiesis. *Nat. Med.* **2014**, *20*, 159–166. [CrossRef] [PubMed]
94. Thangaraju, M.; Cresci, G.A.; Liu, K.; Ananth, S.; Gnanaprakasam, J.P.; Browning, D.D.; Mellinger, J.D.; Smith, S.B.; Digby, G.J.; Lambert, N.A.; et al. Gpr109a is a G-protein-coupled receptor for the bacterial fermentation product butyrate and functions as a tumor suppressor in colon. *Cancer Res.* **2009**, *69*, 2826–2832. [CrossRef] [PubMed]
95. Singh, N.; Gurav, A.; Sivaprakasam, S.; Brady, E.; Padia, R.; Shi, H.; Thangaraju, M.; Prasad, P.D.; Manicassamy, S.; Munn, D.H.; et al. Activation of GPR109a, receptor for niacin and the commensal metabolite butyrate, suppresses colonic inflammation and carcinogenesis. *Immunity* **2014**, *40*, 128–139. [CrossRef] [PubMed]
96. Macia, L.; Tan, J.; Vieira, A.T.; Leach, K.; Stanley, D.; Luong, S.; Maruya, M.; Ian McKenzie, C.; Hijikata, A.; Wong, C.; et al. Metabolite-sensing receptors *gpr43* and *gpr109a* facilitate dietary fibre-induced gut homeostasis through regulation of the inflammasome. *Nat. Commun.* **2015**, *6*, 6734. [CrossRef] [PubMed]
97. Tan, J.; McKenzie, C.; Vuillermin, P.J.; Goverse, G.; Vinuesa, C.G.; Mebius, R.E.; Macia, L.; Mackay, C.R. Dietary fiber and bacterial SCFA enhance oral tolerance and protect against food allergy through diverse cellular pathways. *Cell. Rep.* **2016**, *15*, 2809–2824. [CrossRef] [PubMed]
98. Furusawa, Y.; Obata, Y.; Fukuda, S.; Endo, T.A.; Nakato, G.; Takahashi, D.; Nakanishi, Y.; Uetake, C.; Kato, K.; Kato, T.; et al. Commensal microbe-derived butyrate induces the differentiation of colonic regulatory T cells. *Nature* **2013**, *504*, 446–450. [CrossRef] [PubMed]
99. Arpaia, N.; Campbell, C.; Fan, X.; Dikiy, S.; van der Veeken, J.; deRoos, P.; Liu, H.; Cross, J.R.; Pfeffer, K.; Coffer, P.J.; et al. Metabolites produced by commensal bacteria promote peripheral regulatory T-cell generation. *Nature* **2013**, *504*, 451–455. [CrossRef] [PubMed]
100. Fukuda, S.; Toh, H.; Hase, K.; Oshima, K.; Nakanishi, Y.; Yoshimura, K.; Tobe, T.; Clarke, J.M.; Topping, D.L.; Suzuki, T.; et al. Bifidobacteria can protect from enteropathogenic infection through production of acetate. *Nature* **2011**, *469*, 543–547. [CrossRef] [PubMed]

101. Von Mutius, E.; Schwartz, J.; Neas, L.M.; Dockery, D.; Weiss, S.T. Relation of body mass index to asthma and atopy in children: The national health and nutrition examination study III. *Thorax* **2001**, *56*, 835–838. [CrossRef] [PubMed]
102. Gilliland, F.D.; Berhane, K.; Islam, T.; McConnell, R.; Gauderman, W.J.; Gilliland, S.S.; Avol, E.; Peters, J.M. Obesity and the risk of newly diagnosed asthma in school-age children. *Am. J. Epidemiol.* **2003**, *158*, 406–415. [CrossRef] [PubMed]
103. Flaherman, V.; Rutherford, G.W. A meta-analysis of the effect of high weight on asthma. *Arch. Dis. Child.* **2006**, *91*, 334–339. [CrossRef] [PubMed]
104. Visness, C.M.; London, S.J.; Daniels, J.L.; Kaufman, J.S.; Yeatts, K.B.; Siega-Riz, A.M.; Calatroni, A.; Zeldin, D.C. Association of childhood obesity with atopic and nonatopic asthma: Results from the national health and nutrition examination survey 1999–2006. *J. Asthma* **2010**, *47*, 822–829. [CrossRef] [PubMed]
105. Johnston, R.A.; Zhu, M.; Rivera-Sanchez, Y.M.; Lu, F.L.; Theman, T.A.; Flynt, L.; Shore, S.A. Allergic airway responses in obese mice. *Am. J. Respir. Crit. Care Med.* **2007**, *176*, 650–658. [CrossRef] [PubMed]
106. Calixto, M.C.; Lintomen, L.; Schenka, A.; Saad, M.J.; Zanesco, A.; Antunes, E. Obesity enhances eosinophilic inflammation in a murine model of allergic asthma. *Br. J. Pharmacol.* **2010**, *159*, 617–625. [CrossRef] [PubMed]
107. Dietze, J.; Bocking, C.; Heverhagen, J.T.; Voelker, M.N.; Renz, H. Obesity lowers the threshold of allergic sensitization and augments airway eosinophilia in a mouse model of asthma. *Allergy* **2012**, *67*, 1519–1529. [CrossRef] [PubMed]
108. Kim, H.Y.; Lee, H.J.; Chang, Y.J.; Pichavant, M.; Shore, S.A.; Fitzgerald, K.A.; Iwakura, Y.; Israel, E.; Bolger, K.; Faul, J.; et al. Interleukin-17-producing innate lymphoid cells and the NLRP3 inflammasome facilitate obesity-associated airway hyperreactivity. *Nat. Med.* **2014**, *20*, 54–61. [CrossRef] [PubMed]
109. Sideleva, O.; Dixon, A.E. The many faces of asthma in obesity. *J. Cell. Biochem.* **2014**, *115*, 421–426. [CrossRef] [PubMed]
110. Baffi, C.W.; Winnica, D.E.; Holguin, F. Asthma and obesity: Mechanisms and clinical implications. *Asthma Res. Pract.* **2015**, *1*, 1. [CrossRef] [PubMed]
111. Leiria, L.O.; Martins, M.A.; Saad, M.J. Obesity and asthma: Beyond TH2 inflammation. *Metabolism* **2015**, *64*, 172–181. [CrossRef] [PubMed]
112. Cho, Y.; Shore, S.A. Obesity, asthma, and the microbiome. *Physiology* **2016**, *31*, 108–116. [CrossRef] [PubMed]
113. Wood, L.G.; Garg, M.L.; Gibson, P.G. A high-fat challenge increases airway inflammation and impairs bronchodilator recovery in asthma. *J. Allergy Clin. Immunol.* **2011**, *127*, 1133–1140. [CrossRef] [PubMed]
114. Myles, I.A.; Fontecilla, N.M.; Janelsins, B.M.; Vithayathil, P.J.; Segre, J.A.; Datta, S.K. Parental dietary fat intake alters offspring microbiome and immunity. *J. Immunol.* **2013**, *191*, 3200–3209. [CrossRef] [PubMed]
115. Fritsche, K.L. The science of fatty acids and inflammation. *Adv. Nutr.* **2015**, *6*, 293S–301S. [CrossRef] [PubMed]
116. Bilal, S.; Haworth, O.; Wu, L.; Weylandt, K.H.; Levy, B.D.; Kang, J.X. *Fat-1* transgenic mice with elevated omega-3 fatty acids are protected from allergic airway responses. *Biochim. Biophys. Acta* **2011**, *1812*, 1164–1169. [CrossRef] [PubMed]
117. Yokoyama, A.; Hamazaki, T.; Ohshita, A.; Kohno, N.; Sakai, K.; Zhao, G.D.; Katayama, H.; Hiwada, K. Effect of aerosolized docosahexaenoic acid in a mouse model of atopic asthma. *Int. Arch. Allergy Immunol.* **2000**, *123*, 327–332. [CrossRef] [PubMed]
118. Morin, C.; Fortin, S.; Cantin, A.M.; Rousseau, E. Docosahexaenoic acid derivative prevents inflammation and hyperreactivity in lung: Implication of PKC-potentiated inhibitory protein for heterotrimeric myosin light chain phosphatase of 17 Kd in asthma. *Am. J. Respir. Cell. Mol. Biol.* **2011**, *45*, 366–375. [CrossRef] [PubMed]

7

Effect of Processing Intensity on Immunologically Active Bovine Milk Serum Proteins

Tabea Brick [1], Markus Ege [1,2,*], Sjef Boeren [3], Andreas Böck [1], Erika von Mutius [1,2,4], Jacques Vervoort [3] and Kasper Hettinga [5]

1 Dr. von Hauner Children's Hospital, Ludwig Maximilians University Munich, Lindwurm Str. 4, 80337 Munich, Germany; tabea.brick@med.uni-muenchen.de (T.B.); A.Boeck@med.uni-muenchen.de (A.B.); Erika.Von.Mutius@med.uni-muenchen.de (E.v.M.)
2 Comprehensive Pneumology Centre Munich (CPC-M), Member of the German Center of Lung Reseach (DZL), 80337 Munich, Germany
3 Laboratory of Biochemistry, Wageningen University, 6708 WE Wageningen, The Netherlands; sjef.boeren@wur.nl (S.B.); jacques.vervoort@wur.nl (J.V.)
4 Helmholtz Zentrum München—German Research Center for Environmental Health, Institute for Asthma and Allergy Prevention, Ingolstädter Landstr. 1, 85764 Neuherberg, Germany
5 Dairy Science and Technology, Food Quality and Design Group, Wageningen University, 6708 PB Wageningen, The Netherlands; kasper.hettinga@wur.nl
* Correspondence: Markus.Ege@med.uni-muenchen.de

Abstract: Consumption of raw cow's milk instead of industrially processed milk has been reported to protect children from developing asthma, allergies, and respiratory infections. Several heat-sensitive milk serum proteins have been implied in this effect though unbiased assessment of milk proteins in general is missing. The aim of this study was to compare the native milk serum proteome between raw cow's milk and various industrially applied processing methods, i.e., homogenization, fat separation, pasteurization, ultra-heat treatment (UHT), treatment for extended shelf-life (ESL), and conventional boiling. Each processing method was applied to the same three pools of raw milk. Levels of detectable proteins were quantified by liquid chromatography/tandem mass spectrometry following filter aided sample preparation. In total, 364 milk serum proteins were identified. The 140 proteins detectable in 66% of all samples were entered in a hierarchical cluster analysis. The resulting proteomics pattern separated mainly as high (boiling, UHT, ESL) versus no/low heat treatment (raw, skimmed, pasteurized). Comparing these two groups revealed 23 individual proteins significantly reduced by heating, e.g., lactoferrin (log2-fold change = −0.37, p = 0.004), lactoperoxidase (log2-fold change = −0.33, p = 0.001), and lactadherin (log2-fold change = −0.22, p = 0.020). The abundance of these heat sensitive proteins found in higher quantity in native cow's milk compared to heat treated milk, renders them potential candidates for protection from asthma, allergies, and respiratory infections.

Keywords: proteomics; heat stability; milk serum proteins; immune-active proteins

---

1. Introduction

Consuming raw milk has been associated with a reduction in risk of childhood asthma and atopy [1,2] as well as respiratory infections [3]. However, consumption of raw milk poses significant risks, due to potential presence of pathogens in raw milk [3]. As an alternative to raw milk, specific milk ingredients for supplementing heat treated milk have become the focus of recent research, and a wide range of components have been hypothesized to be related to the allergy and asthma protective potential of raw milk versus commercially available milk [4].

After industrial processing, cow's milk considerably differs from raw milk in several aspects, with fat content and heat-treatment being the most obvious. Although the effects of fat content and heat treatment on reduction of asthma partially overlap, both factors exert strong independent effects [2]. The effect of fat content was mainly attributed to the levels of ω-3 polyunsaturated fatty acids [2]. Similarly, heat treatment reduced the levels of milk serum proteins such as β-lactoglobulin and α-lactalbumin, which in turn were found to be inversely related to asthma risk in children of the GABRIELA study with statistical significance [1].

Although it remains open whether these proteins actually reduce the asthma risk themselves, these findings suggest an allergy preventive potential by heat-sensitive proteins in general. Generally whey proteins are susceptible to heat treatment [5,6], particularly immunoactive proteins such as lactoferrin or lactadherin [7]. Heating of heat-labile proteins results in denaturation and aggregation processes [8] and thereby leads to a loss of biological functionality (e.g., lactoferrin [9]). Denatured and aggregated proteins can be extracted from the milk with a combination of pH reduction and ultracentrifugation [10], after which remaining levels of non-aggregated milk serum proteins can be determined [7]. Besides denaturation and aggregation, heating may also lead to chemical modifications, especially the Maillard reaction [11]. During industrial milk processing, relatively short heating times are applied, thus we expect relatively low levels of such chemical modifications, although especially for UHT processing a certain level of chemical modifications has previously been observed [12]. The aim of this study was to assess the native protein profile of bovine milk serum after different industrially applied processing steps with varying heating intensity for the identification of potential asthma- and allergy-protective candidate proteins.

2. Materials and Methods

2.1. Milk Samples

The milk samples used for this analysis were derived from three different farms located in Southern Germany. The origins and characteristics of these three milk batches are shown in Table 1. Each milk batch was processed on three consecutive days in a pilot plant. From milk collection to the last processing step, milk samples were stored at 1 °C. After processing, the milk samples were stored at −20 °C until proteomics analysis. The milk types resulting from the various processing procedures are listed in Table 2. Industrial milk processing was not done with technical replicates because these procedures are laborious, expensive, and time-consuming and there were biological replicates represented by the three milk batches from the respective farms. In total, eight milk samples from each of the three milk batches were assessed for proteomics. The same 24 milk samples were previously used to assess the effect of different processing methods on microRNA (miRNA) levels [13].

The subsequent proteomics analyses of the 24 samples including sample preparation and mass spectrometry were performed without technical replicates since technical reproducibility proved to be high in previous experiments [14] and most of the variation was expected to come from the three separate batches of milk.

Table 1. Sources of raw milk.

Sample Origin	Farms (in Bavaria)		
	Traunstein	**Freising**	**Starnberg**
No. of cows	13	60	30
Time point of milking for pooled samples	Morning and evening	Morning and evening	Morning and evening
No. of detectable milk serum proteins in raw milk samples	143	153	158

Table 2. Processing details of the milk samples.

Code	Milk Fraction	Processing Conditions	Day of Processing *	Grouping of Milk Types **
RAW	Native raw milk	-	Wednesday	No-low heat
PAS	Pasteurized	72 °C for 20 s Total processing time *** 60 s	Wednesday	No-low heat
SKI	Skim milk	Separation at 50 °C	Tuesday	No-low heat
FAT	Fat fraction/cream	Separation at 50 °C	Tuesday	-
HOM	Homogenized milk	Preheating to 55 °C, 2-stage homogenization at 250/50 bar	Tuesday	-
ESL	Extended shelf life milk	Preheating at 95 °C for 20 s, direct steam injection at 127 °C for 5 s Total processing time *** 60 s	Monday	High heat
UHT	Ultra-high heat treated	Preheating at 93 °C for 23 s, direct steam injection at 142 °C for 5 s Total processing time *** 85 s	Monday	High heat
BOI	Boiled milk	Preheating at >80 °C for >300 s, boiling at 100 °C for 30 s Total processing time *** 2000 s	Tuesday	High heat

* Milk samples were collected on a Monday and stored at 1 °C until they were processed. Processing occurred on the same day or the two subsequent days. After processing samples were frozen to −20 °C and stored until analysis. ** For further analysis of heat treatment on milk proteins, grouping of milk types according to the heat treatment was conducted; homogenized milk was excluded due to additional treatment with pressure; cream was excluded because it contains only the milk fat fraction. *** Total processing time includes heating and cooling stage.

2.2. Removal of Fat and Denatured Protein

All samples were centrifuged at 1500× g for 10 min at 10 °C (with a rotor 25.15, Avanti Centrifuge J-26 XP, Beckman Coulter, Miami, FL, USA). After centrifugation, all skimmed milk samples were acidified by drop-wise addition of 1 M HCl under stirring, until a pH of 4.6 was reached. The samples were then kept at 4 °C for 30 min to equilibrate. When needed, pH was adjusted before the final pH reading. This pH adjustment was done to separate the denatured serum proteins from the native serum proteins during ultracentrifugation, as previously described [7,10]. The acidified skim milk was transferred to ultracentrifuge tubes followed by ultracentrifugation at 100,000× g for 90 min at 30 °C (Beckman L-60, rotor 70 Ti). After ultracentrifugation, samples were separated into three phases. The top layer was remaining milk fat, the middle layer was milk serum, and the bottom layer (pellet) was casein with denatured proteins. Milk serum was used for filter aided sample preparation (FASP) as described below.

2.3. Filter Aided Sample Preparation (FASP)

FASP method was carried out according to Wisniewski et al., 2009 [15], with adaptations according to Zhang et al., 2016 [7]. Milk serum samples (20 μL) were diluted in SDT-lysis buffer (4% SDS with 0.1 M dithiotreitol and 100 mM Tris/HCl pH 8.0) to get a 1 μg/μL protein solution. Samples were then incubated for 10 min at 95 °C. They were centrifuged at 21,540× g for 10 min after being cooled down to room temperature. Of each sample 20 μL were directly added to the middle of 180 μL 0.05 M iodoacetamide (IAA) in 8 M urea with 100 mM Tris/HCl pH 8.0 (called UT) in a low binding Eppendorf tube and incubated for 10 min while mildly shaking at room temperature. The entire volume of the sample (200 μL) was transferred to a Pall 3K omega filter (10–20 kDa cutoff, OD003C34; Pall, Washington, NY, USA) and centrifuged at 20,000× g for 30 min. Another three centrifugations at 20,000× g for 30 min were carried out after adding three times 100 μL UT. Afterwards 110 μL 0.05 M NH_4HCO_3 (ABC) in water was added to the filter unit and centrifuged at 20,000× g for 30 min. Then, the filter was transferred to a new low-binding Eppendorf tube. On the filter, 100 μL ABC containing 0.5 μg trypsin was added and centrifuged at 20,000× g for 30 min after incubation overnight. Finally, the filter was removed and 5 μL 10% trifluoroacetic acid (TFA) was added to adjust the pH of the sample to around 2. These samples were ready for analysis by liquid chromatography/tandem mass spectrometry (LC-MS/MS).

2.4. LC-MS/MS Analysis

A volume of 18 µL of the trypsin digested milk fractions was injected in a 0.10 × 30 mm Magic C18AQ 200A 5 µm beads (Bruker Nederland B.V., Leiderdorp, The Netherlands) pre-concentration column (prepared in house) at a maximum pressure of 270 bar. Peptides were eluted from the pre-concentration column onto a 0.10 × 200 mm Magic C18AQ 200A 3 µm beads analytical column with an acetonitrile gradient at a flow of 0.5 µL/min, using gradient elution from 8 to 33% acetonitrile in water with 0.5 v/v % acetic acid in 50 min. The column was washed using an increase in the percentage of acetonitrile to 80% (with 20% water and 0.5 v/v % acetic acid in the acetonitrile and the water) in 3 min. Between the pre-concentration and analytical columns, an electrospray potential of 3.5 kV was applied directly to the eluent via a stainless steel needle fitted into the waste line of a P777 Upchurch microcross. Full scan positive mode FTMS spectra were measured between m/z 380 and 1400 on a LTQ-Orbitrap XL (Thermo electron, San Jose, CA, USA) in the Orbitrap at high resolution (60,000). IT and FT AGC targets were set to 10,000 and 500,000, respectively, or maximum ion times of 100 µs (IT) and 500 ms (FT) were used. Collision-induced dissociation (CID) fragmented MS/MS scans (isolation width 2 m/z, 30% normalized collision energy, activation Q 0.25 and activation time 15 ms) of the four most abundant 2+ and 3+ charged peaks in the FTMS scan were recorded in data dependent mode in the linear trap (MS/MS threshold = 5.000, 45 s exclusion duration for the selected m/z ±25 ppm).

2.5. Data Analysis

Each run with all MS/MS spectra obtained was analysed with Maxquant 1.3.0.5 with Andromeda search engine [16]. Carbamidomethylation of cysteines was set as a fixed modification (enzyme = trypsin, maximally 2 missed cleavages, peptide tolerance for the first search 20 ppm, fragment ions tolerance 0.5 amu). Oxidation of methionine, N-terminal acetylation and de-amidation of asparagine or glutamine were set as variable modification for both identification and quantification. The bovine reference database for peptides and protein searches was downloaded as fasta file from Uniprot with reverse sequences generated by Maxquant (fasta file downloaded from Uniprot 2013 [17]). A set of 31 protein sequences of common contaminants was used as well, which included Trypsin (P00760, bovine), Trypsin (P00761, porcine), Keratin K22E (P35908, human), Keratin K1C9 (P35527, human), Keratin K2C1 (P04264, human), and Keratin K1C1 (P35527, human). A maximum of two missed cleavages were allowed and a mass deviation of 0.5 Da was set as limit for MS/MS peaks and maximally 6 ppm deviation on the peptide m/z during the main search. The false discovery rate (FDR) was set to 1% on both peptide and protein levels. The length of peptides was set to at least seven amino acids. Finally, proteins were displayed based on minimally 2 distinct peptides of which at least one unique and at least one unmodified. Match between runs was used with a time window of 10 min. Both unmodified and modified peptides were used for quantification. Only unique or razor peptides were used for quantification. Minimum ratio count for label-free quantification (LFQ) was set as 2.

The quantification of the full proteome is based on the extracted ion current and is taking the whole three-dimensional isotope pattern into account, using peak volumes of all measured isotopes for quantification [16]. At least two quantitation events were required for a quantifiable protein. MaxQuant was used with the Intensity based absolute quantification (IBAQ) algorithms for quantification [18]. The IBAQ algorithm estimates the absolute amount of a protein as the sum of the intensities of all peptides (based on peak volumes), divided by the number of tryptic peptides that can theoretically be generated. Proteins had to have at least three valid IBAQ intensities in the individual samples for counting of the number of identified proteins.

The function of the identified proteins was checked in the UniprotKB database released February 2014 [17].

2.6. Statistical Analysis

Statistical analysis was performed with R 3.3.2 software [19]. The average number of measurable proteins in raw milk was calculated and related to the respective numbers of milks after different processing methods.

Proteins with ≤33% non-detects were included in further analysis. Non-detects of these proteins were either simply replaced by zero or imputed by simple imputation. For the imputation firstly the mean and standard deviation of each protein was estimated including the non-detected values as censored observations by a linear Tobit model to determine protein specific distributions. Subsequently, non-detects were replaced by random samples from the lower tail of the respective distribution, i.e., below the protein specific detection limit as defined by the minimum of the measured protein levels. The quality of imputation was examined via Wilcoxon tests, comparing median protein levels of the imputed data against the raw data. For subsequent analyses, the imputed data were used.

Hierarchical clustering of milk samples was based on Pearson's correlation of the specific protein profiles following imputation.

For assessment of the effect of heating, milks were categorized in two groups by temperatures above and below 80 °C [20]; high heated milk samples, defined as UHT, ESL and boiled milk and no-/low heat treated milks, represented by pasteurized, skimmed and raw milk samples (Table 2).

A logistic regression model adjusted for the milk origin (Traunstein, Freising, Starnberg) was used to calculate the differences in high vs. low heat treated milks. The log2 fold-changes of the protein levels in low versus high heat treated milks were calculated to rank the proteins according to their heat sensitivity, and plotted against the corresponding negative decadic logarithm of the p-values in a volcano plot. Resulting p-values were adjusted for the false discovery rate according to Benjamini–Hochberg, and a corrected p-value < 0.05 was considered statistically significant.

3. Results

A total of 364 milk serum proteins were identified and quantified in at least one of the 24 milk samples, of which 44 could be quantified in all 24 samples. Subsequent analyses were based on the 169 proteins found in at least three different milk samples; 130 of those proteins were detected in all three raw milk samples and further 28 proteins in two raw milk samples. The average LFQ levels of proteins in the raw milk samples did not differ significantly between the three farms ($p = 0.49$), thereby ruling out major differences in original milk batches.

Figure 1 shows a substantial loss of detectable proteins after the various processing procedures.

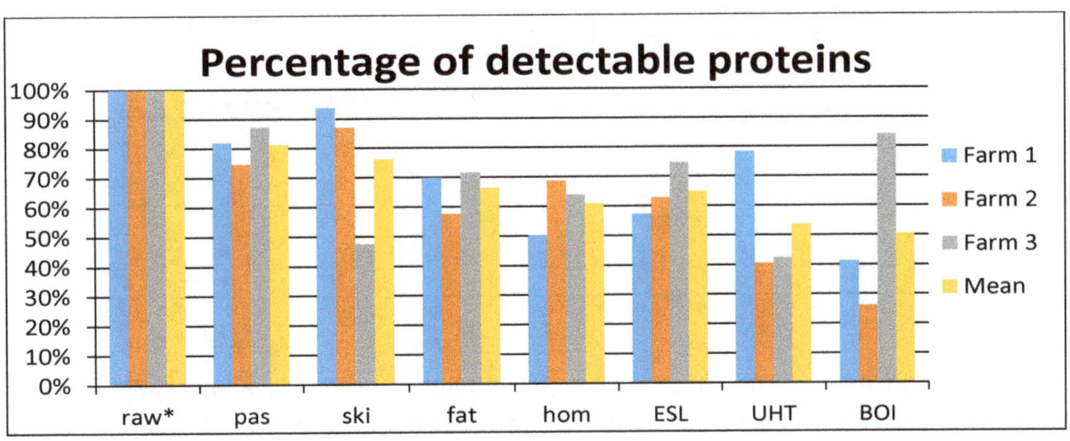

Figure 1. Proportion of number of detectable proteins in milk samples (each sample per farm individually and averaged over the three different samples) after different processing compared to raw cow's milk. * No. of detectable native proteins in raw milk is the reference, i.e., 151 distinct proteins were detected in the three raw milk samples on average.

For further statistical analysis, proteins with >33% non-detects were excluded. Non-detects in the remaining proteins (n = 140) were either replaced by imputed values below detection limit or simply by zeros. Figure 2 shows the superiority of the imputation method in contrast to the simple replacement of missing values by zero. The median of the individual protein LFQ levels averaged over all 24 samples is solely slightly reduced after imputation compared to the raw data set (median value was calculated after exclusion of missing values). In contrast, replacement of non-detects by zero resulted in a clear distortion of the distribution and was not considered for further analysis.

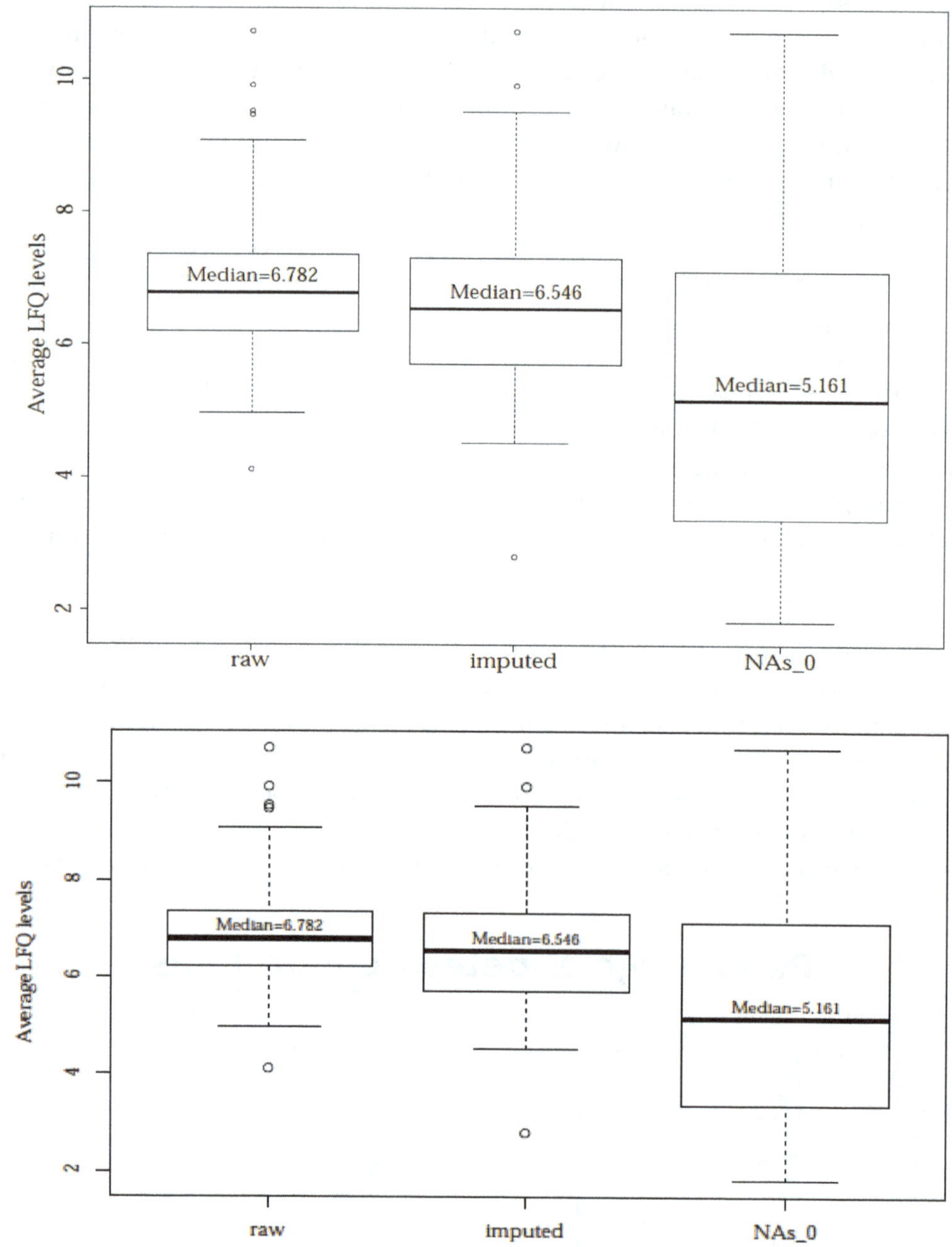

Figure 2. Boxplots of average protein LFQ levels after different NA replacement. Comparison of mean LFQ protein values in different data (raw, imputed, and NAs replaced by 0). Replacement by 0 differed significantly from the raw data ($p < 0.0001$).

Similar protein patterns resulted from similar heating temperatures of the milk samples as demonstrated by hierarchical clustering of the specific protein profiles (Figure 3): raw, skimmed and pasteurized milk samples formed one cluster, whereas UHT, ESL, and boiled milk samples formed another cluster with the exception of one boiled milk sample, which differed substantially from both main clusters. Under the assumption that this milk was partially overcooked, it was excluded from subsequent analyses.

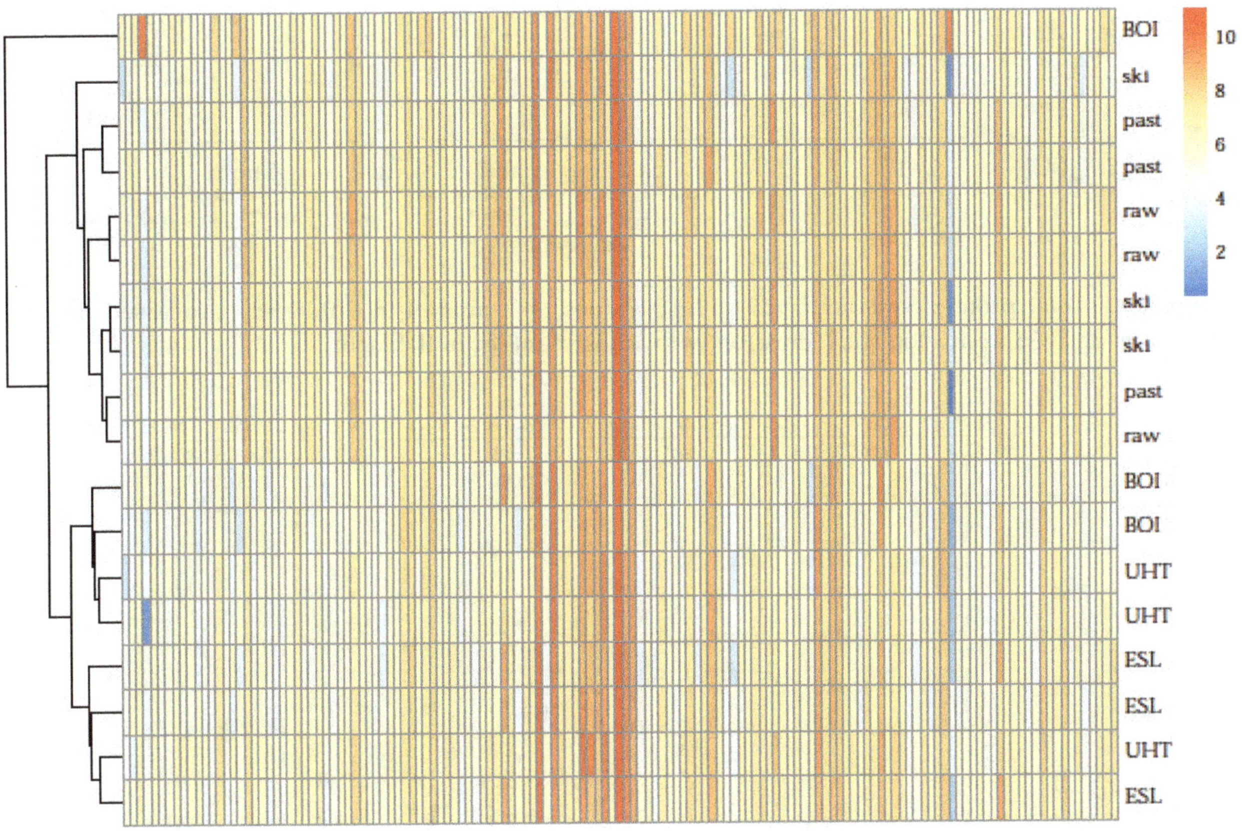

Figure 3. Heat map for protein levels and milk types. Rows reflect individual samples, whereas individual proteins are given in columns. Their LFQ values are represented by different colors according to the color code from low (blue) to high (red) expression.

Comparison of milks in the high heat versus the low heat treated group revealed a significant reduction of the total protein LFQ levels in high heated milks compared to no/low heat treated milks, as shown in Figure 4. Boiled milk showed the lowest protein levels; other heat treated milks contained total protein LFQ levels ranging between boiled and raw milk and were inversely related to heating temperatures (Figure 4).

When focusing on individual proteins, a significant reduction in quantity of at least 10% was found in 23 proteins after high heat treatment compared to low heat treatment (Figure 5).

Ten of these proteins were related to immune functions (Table 3).

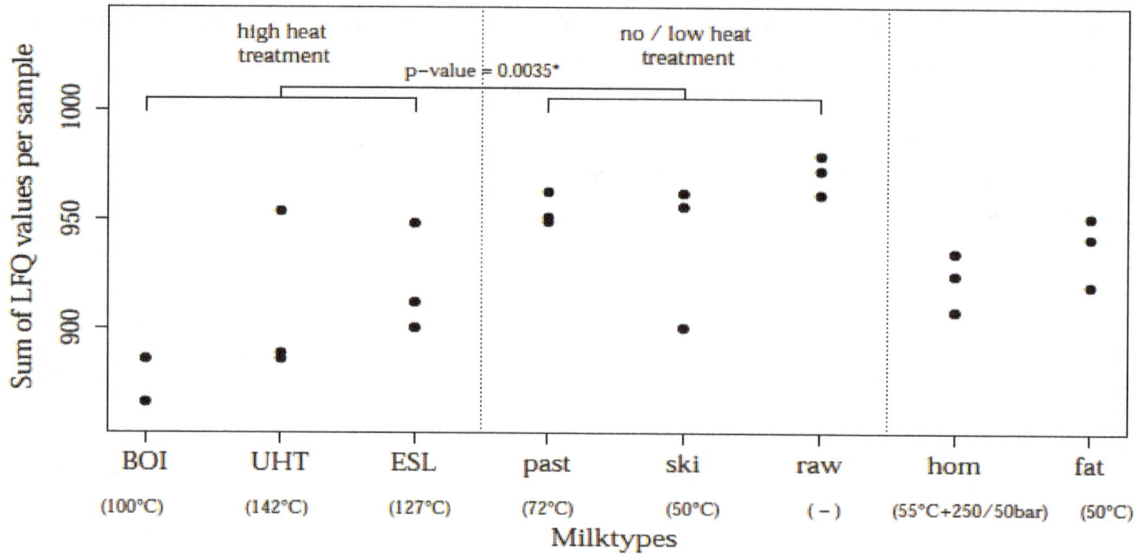

Figure 4. Total protein contents (sum of LFQ values per sample) in differently processed milks. * p-value derived from a logistic regression with adjustment for milk batch.

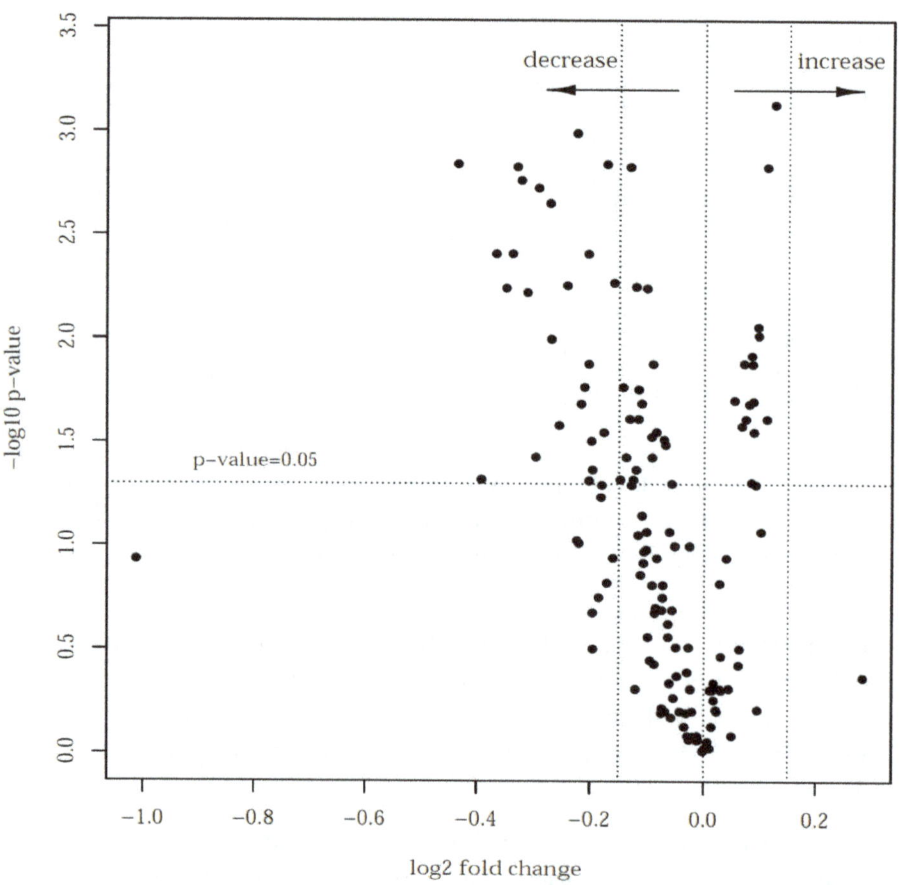

Figure 5. Volcano plot for the comparison of proteins in low- versus high-heat treated milk samples. The log two-fold change of protein expression between low- and high-heat treated milk samples is plotted against the corresponding p-values from a t-test given as negative decadic logarithm. A negative log two-fold change indicates a decrease in LFQ levels.

Table 3. Significantly differing proteins between high and no/low heat treated milk-types with a change of ≥10%.

Protein Code	Number of Peptides	*p*-Value *	Log2 Fold Change (95% CI)	Protein Name	Protein Function
P80457	67	0.001	−0.44 (−0.56; −0.31)	Xanthine dehydrogenase/oxidase	immunity
P24627	71	0.004	−0.37 (−0.51; −0.22)	Lactoferrin	immunity
G3X6N3	57	0.006	−0.35 (−0.50; −0.20)	Serotransferrin	transport
F1MR22	42	0.004	−0.34 (−0.47; −0.21)	Polymeric immunoglobulin receptor	immunity
P80025	37	0.001	−0.33 (−0.43; −0.23)	Lactoperoxidase	immunity
G3N1R1	4	0.002	−0.32 (−0.44; −0.21)	Uncharacterized protein	unknown
F1MGU7	7	0.04	−0.30 (−0.52; −0.07)	Fibrinogen gamma-B chain	Blood coagulation
G3X7A5	80	0.002	−0.29 (−0.41; −0.18)	Complement C3	immunity
F1MZ96	10	0.002	−0.27 (−0.36; −0.18)	Uncharacterized protein	unknown
F1MX50	4	0.01	−0.27 (−0.40; −0.13)	Uncharacterized protein	cell
F1MM32	8	0.026	−0.26 (−0.43; −0.08)	Sulfhydryl oxidase	enzyme
P81265	42	0.006	−0.24 (−0.35; −0.14)	Polymeric immunoglobulin receptor	immunity
F1N076	12	0.001	−0.23 (−0.30; −0.15)	Ceruloplasmin	cell
F1MXX6	26	0.02	−0.22 (−0.35; −0.08)	Lactadherin	cell
Q08DQ0	6	0.017	−0.21 (−0.34; −0.08)	Plakophilin-3	cell
P07589	6	0.004	−0.20 (−0.30; −0.11)	Fibronectin	immunity
A6QNL0	6	0.01	−0.20 (−0.32; −0.09)	Monocyte differentiation antigen CD 14	immunity
P10152	11	0.048	−0.20 (−0.37; −0.04)	Angiogenin-1 (ribonuclease 5)	cell
F1MMD7	5	0.031	−0.20 (−0.34; −0.06)	Inter-alpha-trypsin inhibitor heavy chain H4	Protease inhibitor
Q3MHN2	6	0.043	−0.20 (−0.35; −0.04)	Complement component C9	immunity
P00735	7	0.028	−0.18 (−0.30; −0.05)	Prothrombin	immunity
F1MCF8	9	0.001	−0.17 (−0.22; −0.12)	Uncharacterized protein	immunity
P17690	9	0.005	−0.16 (−0.23; −0.09)	Beta-2-glycoprotein 1	Blood coagulation

* *p*-values are adjusted for multiple testing.

4. Discussion

Heat treatment of milk led to a considerable decrease in number of detectable proteins and their levels of quantification with a clear relationship to the applied heat load. The most intensive treatment, i.e., boiling, reduced the number of proteins that could be detected by about 50% compared to raw milk, with the other heating types ranging in between. The various processing methods led to specific proteomic patterns covering 140 individual proteins as demonstrated by a cluster analysis. Of these, 23 distinct proteins were found to be substantially diminished in high heat treated milks. The majority of these heat-sensitive proteins were related to immune functions.

Typically, people in Westernized countries consume industrially processed milk and, increasingly, milk types with an extended shelf life. In addition, UHT milk with its very long storage duration of three months or more is nowadays very popular. Traditionally, commercially available milk had been pasteurized, i.e., heated at 72 °C for 20 s to inactivate potential hazardous microorganisms with only small gain in shelf life.

Despite the potential risk of life-threatening infections, a minority of people still consume raw cow's milk, which has repeatedly been reported to protect against asthma, allergies, and respiratory infections in childhood [1,3,21,22]. The wide consumption of cow's milk thus renders it an attractive strategy for prevention if the risk of infections were to be overcome. An option might be the isolation and purification of the protective milk ingredients, and various studies have focused on the impact of industrial processing on the potentially beneficial molecules. At the same time, reducing heat load of commercially available dairy products may already lead to an increase in the availability of potentially immunoactive proteins.

Of the industrially applied processing steps, predominantly fat separation for adjusting milk fat levels, and homogenization for preventing fat creaming, affect the milk lipid fraction. However, homogenization also leads to a massive increase in fat globule surface, which will be covered by milk proteins, leading to a reduction of milk proteins in serum.

Waser at al., 2007 [23] found an asthma and wheeze protective effect of milk fat containing products such as full cream milk and butter. In addition, Brick et al., 2016 [2] implied the higher fat content and more precisely the higher content of anti-inflammatory omega-3 fatty acids in raw milk in the asthma protective effect of full cream milk obtained directly from a farm. Despite mild heating to

55 °C, high pressure treatment of milk (250 bar) used during the homogenization process has been found to profoundly rearrange protein quantity and structure [22,24,25]. In addition, in the present study homogenization reduced total protein LFQ levels and specific protein detectability markedly.

Another major processing step is heating for destroying hazardous microorganisms and increasing shelf life. Thermo-labile milk components such as miRNAs [13] and proteins may thus be involved in the protective effect of raw milk. Particularly protein functionality, solubility and quantity are all affected by intensity of heat treatment [7,8,18,26]. Previously specific miRNA species were identified as possible contributors to the asthma-protective effect of farm milk [11]. This notion is not in conflict with our current findings; rather both molecule classes might add to the effect or might even interact.

Loss et al., 2011 [1] found inverse associations of asthma with higher levels of several milk whey proteins, i.e., bovine serum albumin, alpha-lactalbumin and beta-lactoglobulin. However, it remains unclear whether these specific proteins confer the effect themselves or whether they are proxies of heat labile proteins in general. Therefore, we quantified heat-induced alterations of the entire milk proteome by a comprehensive, standardized, and unbiased approach, i.e., without preselection of proteins.

First, we observed a considerable decrease of detectable proteins after heat treatment in a dose-dependent manner. Boiled cow's milk contained the lowest number of detectable proteins, which is explained by the high heat load applied. The lower temperature of boiling compared to ESL or UHT is more than compensated by the much longer duration of the heating (Table 2). In addition, the long heating time of boiling may also lead to more extensive chemical modification compared to industrial processes [11], further reducing protein levels in these samples.

For further investigation in the impact of heating on the protein quantity and heat sensitivity, milk samples were categorized into high heat and no/low heat treated milk groups according to the clusters presented in the heat map (Figure 3). This dichotomization was in line with findings on the first marginal transition of bovine whey proteins at about 81 °C [20]. Actually, the difference between high and no/low heat treated samples was more than 25 °C with pasteurization not exceeding 72 °C and high heat treatment starting with 100 °C.

Figures 1 and 4 describe some variance within milk types between the three farms, e.g., one of the UHT samples had a higher percentage of detectable proteins and a higher summed LFQ value than the respective other two UHT samples. Nevertheless, the heat map (Figure 3) still groups all the high-heated samples together. Even though this UHT sample contains a higher overall protein intensity, and a higher number of identified proteins, the proteome profile still reflects a high heated sample. This might be due to a similar pattern in decrease of individual, heat sensitive proteins. The exact underlying mechanisms for these individual variations however cannot be explained in this study. Further investigations on a larger scale are needed to better understand the variability in proteome profile after heat processing.

The sum over all proteins, and more specifically the levels of 23 individual proteins were substantially lower in high heat treated samples as expected by previous work from Zhang et al., 2016 [7]. Interestingly, most of these 23 particularly heat-sensitive proteins were related to immune functions (Table 3), and several proteins have already been mentioned in the context of asthma and allergies. Under the assumption that some proteins withstand the acidity of the stomach milieu, they may be resorbed in the gut and exert physiologic functions. At least this has been suggested for e.g., lactoferrin (LTF) [27], protease inhibitors [28] and IgG [29].

Among the most promising candidates was lactoferrin, which is known to stimulate the immune system by counteracting pathogenic invaders and injuries and preventing harmful overreactions of the immune system [30,31].

Lactoperoxidase is a peroxidase enzyme secreted from the mammary gland that operates as a natural antibacterial agent [32]. Asthmatic patients who were treated with lactoperoxidase aerosol showed lower disease activity and reduced damaging effects of hydrogen peroxide (H_2O_2), which is mainly generated by neutrophils and eosinophils in asthma and contributes to airway damages and inflammation [33].

Xanthine dehydrogenase/oxidase (XOR) might contribute to the formation of NO in the intestinal lumen and thereby exert antimicrobial properties [34]. In our study we were unable to differentiate the rather similar variants, dehydrogenase and oxidase, as the only difference is an intramolecular change of two cysteines in the disulfide bond, whereas the amino acid chain, analyzed with the LC-MS/MS analysis, is identical.

In addition, a number of acute phase proteins such as fibrinogen, prothrombin, complement C3 and C9 were found to be highly heat-sensitive. How they may be involved in the anti-inflammatory effects ascribed to raw milk remains unclear, although the complement pathway, and specifically C3, has been implied in the development of allergy and asthma [35–37].

Plakophilin-3 acts protective in both local and systemic inflammatory diseases [38] and inter-alpha-trypsin inhibitor has anti-inflammatory, anti-scarring and anti-angiogenic properties [39]. Protease inhibitors, including several inter alpha-trypsin inhibitors, have been found to be upregulated in the breast milk of allergic mothers and have been related to the pathogenesis of allergy and asthma [40,41].

Lactadherin expression is found to be markedly reduced in asthmatic patients compared to healthy subjects, and suppresses airway smooth muscle hypercontractility [42].

Polymeric immunoglobulin receptor may influence eosinophilic inflammation by binding secretory immunoglobulins [43]. In addition, secretory components, which are part of the polymeric immunoglobulin receptor that can be cleaved off, have shown individual effects in mucosal immunity [44].

Ultimately, the discovery of the CD14 molecule, a receptor of bacterial endotoxin, is interesting as gene–environment interactions of raw milk consumption and polymorphisms associated with this gene have been discussed controversially for childhood onset asthma [45,46]. Similar to the human CD14 molecule, its bovine counterpart might transmit signals elicited by endotoxin, and thereby have an effect on the development or prevention of allergy and asthma.

Despite the plausible involvement of several proteins in the beneficial health effects we have to acknowledge that we cannot provide a direct link to disease status in this study. However, the palette of immune-active milk components detected in the present study can be seen as an extension to the findings by Loss et al., 2011 [1], which explicitly linked protein levels to disease. In addition, this study only shows a decrease in native proteins, due to either denaturation or heat-induced chemical modification, without direct evidence for a loss-of-function. However, heating of milk has been shown to reduce biological activity of milk, including antibacterial capacity [6] and previous studies showed a loss-of-function of milk immune proteins upon denaturation (e.g., Paulson, 1993 [47]; Marin et al., 2003 [48]). However, future studies are needed to investigate in the biological function of milk's immunoactive proteins after applying heat treatments.

Another limitation of this analysis is the omission of the milk fat globule membrane (MFGM) fraction [49]; their relatively low abundance in cow's milk, however, precludes a major contribution to the effects by the entirety of immunoactive proteins present in milk. Our analyses were made after one freezing cycle; resulting alterations, however, seem to be very limited [7,50].

5. Conclusions

Taken together, we have performed a comprehensive search for proteins most likely to be affected by industrial processing methods. Their higher abundance in native cow's milk as compared to industrially processed milks renders them potential candidates for protection from asthma, allergies, and respiratory infections. However, in this study, we solely analyzed protein patterns of differently processed milks, thus associations of found potential protein candidates with disease status have to be investigated in population based studies.

Acknowledgments: This study was supported by the Leibniz Award 2013 of the Deutsche Forschungsgemeinsacht (DFG) awarded to EvM.

Author Contributions: T.B. statistical analyses and preparation of the manuscript, M.E. design of the study, supervision of statistical analyses, and preparation of the manuscript, S.B. laboratory analyses, A.B. statistical analyses, E.v.M. design of the study and preparation of the manuscript, J.V. laboratory analyses, K.H. design of the study, supervision of laboratory analyses, and preparation of the manuscript.

References

1. Loss, G.; Apprich, S.; Waser, M.; Kneifel, W.; Genuneit, J.; Buchele, G.; Weber, J.; Sozanska, B.; Danielewicz, H.; Horak, E.; et al. The protective effect of farm milk consumption on childhood asthma and atopy: The gabriela study. *J. Allergy Clin. Immunol.* **2011**, *128*, 766–773. [CrossRef] [PubMed]
2. Brick, T.; Schober, Y.; Bocking, C.; Pekkanen, J.; Genuneit, J.; Loss, G.; Dalphin, J.C.; Riedler, J.; Lauener, R.; Nockher, W.A.; et al. Omega-3 fatty acids contribute to the asthma-protective effect of unprocessed cow's milk. *J. Allergy Clin. Immunol.* **2016**, *137*, 1699–1706. [CrossRef] [PubMed]
3. Loss, G.; Depner, M.; Ulfman, L.H.; van Neerven, R.J.; Hose, A.J.; Genuneit, J.; Karvonen, A.M.; Hyvarinen, A.; Kaulek, V.; Roduit, C.; et al. Consumption of unprocessed cow's milk protects infants from common respiratory infections. *J. Allergy Clin. Immunol.* **2015**, *135*, 56–62. [CrossRef] [PubMed]
4. Van Neerven, R.J.; Knol, E.F.; Heck, J.M.; Savelkoul, H.F. Which factors in raw cow's milk contribute to protection against allergies? *J. Allergy Clin. Immunol.* **2012**, *130*, 853–858. [CrossRef] [PubMed]
5. Li-Chan, E.; Kummer, A.; Losso, J.N.; Kitts, D.D.; Nakai, S. Stability of bovine immunoglobulins to thermal treatment and processing. *Food Res. Int.* **1995**, *28*, 9–16. [CrossRef]
6. Van Gysel, M.; Cossey, V.; Fieuws, S.; Schuermans, A. Impact of pasteurization on the antibacterial properties of human milk. *Eur. J. Pediatr.* **2012**, *171*, 1231–1237. [CrossRef] [PubMed]
7. Zhang, L.; Boeren, S.; Smits, M.; Hooijdonk, T.V.; Vervoort, J.; Hettinga, K. Proteomic study on the stability of proteins in bovine, camel, and caprine milk sera after processing. *Food Res. Int.* **2016**, *82*, 104–111. [CrossRef]
8. Anema, S.G. Chapter 8—The whey proteins in milk: Thermal denaturation, physical interactions and effects on the functional properties of milk a2—Thompson, abby. In *Milk Proteins*; Boland, M., Singh, H., Eds.; Academic Press: San Diego, CA, USA, 2008; pp. 239–281.
9. Navarro, F.; Harouna, S.; Calvo, M.; Perez, M.D.; Sanchez, L. Kinetic and thermodynamic parameters for thermal denaturation of ovine milk lactoferrin determined by its loss of immunoreactivity. *J. Dairy Sci.* **2015**, *98*, 4328–4337. [CrossRef] [PubMed]
10. Spiegel, T. Whey protein aggregation under shear conditions—Effects of lactose and heating temperature on aggregate size and structure. *Int. J. Food Sci. Technol.* **1999**, *34*, 523–531. [CrossRef]
11. Van Boekel, M.A.J.S. Effect of heating on maillard reactions in milk. *Food Chem.* **1998**, *62*, 403–414. [CrossRef]
12. Milkovska-Stamenova, S.; Hoffmann, R. Identification and quantification of bovine protein lactosylation sites in different milk products. *J. Proteom.* **2016**, *134*, 112–126. [CrossRef] [PubMed]
13. Kirchner, B.; Pfaffl, M.W.; Dumpler, J.; von Mutius, E.; Ege, M.J. Microrna in native and processed cow's milk and its implication for the farm milk effect on asthma. *J. Allergy Clin. Immunol.* **2016**, *137*, 1893–1895. [CrossRef] [PubMed]
14. Lu, J.; Boeren, S.; de Vries, S.C.; van Valenberg, H.J.; Vervoort, J.; Hettinga, K. Filter-aided sample preparation with dimethyl labeling to identify and quantify milk fat globule membrane proteins. *J. Proteom.* **2011**, *75*, 34–43. [CrossRef] [PubMed]
15. Wisniewski, J.R.; Zougman, A.; Nagaraj, N.; Mann, M. Universal sample preparation method for proteome analysis. *Nat. Methods* **2009**, *6*, 359–362. [CrossRef] [PubMed]
16. Cox, J.; Mann, M. Maxquant enables high peptide identification rates, individualized p.P.B.-range mass accuracies and proteome-wide protein quantification. *Nat. Biotechnol.* **2008**, *26*, 1367–1372. [CrossRef] [PubMed]
17. UniProt, C. Universal Protein Resource (Uniprot). Avaliable online: http://www.uniprot.org/ (accessed on 31 August 2017).
18. Schwanhausser, B.; Busse, D.; Li, N.; Dittmar, G.; Schuchhardt, J.; Wolf, J.; Chen, W.; Selbach, M. Corrigendum: Global quantification of mammalian gene expression control. *Nature* **2013**, *495*, 126–127. [CrossRef] [PubMed]

19. The R Development Core Team. R: A Language and Environment for Statistical Computing. Avaliable online: https://www.R-project.org/ (accessed on 31 August 2017).
20. Laleye, L.C.; Jobe, B.; Wasesa, A.A. Comparative study on heat stability and functionality of camel and bovine milk whey proteins. *J. Dairy Sci.* **2008**, *91*, 4527–4534. [CrossRef] [PubMed]
21. Riedler, J.; Eder, W.; Oberfeld, G.; Schreuer, M. Austrian children living on a farm have less hay fever, asthma and allergic sensitization. *Clin. Exp. Allergy* **2000**, *30*, 194–200. [CrossRef] [PubMed]
22. Sharma, S.K.; Dalgleish, D.G. Interactions between milk serum proteins and synthetic fat globule membrane during heating of homogenized whole milk. *J. Agric. Food Chem.* **1993**, *41*, 1407–1412. [CrossRef]
23. Waser, M.; Michels, K.B.; Bieli, C.; Floistrup, H.; Pershagen, G.; von Mutius, E.; Ege, M.; Riedler, J.; Schram-Bijkerk, D.; Brunekreef, B.; et al. Inverse association of farm milk consumption with asthma and allergy in rural and suburban populations across europe. *Clin. Exp. Allergy* **2007**, *37*, 661–670. [CrossRef] [PubMed]
24. Corredig, M.; Dalgleish, D.G. Effect of temperature and ph on the interactions of whey proteins with casein micelles in skim milk. *Food Res. Int.* **1996**, *29*, 49–55. [CrossRef]
25. Lee, S.J.; Sherbon, J.W. Chemical changes in bovine milk fat globule membrane caused by heat treatment and homogenization of whole milk. *J. Dairy Res.* **2002**, *69*, 555–567. [CrossRef] [PubMed]
26. Dewit, J.N.; Klarenbeek, G. Effects of various heat treatments on structure and solubility of whey proteins. *J. Dairy Sci.* **1984**, *67*, 2701–2710. [CrossRef]
27. Troost, F.J.; Steijns, J.; Saris, W.H.; Brummer, R.J. Gastric digestion of bovine lactoferrin in vivo in adults. *J. Nutr.* **2001**, *131*, 2101–2104. [PubMed]
28. Davidson, L.A.; Lonnerdal, B. Fecal alpha 1-antitrypsin in breast-fed infants is derived from human milk and is not indicative of enteric protein loss. *Acta Paediatr. Scand.* **1990**, *79*, 137–141. [CrossRef] [PubMed]
29. Jasion, V.S.; Burnett, B.P. Survival and digestibility of orally-administered immunoglobulin preparations containing igg through the gastrointestinal tract in humans. *Nutr. J.* **2015**, *14*, 22. [CrossRef] [PubMed]
30. Giansanti, F.; Panella, G.; Leboffe, L.; Antonini, G. Lactoferrin from milk: Nutraceutical and pharmacological properties. *Pharmaceuticals (Basel)* **2016**, *9*, 61. [CrossRef] [PubMed]
31. Drago-Serrano, M.E.; Campos-Rodriguez, R.; Carrero, J.C.; de la Garza, M. Lactoferrin: Balancing ups and downs of inflammation due to microbial infections. *Int. J. Mol. Sci.* **2017**, *18*, 501. [CrossRef] [PubMed]
32. Kussendrager, K.D.; van Hooijdonk, A.C. Lactoperoxidase: Physico-chemical properties, occurrence, mechanism of action and applications. *Br. J. Nutr.* **2000**, *84* (Suppl. 1), S19–S25. [CrossRef] [PubMed]
33. Al Obaidi, A.H. Role of airway lactoperoxidase in scavenging of hydrogen peroxide damage in asthma. *Ann. Thorac. Med.* **2007**, *2*, 107–110. [CrossRef] [PubMed]
34. Setiawan, H.; Nagaoka, K.; Kubo, M.; Fujikura, Y.; Ogino, K. Involvement of xanthine oxidoreductase-related oxidative stress in a dermatophagoides farinae-induced asthma model of nc/nga mice. *Acta Med. Okayama* **2016**, *70*, 175–182. [PubMed]
35. Varga, L.; Farkas, H.; Fust, G. Role of complement in allergy. In *The Complement System: Novel Roles in Health and Disease*; Szebeni, J., Ed.; Springer: Boston, MA, USA, 2004; pp. 345–360.
36. Zhang, X.; Kohl, J. A complex role for complement in allergic asthma. *Exp. Rev. Clin. Immunol.* **2010**, *6*, 269–277. [CrossRef]
37. Drouin, S.M.; Corry, D.B.; Kildsgaard, J.; Wetsel, R.A. Cutting edge: The absence of c3 demonstrates a role for complement in th2 effector functions in a murine model of pulmonary allergy. *J. Immunol.* **2001**, *167*, 4141–4145. [CrossRef] [PubMed]
38. Sklyarova, T.; van Hengel, J.; Van Wonterghem, E.; Libert, C.; van Roy, F.; Vandenbroucke, R.E. Hematopoietic plakophilin-3 regulates acute tissue-specific and systemic inflammation in mice. *Eur. J. Immunol.* **2015**, *45*, 2898–2910. [CrossRef] [PubMed]
39. Zhang, S.; He, H.; Day, A.J.; Tseng, S.C. Constitutive expression of inter-alpha-inhibitor (ialphai) family proteins and tumor necrosis factor-stimulated gene-6 (tsg-6) by human amniotic membrane epithelial and stromal cells supporting formation of the heavy chain-hyaluronan (hc-ha) complex. *J. Biol. Chem.* **2012**, *287*, 12433–12444. [CrossRef] [PubMed]
40. Hettinga, K.A.; Reina, F.M.; Boeren, S.; Zhang, L.; Koppelman, G.H.; Postma, D.S.; Vervoort, J.J.; Wijga, A.H. Difference in the breast milk proteome between allergic and non-allergic mothers. *PLoS ONE* **2015**, *10*, e0122234. [CrossRef] [PubMed]

41. Gregory, L.G.; Lloyd, C.M. Orchestrating house dust mite-associated allergy in the lung. *Trends Immunol.* **2011**, *32*, 402–411. [CrossRef] [PubMed]
42. Kudo, M.; Khalifeh Soltani, S.M.; Sakuma, S.A.; McKleroy, W.; Lee, T.H.; Woodruff, P.G.; Lee, J.W.; Huang, K.; Chen, C.; Arjomandi, M.; et al. Mfge8 suppresses airway hyperresponsiveness in asthma by regulating smooth muscle contraction. *Proc. Natl. Acad. Sci. USA* **2013**, *110*, 660–665. [CrossRef] [PubMed]
43. Hupin, C.; Rombaux, P.; Bowen, H.; Gould, H.; Lecocq, M.; Pilette, C. Downregulation of polymeric immunoglobulin receptor and secretory iga antibodies in eosinophilic upper airway diseases. *Allergy* **2013**, *68*, 1589–1597. [CrossRef] [PubMed]
44. Kaetzel, C.S. The polymeric immunoglobulin receptor: Bridging innate and adaptive immune responses at mucosal surfaces. *Immunol. Rev.* **2005**, *206*, 83–99. [CrossRef] [PubMed]
45. Ege, M.J.; Strachan, D.P.; Cookson, W.O.; Moffatt, M.F.; Gut, I.; Lathrop, M.; Kabesch, M.; Genuneit, J.; Buchele, G.; Sozanska, B.; et al. Gene-environment interaction for childhood asthma and exposure to farming in central europe. *J. Allergy Clin. Immunol.* **2011**, *127*, 138–144. [CrossRef] [PubMed]
46. Bieli, C.; Eder, W.; Frei, R.; Braun-Fahrlander, C.; Klimecki, W.; Waser, M.; Riedler, J.; von Mutius, E.; Scheynius, A.; Pershagen, G.; et al. A polymorphism in cd14 modifies the effect of farm milk consumption on allergic diseases and *cd14* gene expression. *J. Allergy Clin. Immunol.* **2007**, *120*, 1308–1315. [CrossRef] [PubMed]
47. Paulsson, M.A.; Svensson, U.; Kishore, A.R.; Naidu, A.S. Thermal behavior of bovine lactoferrin in water and its relation to bacterial interaction and antibacterial activity. *J. Dairy Sci.* **1993**, *76*, 3711–3720. [CrossRef]
48. Marín, E.; Sánchez, L.; Pérez, M.D.; Puyol, P.; Calvo, M. Effect of heat treatment on bovine lactoperoxidase activity in skim milk: Kinetic and thermodynamic analysis. *J. Food Sci.* **2003**, *68*, 89–93. [CrossRef]
49. Hettinga, K.; van Valenberg, H.; de Vries, S.; Boeren, S.; van Hooijdonk, T.; van Arendonk, J.; Vervoort, J. The host defense proteome of human and bovine milk. *PLoS ONE* **2011**, *6*, e19433. [CrossRef] [PubMed]
50. Garcia-Lara, N.R.; Escuder-Vieco, D.; Garcia-Algar, O.; De la Cruz, J.; Lora, D.; Pallas-Alonso, C. Effect of freezing time on macronutrients and energy content of breastmilk. *Breastfeed. Med.* **2012**, *7*, 295–301. [CrossRef] [PubMed]

8

Immune Components in Human Milk are Associated with Early Infant Immunological Health Outcomes: A Prospective Three-Country Analysis

Daniel Munblit [1,2,3,*], Marina Treneva [3,4], Diego G. Peroni [3,5], Silvia Colicino [6], Li Yan Chow [1], Shobana Dissanayeke [7], Alexander Pampura [3,4], Attilio L. Boner [8], Donna T. Geddes [3,9], Robert J. Boyle [1,3,†] and John O. Warner [1,3,10,†]

1 Department of Paediatrics, Imperial College London, London W2 1NY, UK; lychow8@gmail.com (L.Y.C.); r.boyle@nhs.net (R.J.B.); j.o.warner@imperial.ac.uk (J.O.W.)

2 Faculty of Pediatrics, Federal State Autonomous Educational Institution of Higher Education I.M. Sechenov First Moscow State Medical University of the Ministry of Health of the Russian Federation., Moscow 119991, Russia

3 International Inflammation (in-FLAME) network of the World Universities Network, Perth 6000, WA, Australia

4 Allergy Department, Veltischev Clinical Pediatric Research Institute of Pirogov Russian National Research Medical University, Moscow 125412, Russia; trenevamarina@mail.ru (M.T.); apampura1@mail.ru (A.P.)

5 Department of Clinical and Experimental Medicine, Section of Paediatrics, University of Pisa, Pisa 56126, Italy; diego.peroni@unipi.it

6 National Heart and Lung Institute, Imperial College London, London SW3 6NP, UK; s.colicino@imperial.ac.uk

7 Royal Holloway University of London School of Biological Sciences, Biomedical Sciences, London TW20 0EX, UK; shobanadis@hotmail.com

8 Department of Life and Reproduction Sciences, Section of Paediatrics, University of Verona, Verona 37124, Italy; attilio.boner@univr.it

9 School of Molecular Sciences, The University of Western Australia, Perth, WA 6009, Australia; donna.geddes@uwa.edu.au

10 National Institute of Health Research Collaboration for Leadership in Applied Health Research and Care for NW London, London SW10 9NH, UK

* Correspondence: daniel.munblit08@imperial.ac.uk

† These authors contributed equally to this work.

Abstract: The role of breastfeeding in improving allergy outcomes in early childhood is still unclear. Evidence suggests that immune mediators in human milk (HM) play a critical role in infant immune maturation as well as protection against atopy/allergy development. We investigated relationships between levels of immune mediators in colostrum and mature milk and infant outcomes in the first year of life. In a large prospective study of 398 pregnant/lactating women in the United Kingdom, Russia and Italy, colostrum and mature human milk (HM) samples were analysed for immune active molecules. Statistical analyses used models adjusting for the site of collection, colostrum collection time, parity and maternal atopic status. Preliminary univariate analysis showed detectable interleukin (IL) 2 and IL13 in HM to be associated with less eczema. This finding was further confirmed in multivariate analysis, with detectable HM IL13 showing protective effect OR 0.18 (95% CI 0.04–0.92). In contrast, a higher risk of eczema was associated with higher HM concentrations of transforming growth factor β (TGFβ) 2 OR 1.04 (95% CI 1.01–1.06) per ng/mL. Parental-reported food allergy was reported less often when IL13 was detectable in colostrum OR 0.10 (95% CI 0.01–0.83). HM hepatocyte growth factor (HGF) was protective for common cold incidence at 12 months OR 0.19

(95% CI 0.04–0.92) per ng/mL. Data from this study suggests that differences in the individual immune composition of HM may have an influence on early life infant health outcomes. Increased TGFβ2 levels in HM are associated with a higher incidence of reported eczema, with detectable IL13 in colostrum showing protective effects for food allergy and sensitization. HGF shows some protective effect on common cold incidence at one year of age. Future studies should be focused on maternal genotype, human milk microbiome and diet influence on human milk immune composition and both short- and long-term health outcomes in the infant.

Keywords: colostrum; human milk; immune modulators; immunologically active molecules; cytokines; growth factors; health outcomes; immunological outcomes

1. Introduction

Increasing rates of allergy/atopy are of great concern with children bearing the greatest burden of this increase [1]. Long-term disease and health outcomes have been associated with multiple factors but, in particular, maturation of the immune system and immune-mediated diseases have been linked to later metabolic disorders such as cardiovascular disease [2]. Whilst there is evidence to suggest that the maternal environment in pregnancy has an impact on subsequent development of immune system in their offspring [3], early nutrition in the first two years of life, a rapid period of infant growth and development, is also believed to impact short- and long-term health. A plethora of evidence exists describing the multiple benefits of breastfeeding for both the mother and the infant, yet the mechanisms by which they confer these benefits remain to be fully elucidated.

Human milk (HM) contains a large variety of active immune components [4], which are present in differing concentrations [5], yet no comprehensive study has delved into the influences of maternal characteristics on immune composition of HM. We may expect HM to contain all necessary immunological components in the amounts needed for an appropriate infant immune development. Abundance of immune active molecules in HM represents a major difference when compared with any formula milk available. Further, little is known about the immune composition's influence on short- and long-term health outcomes.

It can be expected that HM composition may naturally change as a response to a number of environmental and genetic factors. HM immune components may influence immunological health outcomes but linear relationships between HM composition and subsequent health outcomes should be evaluated with care, due to potential confounding. Previously reported differences in HM immune composition between the countries and within the same populations provide evidence of volatility and reasons behind it remain unclear.

Amongst immunologically active molecules studied in HM, transforming growth factor β (TGFβ) is the most well described. HM contains all the isoforms of TGFβ, with TGFβ2 being the most dominant; accounting for 95% of the total TGFβ [6]. Protective effects of TGFβ on gut mucosal inflammation have been shown in animal models [7]. This protective effect may be explained by promotion of IgA production and induction of oral tolerance [8,9]. Oddy and Rosales systematically reviewed human milk TGFβ ability to influence infantile immunological outcomes [10]. Most of the studies included in the analysis found a statistically significant association between higher TGFβ concentration in HM and reduced risk of atopic diseases in the child. The authors suggested that TGFβ found in the milk may play a role in homeostasis maintenance in the intestine, regulating inflammation and subsequently promoting oral tolerance which may reduce the risk of allergy development.

Cytokines are one of the major classes of immune components in HM [11] but they are present in low concentrations; therefore, there is some doubt as to whether they have significant biological activity sufficient to modify health outcomes. On the other hand, growth factors are detected in much higher quantities in both colostrum and mature milk [12] and may therefore have a more potent influence in facilitating immunity maturation, as has been shown in both animal models [13] and human studies [14,15].

Hepatocyte growth factor (HGF) is a less-studied component that is also present in HM in high amounts, comparable with those of TGFβ [12,16,17], but has received less attention. HGF levels in human colostrum are 20 to 30 times higher when compared to paired maternal serum [16], suggesting that this growth factor is actively secreted into breast milk and may have an important role in early immune development. HGF is assumed to be in such high concentrations to facilitate proliferation, angiogenesis and intestinal tissue maturation via paracrine and endocrine signaling [12,17]. Accumulated knowledge from animal model studies suggests that HGF may also play a role in airway hyper-responsiveness and airway remodeling in allergic asthma [18–20] which highlights potential importance of this immune active molecule for human milk research.

We aimed to assess the impact of maternal and environmental factors in relation to colostrum and mature human milk immune active components composition and health outcomes at the age of six and twelve months.

2. Materials and Methods

2.1. Study Setting, Eligibility Criteria, and Ethics

The investigations and sample collection have been conducted following ethical approval by Ethics committees in three countries participating in the study: West London Rec 3 (UK) (Ref. number 10/H0706/32) and all paperwork has been completed according to the hospital R & D Joint Research Office (UK) (JROSM0072) policy; the Ethical Committee of the Azienda Ospedaliera di Verona (Italy) (approval No. 1288), and the Moscow Institute of Paediatrics and Child Health of the Ministry of Health of the Russian Federation (Russia) (approval No. 1-MS/11). All women provided written informed consent.

Women were enrolled at antenatal and postnatal units of 3 participating centers: Maternity Hospital No. 1, Moscow, Russia; St. Mary's Hospital, London, UK; G.B. Rossi Hospital, Verona, Italy. Details of recruitment are described in full elsewhere [21].

2.2. Medical Records and Interview

Following enrolment, participants underwent allergy skin prick testing (SPT) and answered a 10-minute interview-based questionnaire regarding their medical history. Exposure variables recorded were selected based on a detailed review of known determinants of HM composition [22]. Information collected from the recruited women included: parity; age; mode of delivery; details of residence environment, such as mould presence at home, regular contact with animals and/or pets at home; exposure to tobacco smoke (smoker or living in household with smoker or self-reported passive smoker); any reports of infections during pregnancy. We also obtained information on maternal dietary preferences—fish, fresh fruit, and probiotic intake. Participant medical records were reviewed by study personnel to extract relevant health information which was not available from questionnaires, prior to breast milk analysis. SPT was undertaken using the following solutions: Histamine 1% Positive Control, Glycerol Negative Control, House Dust Mite (*Dermatophagoides pteronyssinus*), Cat (*Felix domesticus*), Grass Pollen, Birch pollen, Peanut, Hazelnut, Egg (all from Stallergenes, SA 92160 Anthony, France), and Cow's milk (ALK-Abello, Hørsholm, Denmark). SPT was performed by standard technique using 1 mm lancets (ALK-Abello, Hørsholm, Denmark), and were read at 15 min. Allergic sensitization was defined as a wheal $\geq$3 mm to at least one allergen, in the context of a wheal $\geq$3 mm to histamine and no wheal to the negative control.

2.3. Human Milk Sampling

Participants were given sterile tubes to collect their own colostrum (once in the first 6 days of life) and mature HM (once at 4–6 weeks postpartum). Instructions were given for collection of samples by manual expression or by collecting the drip from the contra-lateral breast during feeding [23]. Colostrum samples were frozen at −50 °C to −80 °C within 12 h of collection. HM samples were collected at home, transported to participating units by study staff, and frozen at −50 °C to −80 °C within 12 h of collection. It has been previously demonstrated that storage for 6 months at either −20 °C or −80 °C did not influence the concentration of immune active factors in human milk [24]. After thawing, samples were centrifuged at 1500× g for 15 min at 4 °C. The lipid layer was removed with a pipette and aqueous fraction was analysed for immune modulators [25]. All milk samples were transported to London at −70 °C where the samples were stored at −80 °C until analysis.

2.4. Electro-Chemiluminescence

We used electro-chemiluminescence to measure immune mediators in colostrum and breast milk samples for Th1 and Th2 cytokines, HGF, and TGFβ1-3 (MesoScale Discovery, Rockville, MD, USA). Laboratory experiments were run according to manufacturer's protocol, using an eight-point standard curve. Assays were run in duplicate with no dilution used for Th1 and Th2 cytokines (IL2, IL4, IL5, IL10, IFNγ, IL12, IL13) and HGF, and 1:2 dilution for TGFβ assays, following pilot experiments which showed that TGFβ2 levels in undiluted milk samples were often greater than the upper limit of detection. For TGFβ analysis, samples were acidified by the addition of 1N HCl to colostrum or mature milk. Acidified samples were then neutralised by addition of 20 μL of 1.2 NaOH, 0.5 HEPES. Assays were run in duplicate, and mediator levels were excluded where the CV was >25%.

2.5. Health Outcomes

The infants' health outcomes were assessed at the age of 6 months by means of a phone questionnaire and at one year of age by a questionnaire during the follow-up visit. All questions were carefully explained to the mothers. All health outcomes were self-reported by the mother except atopic sensitization which was assessed by skin prick test. Information on fever, wheeze, common cold, eczematous rash, reflux and vomiting cumulative incidence, food allergy/sensitivity or intolerance incidence were solicited.

Common cold was defined as at least one episode of runny nose or cold lasting for a minimum of 3 days. Cough/wheeze outcome was defined as at least one episode of recurrent cough or wheezing prior to assessment at one year of age. Eczema symptoms were considered present if the child had ever had a characteristic itchy eczematous rash intermittently at any time during the last 6 months. Parental-reported food allergy was defined as food allergy/sensitivity or intolerance incidence reported by the parents within the first 12 months of life. An infant was considered to be atopic if s/he had positive control wheal of ≥3 mm and any of the allergen-induced wheals being ≥3 mm greater than negative control.

For exclusive breastfeeding, the World Health Organisation (WHO) recommended definition "that the infant receives only breast milk" was used. No other liquids or solids are given—not even water—with the exception of oral rehydration solution, or drops/syrups of vitamins, minerals or medicines" [26].

2.6. Statistical Analysis

We assessed the probability of infants to develop particular health outcomes (presented as a binary variables) depending on potential determinant, using a binomial GLmulti (GLM) and LASSO (Least Absolute Shrinkage and Selection Operator) analyses. The resulting term importance was plotted in order to graphically visualize the effects of determinants. Such plots provide a graphical representation of importance estimate or relative evidence weight of candidate determinants. These weights are computed as the sum of the relative evidence weights of all possible models in which the term appears. Sensitivity analysis was performed for both methods and all models; a different number of variables were included to make sure that those selected had a real and credible effect on the outcome.

Health outcomes assessed using models were: fever, eczema, food allergy/sensitivity/intolerance assessed at 6 months. Common cold incidence, reflux and/or vomiting, and cough/wheeze were assessed both at 6 and 12 months. Influence of immune active molecules level in colostrum and mature

HM in conjunction with potential confounding factors was analysed in relation to health outcomes at the age of 6 and 12 months. The most reliable information was available for eczema, cough/wheeze and food allergy at 6 months and common cold at 12 months, these data were used as health outcomes for the statistical modelling.

The following determinants of health outcomes were included into the models: levels of growth factors in colostrum and mature human milk, detectability of cytokines in colostrum and breast milk, site of collection, colostrum collection time, maternal atopic status, delivery type, infant gender. Prior to inclusion, descriptive statistics, cross-tables, correlation and descriptive statistical tests were performed on each determinant to describe the importance of each variable and identify which may be the most useful in explaining and predicting a particular health outcome. Human milk immune active molecules assessed were presented as levels of HGF, TGFβ1, TGFβ2, TGFβ3, and cytokines (IL2, IL4, IL5, IL10, IFNγ, IL12, IL13) detectability. As cytokines are detected in human milk in low concentrations, data were transformed into binary variable (detectable vs. undetectable) to increase statistical analysis power. Data on cytokine detectability can be found elsewhere [21].

Statistical analysis was performed using R statistical package version 3.1.0 (R Core Team. R: A language and environment for statistical computing. R Foundation for Statistical Computing, Vienna, Austria). As a first step, univariate analysis and correlation matrix were used, followed by multivariate analysis which included modelling, using LASSO and GLM.

3. Results

3.1. Study Population

A total of 481 mothers were recruited into the study from June 2011 to March 2012 from the birth centres and antenatal and postnatal units of secondary and tertiary hospitals from three countries, located in Northern Europe, Eastern Europe, and the Mediterranean area. Of 481 women, 398 (UK $n = 101$, Russia $n = 221$, Italy $n = 76$) provided samples and were included in this study. The 83 mothers unwilling or unable to provide colostrum samples were not evaluated further.

Demographic data of the participants is described in full elsewhere [21]. Data on co-variates included into multivariate statistical analysis and health outcomes is presented in Table 1. Significant differences between groups were seen for most variables recorded. Maternal allergic sensitization (highest in UK), tobacco smoke exposure (highest in Russia), rate of infant allergic sensitisation (highest in Italy), parental-reported food allergy and common cold (highest in Russia), and parental-reported cough and wheeze (highest in UK), all differed significantly. Rates of maternal atopy, parity and infant gender did not differ for health outcomes assessed (Tables A1, A3, A5 and A7).

Table 1. Characteristics of study participants and health outcomes between sites of collection.

Characteristics	UK	Russia	Italy	p-Value (Three Countries)
Maternal allergic sensitisation *	35/94 (37)	22/156 (14)	9/40 (23)	<0.01 [a]
Male gender	54/101 (53)	118/216 (55)	41/76 (54)	0.98 [a]
Primiparous women	55/100 (55)	93/216 (43)	29/75 (39)	0.06 [a]
Household tobacco smoke exposure	30/99 (30)	135/218 (62)	25/76 (33)	<0.01 [a]
Parent-reported eczema	20/81 (25)	69/210 (33)	5/47 (11)	<0.01 [a]
Infant allergic sensitisation *	3/43 (7)	4/156 (3)	7/35 (20)	<0.01 [a]
Parent-reported food allergy	15/80 (19)	103/210 (49)	3/47 (6)	<0.01 [a]
Parent-reported common cold	50/101 (50)	117/221 (53)	28/74 (38)	<0.01 [a]
Parental-reported cough/wheeze	29/101 (37)	43/221 (21)	13/74 (28)	0.02 [a]

[a] Pearson χ^2 test has been used. Data shown are (n/(%)) for all binary variables presented; * Defined as skin prick test wheal $\geq$3 mm to at least one of a panel of common allergens.

3.2. Associations between Determinants and Infant Health Outcomes

When unadjusted levels of growth factors and detectability of cytokines were assessed, we found that detectable IL13 and IL2 in breast milk were significantly less often associated with eczema at 6 months. In contrast, TGFβ2 in breast milk was associated with eczema, but this did not reach statistical significance. Lower levels of HGF were found in colostrum of the mothers of infants who subsequently developed common cold at 12 months of age. No other factors were found to be associated with any health outcome (Tables A1–A8).

When multivariate analysis was performed, "Best" statistical model for each outcome highlighted those factors having the most significant influence on a particular outcome. All results are adjusted for the site of collection as a potential confounder. The average importance of the variables for a particular health outcome across all possible models visualised is shown in Figure 1. All factors found to be important at least in a single model and any significant associations with health outcomes are presented in Table 2.

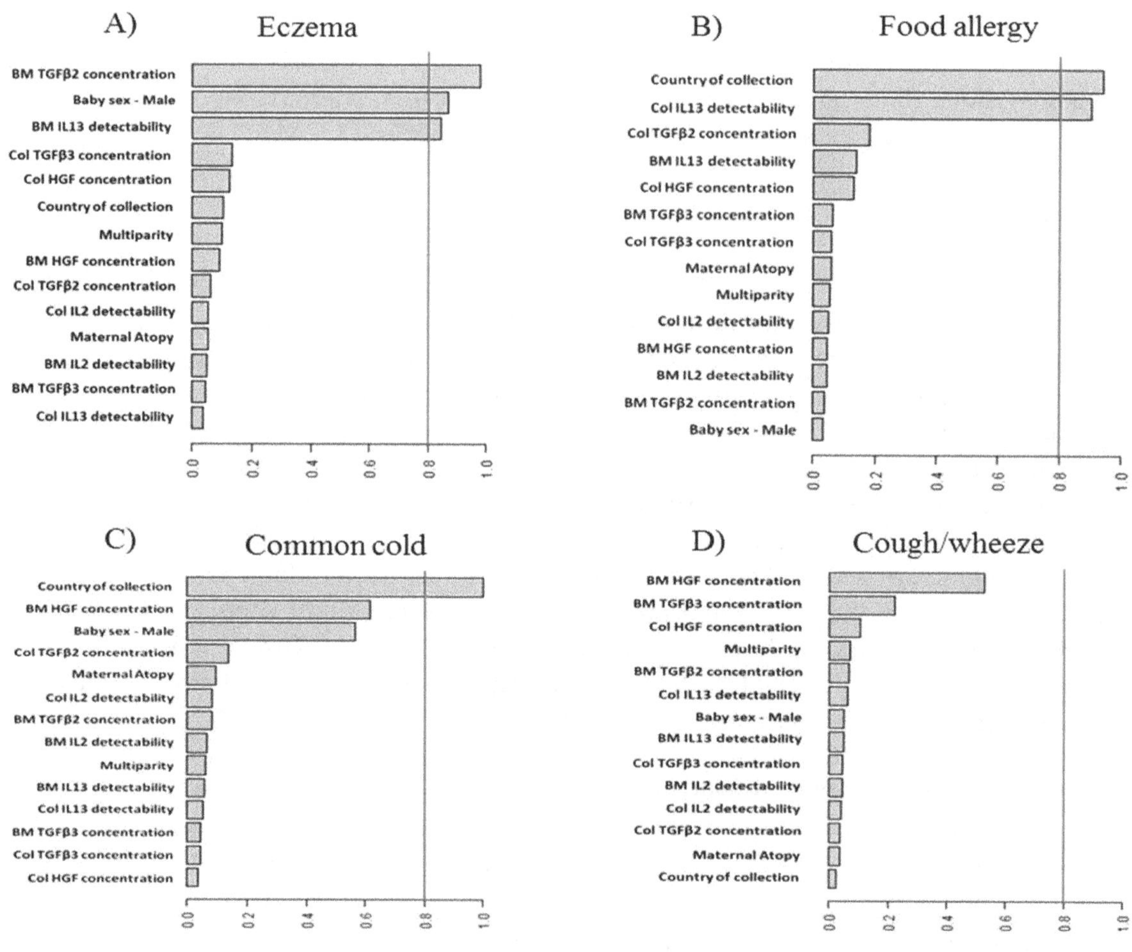

Figure 1. "Best" statistical model for each outcome: (**A**) eczema; (**B**) food allergy; (**C**) common cold; (**D**) cough/wheeze. Each model highlights those factors having the most significant influence on a particular outcome development, out of all determinants assessed. These are relative evidence weights of the covariates, with scale between 0 and 1.0 (equivalent of 0% to 100%). These weights are computed as the sum of the relative evidence weights of all models demonstrating presence of a particular determinant out of all models assessed in which the covariate appears. All results are adjusted. Col. stands for colostrum; BM-mature breast milk.

3.2.1. Associations between Maternal Factors/Environment and Health Outcomes

Maternal/environmental determinants reviewed were not found to be important for health outcomes development. At least one episode of common cold at the age of 12 months was reported less often OR 0.02 (95% CI 0.01–0.23) by mothers living in Moscow. Country of sample collection was not associated with parental-reported food allergy OR 0.13 (95% CI 0.01–1.46) and OR 2.07 (95% CI 0.47–9.02) for Verona and Moscow respectively.

3.2.2. Association between Collection Site and Colostrum/Breast Milk Composition

Among the studied variables, three were associated with eczema development at 6 months postpartum. Infants having breast milk with higher levels of TGFβ2 were at significantly higher risk OR 1.04 (95% CI 1.01–1.06) of eczema development. In contrast, if detectable levels of IL13 were present in HM, it was associated with a reduced risk OR 0.18 (95% CI 0.04–0.92) of eczema development. These results confirm the outcomes of the univariate analysis. In our cohort, boys tended to have eczema less often OR 0.2 (95% CI 0.05–0.84) compared with girls. Children fed colostrum with detectable levels of IL13 in colostrum were found to be less likely OR 0.1 (95% CI 0.01–0.83) associated with parental-reported food allergy at the age of 6 months.

HGF concentration in breast milk was associated with less common cold development OR 0.19 (95% CI 0.04–0.92). No determinants were found to be associated with cough/wheeze development at the age of 12 months. There is some tendency for HGF to be associated with a higher risk of cough or wheeze development, but results did not reach significance OR 1.89 (95% CI 0.94–3.78).

There was no association between any factor and infant allergic sensitisation at one year of age. It may be explained by a very small sample size as only 14 babies from the three cohorts developed allergic sensitisation.

Table 2. Factors found to be important at least in a single GLM model.

Health Outcome	HM TGFβ2 (ng/mL)	HM HGF (ng/mL)	Detectable HM IL13	Detectable Col IL 13	Sex Baby-Male	Verona	Moscow
Eczema (6 months)	**1.04 (1.01–1.06)**	NI	**0.18 (0.04–0.92)**	NI	**0.2 (0.05–0.84)**	NI	NI
Food allergy (6 months)	NI	NI	NI	**0.10 (0.01–0.83)**	NI	0.13 (0.01–1.46)	2.07 (0.47–9.02)
Cough or wheeze (6 months)	NI	1.89 (0.94–3.78)	NI	NI	NI	NI	NI
Common cold (12 months)	NI	**0.19 (0.04–0.92)**	NI	NI	**4.27 (1.08–16.90)**	NI	**0.02 (0.01–0.23)**

Average importance of the determinants for a particular health outcome during the first year of life, across all possible models. Data for exposures shown to be important presented as OR (95% CI). NI-determinant has not been found to be important for the particular health outcomes development. Statistically significant results presented in bold. GLM = GLmulti; HM = human milk; HGF = Hepatocyte growth factor; TGFβ = transforming growth factor β.

4. Discussion

Mothers from the three geographical regions studied live in very different environments, have differences in diet, lifestyle and it is necessary to take into account many factors which may potentially influence human milk composition as well as health outcomes. In contrast to other studies, we included a large number of potential determinants, adjusting the results to the site of collection as a potential confounder making the results more robust.

The aim of the study was to investigate whether peptide regulatory factors in human milk impacted infant health outcomes. Despite limitations, the results suggest that variability of human milk composition has an effect on parental-reported eczema, food allergy, and common cold development. The results support the concept that IL13 and HGF have protective effects and TGFβ2 may act as a risk factor, which may explain the diversity of results from epidemiological studies on the health-promoting effects of breastfeeding with regards to allergic diseases. Further, many studies attempted to evaluate colostrum and human milk composition influence on atopy and/or allergy development in the first years of life and produced conflicting results [23,27–29].

As TGFβ is an important regulatory cytokine suppressing both Th-1 and 2 activity, it appears counter-intuitive that high levels are associated with increased risk of eczema development. However, eczema is primarily a condition of impaired skin barrier function with allergic sensitization being a secondary phenomenon. Our findings suggest that higher concentrations of TGFβ2 in mature human milk are associated with significantly increased risk of eczema reported by the age of 12 months. Some studies support this observation, having found increased TGFβ1 and TGFβ2 in colostrum associated with the eczema onset in infants [6,28,29]. However, conflicting results have come from other studies [23,27,30–32]. It is not known why TGFβ might have an adverse effect on eczema, but it may be related to a particular isoform influence. A known classic example of TGFβ isoform differences has been observed in cutaneous scarring experiments done on animal models [33]. In these experiments mammalian embryos showed healing with no scarring and full skin recovery [34] with the expression of high levels of TGFβ3. In contrast, low levels of TGFβ1 and 2 [35] as well as similar TGFβ3 function have been demonstrated in human scarring physiology [36]. These pathways suppress immune surveillance in the skin such that infections break down the already genetically susceptible tissue. TGFβ family proteins are known for their diversity in biological functions, including migration of normal and abnormal cells, as shown in cancer research [37]. This may be a mechanism behind an association between the levels of TGFβ2 in HM and eczema. High concentrations of TGFβ2 may represent a biomarker that may predict risk of eczema in breastfed infants. This provides the initial inflammatory trigger to establish skin inflammation. Only a small number of children in our cohort were sensitized, which does not allow for an accurate assessment of a decreased barrier function; however, TGFβ may be impacting the skin barrier independent of allergy. However, the most likely explanation is that TGFβ in HM is a key factor, playing an important role in gut integrity maintenance as well as oral tolerance induction [38,39].

Detectable IL13 in mature milk reduced the risk of parent-reported eczematous rash development, whilst detectability of this cytokine in colostrum seems to have a similar association with food allergy/sensitivity/intolerance reported by the mothers at six months of age. This is the first study to report this association between IL13 in colostrum/human milk and eczema and/or food adverse events in children at 12 months of age. Eczema is not primarily an allergic condition but a heterogeneous disease. It may be speculated that a combination of TGFβ and IL13 may lead to TH1 responses impairment. The high IL-13 in colostrum fits well with the presumed impact on Immunoglobulin (Ig) E production but the counter effect of detectable levels in mature milk may be irrelevant as they are so low as to have little if any biological significance. Although maternal-reported events are a subjective measure and risk of bias is increased, these data should be validated on larger cohorts of high-risk infants.

Most studies agree that levels of other human milk immune active molecules, cytokines in particular, are not associated with atopy and/or allergy development in early life [23,27,29,30]. Only 14 infants developed allergic sensitisation in our cohort, which therefore provided insufficient statistical power to analyse for any associations.

Human milk has been shown to be beneficial for infants in part by providing high concentrations of immune active molecules which are associated with a decreased incidence of neonatal respiratory infections as well as long-term outcomes, such as wheeze and/or asthma [40]. Gdalevich and Mimouni provided a meta-analysis suggesting protective effects of exclusive breastfeeding in the first months of life on later asthma development [41]. However, the difficulty in combining data is that the wheeze/asthma phenotype differs between studies. Further, it is known that most early life wheezers do not subsequently develop persistent asthma.

Our data did not show any significant association of colostrum and/or HM immune active molecules with parent-reported cough or wheeze episodes at 12 months of age. It is known that a large proportion of infants suffer asymptomatic infections during the first year of life [42]. There was also no association between human milk composition and common cold reported at 6 months of age. However, when assessed at one year of age, HGF levels in HM were associated with reduced incidence of common cold reported at 12 months of age. HGF is known for its ability to provide protection during inflammatory diseases, directly targeting macrophages or lymphocytes [20]. Animal research showed that HGF administration stimulates intestinal cell proliferation resulting in intestinal growth induction [43]. HGF may well act in a similar fashion when transferred in high amounts into infants' gut. This finding shows that HGF as a component of human milk may not only play a very important role during the very first days of life, providing infant gut immunity development and maturation, but it is also capable of influencing long-term health outcomes. However, we cannot rule out a reversed causative relationship, due to the presence of common cold viruses which may lead woman to express higher quantities of HGF into their milk, in order to protect the offspring.

The main strength of this study is that it is one of the largest to date, assessing immune active molecules in colostrum and mature milk. The main limitation of this study is recruitment of women from the general population. As a consequence, very few babies developed eczema. According to UK working party criteria, recurrent rash development reported by the mother is not the most accurate and precise criteria to use. An apparent weakness of this study is that all immunological outcomes were reported by the parents and not based on healthcare professional diagnosis. Mothers tend to over-report health outcomes, such as food allergy in their children, but childhood eczema can be accurately reported by caregivers [44]. The same applies to common cold symptoms as retrospective parental reporting can be inaccurate. Another weakness is that health outcomes were reported by the parents at 6 and 12 months only, with most of the data coming from 6 months. We also did not collect HM on a multiple occasion at many time points, which would be required for the assessment of the actual intake of immune active molecules depending on the duration of breastfeeding.

Our data suggests that another factor substantially increasing the risk of eczematous rash development is the gender of the baby, with girls at higher risk. This result is in agreement with the International Study of Asthma and Allergies in Childhood (ISAAC) phase three data [45], although usually prevalence of eczema during the first year of life varies slightly when compared with older age groups. Differences in perception of eczema by women living in different countries and participating in our study could also play some role in reporting. Some of the previous studies have shown that gender long term does not seem to play a significant role in risk of developing atopy, eczema [42,46] and allergic rhino-conjunctivitis.

5. Conclusions

In this large international cohort study of HM immune composition, we found an important association between HM constituents and infant health outcome. Our hypothesis is at least in part confirmed but will require more detailed evaluation of environments. We have also confirmed that variations in levels peptide regulatory factors in human milk do associate with different infant health outcomes. As we focused on an un-selected general population cohort, the power to detect effects on allergy outcomes was limited. Despite this, higher TGFβ and IL13 did associate with eczema. This will require confirmation in a high-risk cohort and could indicate targets for trial of interventions to prevent atopic diseases.

Future research assessing human milk composition association with immunological health outcomes should include international collaborative studies with strict harmonisation of sampling, storage and analysis protocols between the sites. There is a need in studies, for evaluating human milk immune composition with samples collected at multiple time points prospectively. The only way forward is to bring different research groups together in an attempt to map human milk composition, highlighting differences between the countries and finding associations between human milk immunology and health outcomes.

Acknowledgments: We are grateful to the staff of birth centres and postnatal units involved, and all the women and their babies, participating in our study. D.M. is grateful to Charlotte's W5 staff for their patience. R.J.B. is supported by a National Institute for Health Research Biomedical Research Centre (BRC). Both J.O.W. and R.J.B. have received research grant income from Danone in relation to studies of the value of prebiotics in allergy prevention, and Airsonette to evaluate Temperature-controlled laminar airflow for asthma. J.O.W. is on a Danone, UCB and Airsonette scientific advisory board and both J.O.W. and R.J.B. have given paid lectures for the companies. D.M. has received consultancy payment from Dairy Goat Co-Operative (NZ) Ltd. and has given paid lectures for the MSD. D.T.G. receives an unrestricted research grant from Medela AG and has received travel funding and support for lectures. J.O.W. is supported by the NIHR CLAHRC for NW London and is its Early years theme lead. The views expressed in this paper are those of the authors and not the NIHR or Department of Health.

Author Contributions: J.O.W., R.J.B. and D.M. conceived and designed the experiments; D.M., S.D., L.Y.C. performed the experiments; D.M., L.Y.C. collected data in London; D.G.P. and A.L.B. collected data in Verona; M.T. and A.P. collected data in Moscow; S.C. analysed the data; D.M., D.T.G., R.J.B. and J.O.W. wrote the paper.

Appendix A

Table A1. Univariate analysis demonstrating demographic data and difference in colostrum and HM cytokine detectability for eczema as a health outcome.

Categorical Variables	No Eczema (n = 244)	Eczema (n = 94)	p-Value
	Demographics		
Positive maternal atopy	42 (22.2%)	16 (35.5%)	0.735
Gender (male)	122 (50.8%)	57 (61.3%)	0.111
Multiparity	137 (57.3%)	47 (98.6%)	0.422
	Immune active molecules		
Detectable HM IL13	45 (37.8%)	9 (23.8%)	0.002
Detectable Col IL13	52 (24.6%)	16 (36.8%)	0.598
Detectable HM IL2	31 (26.1%)	4 (10.6%)	0.001
Detectable Col IL2	33 (15.6%)	8 (18.4%)	0.355

Pearson χ^2 test or Fisher's exact test (if appropriate) were used for this analysis. Statistically significant differences ($p < 0.05$) appear in bold.

Table A2. Difference in crude levels of growth factors (ng/mL) for eczema as a health outcome.

Numeric Variables	No Eczema (n = 244)	Eczema (n = 94)	p-Value
HM TGFβ2, median (IQR)	13.57 (14.717)	17.48 (25.619)	0.087
Col TGFβ3, median (IQR)	1.52 (2.513)	2.04 (2.570)	0.169
Col HGF, median (IQR)	2.11 (5.239)	2.52 (6.540)	0.371
HM HGF, median (IQR)	0.79 (0.602)	0.76 (0.745)	0.834
Col TGFβ2, median (IQR)	41.80 (73.124)	47.69 (81.280)	0.663
HM TGFβ3, median (IQR)	0.254 (0.220)	0.302 (0.200)	0.663

Wilcoxon test was used for this analysis. Statistically significant differences ($p < 0.05$) appear in bold.

Table A3. Univariate analysis demonstrating demographic data and difference in colostrum and HM cytokine detectability for food allergy as a health outcome.

Categorical Variables	No Food Allergy (n = 216)	Food Allergy (n = 121)	p-Value
	Demographics		
Maternal atopy	44 (25.1%)	14 (14.7%)	0.067
Gender (male)	111 (51.9%)	67 (56.8%)	0.457
Multiparity	119 (56.7%)	63 (52.9%)	0.591
	Immune active molecules		
Detectable HM IL13	33 (33.7%)	21 (25.9%)	0.337
Detectable Col IL2	46 (25.1%)	22 (21.4%)	0.565
Detectable HM IL2	22 (22.4%)	13 (16.0%)	0.376
Detectable Col IL13	24 (13.0%)	17 (16.5%)	0.530

Pearson χ^2 test or Fisher's exact test (if appropriate) were used for this analysis. Statistically significant differences ($p < 0.05$) appear in bold.

Table A4. Difference in crude levels of growth factors (ng/mL) for food allergy as a health outcome.

Numeric Variables	No Food Allergy (n = 216)	Food Allergy (n = 121)	p-Value
HM TGFβ2, median (IQR)	13.765 (24.656)	13.616 (12.434)	0.984
Col TGFβ3, median (IQR)	1.718 (2.704)	1.531 (1.854)	0.494
Col HGF, median (IQR)	2.082 (5.436)	2.419 (6.199)	0.437
HM HGF, median (IQR)	0.843 (0.769)	0.731 (0.539)	0.066
Col TGFβ2, median (IQR)	0.289 (0.216)	0.275 (0.207)	0.909
HM_TGFβ3, median (IQR)	0.289 (0.216)	0.275 (0.207)	0.909

Wilcoxon test was used for this analysis. Statistically significant differences ($p < 0.05$) appear in bold.

Table A5. Univariate analysis demonstrating demographic data and difference in colostrum and HM cytokine detectability for cough/wheeze as a health outcome.

Categorical Vars	No Cough/Wheeze (n = 251)	Cough/Wheeze (n = 85)	p-Value
	Demographics		
Positive maternal atopy	38 (19.7%)	18 (24.0%)	0.541
Gender (male)	128 (51.4%)	48 (58.5%)	0.320
Multiparity	132 (54.3%)	50 (58.8%)	0.554
	Immune active molecules		
Detectable HM IL13	40 (29.4%)	14 (33.3%)	0.771
Detectable Col IL2	51 (24.4%)	17 (22.1%)	0.849
Detectable HM IL2	26 (19.1%)	9 (21.4%)	0.825
Detectable Col IL13	31 (14.8%)	10 (13.0%)	0.800

Pearson χ^2 test or Fisher's exact test (if appropriate) were used for this analysis. Statistically significant differences ($p < 0.05$) appear in bold.

Table A6. Difference in crude levels of growth factors (ng/mL) for cough/wheeze as a health outcome.

Numeric Vars	No Cough/Wheeze (n = 251)	Cough/Wheeze (n = 85)	p-Value
HM TGFβ2, median (IQR)	12.891 (15.595)	21.725 (20.910)	0.090
Col TGFβ3, median (IQR)	1.523 (1.932)	1.890 (3.2648)	0.193
Col HGF, median (IQR)	2.115 (5.413)	2.337 (6.36)	0.564
HM HGF, median (IQR)	0.729 (0.615)	0.859 (0.769)	0.153
Col TGFβ2, median (IQR)	41.274 (64.585)	54.094 (96.060)	0.283
HM_TGFβ3, median (IQR)	0.274 (0.200)	0.314 (0.395)	0.283

Wilcoxon test was used for this analysis. Statistically significant differences ($p < 0.05$) appear in bold.

Table A7. Univariate analysis demonstrating demographic data and difference in colostrum and HM cytokine detectability for common cold as a health outcome.

Categorical Vars	No Common Cold (n = 143)	Common Cold (n = 130)	p-Value
	Demographics		
Positive maternal atopy	20 (19.0%)	26 (24.1%)	0.469
Gender (male)	76 (54.3%)	69 (53.9%)	1.000
Multiparity	81 (57.9%)	66 (52.0%)	0.399
	Immune active molecules		
Detectable HM IL13	28 (31.5%)	13 (21.3%)	0.237
Detectable Col IL2	27 (22.5%)	28 (25.9%)	0.862
Detectable HM IL2	16 (18.0%)	8 (13.1%)	0.501
Detectable Col IL13	20 (16.5%)	16 (14.8%)	0.654

Pearson χ^2 test or Fisher's exact test (if appropriate) were used for this analysis. Statistically significant differences ($p < 0.05$) appear in bold.

Table A8. Difference in crude levels of growth factors (ng/mL) for common cold as a health outcome.

Numeric Vars	No Common Cold (n = 143)	Common Cold (n = 130)	p-Value
HM TGFβ2, median (IQR)	13.0121 (11.823)	15.67338 (24.983)	0.324
Col TGFβ3, median (IQR)	1.9393452 (2.453)	1.7625169 (4.183)	0.977
Col HGF, median (IQR)	3.4656324 (8.459)	1.997605 (5.249)	0.009
HM HGF, median (IQR)	0.7281423 (0.660)	0.8027212 (0.556)	0.910
Col TGFβ2, median (IQR)	44.1042 (71.380)	42.36296 (77.730)	0.462
HM_TGFβ3, median (IQR)	0.288506 (0.216)	0.2748667 (0.207)	0.909

Wilcoxon test was used for this analysis. Statistically significant differences ($p < 0.05$) appear in bold.

References

1. Mallol, J.; Crane, J.; von Mutius, E.; Odhiambo, J.; Keil, U.; Stewart, A. The international study of asthma and allergies in childhood (ISAAC) phase three: A global synthesis. *Allergol. Immunopathol.* **2013**, *41*, 73–85. [CrossRef] [PubMed]
2. Prescott, S.L. *The Allergy Epidemic: A Mystery of Modern Life*; UWA Publishing: Perth, Australia, 2011.
3. Thorburn, A.N.; Macia, L.; Mackay, C.R. Diet, metabolites, and "western-lifestyle" inflammatory diseases. *Immunity* **2014**, *40*, 833–842. [CrossRef] [PubMed]
4. D'Alessandro, A.; Scaloni, A.; Zolla, L. Human milk proteins: An interactomics and updated functional overview. *J. Rroteome Res.* **2010**, *9*, 3339–3373. [CrossRef] [PubMed]
5. Agarwal, S.; Karmaus, W.; Davis, S.; Gangur, V. Immune markers in breast milk and fetal and maternal body fluids: A systematic review of perinatal concentrations. *J. Hum. Lact.* **2011**, *27*, 171–186. [CrossRef] [PubMed]
6. Kalliomaki, M.; Ouwehand, A.; Arvilommi, H.; Kero, P.; Isolauri, E. Transforming growth factor-beta in breast milk: A potential regulator of atopic disease at an early age. *J. Allergy Clin. Immunol.* **1999**, *104*, 1251–1257. [CrossRef]
7. Penttila, I.A.; Flesch, I.E.; McCue, A.L.; Powell, B.C.; Zhou, F.H.; Read, L.C.; Zola, H. Maternal milk regulation of cell infiltration and interleukin 18 in the intestine of suckling rat pups. *Gut* **2003**, *52*, 1579–1586. [CrossRef] [PubMed]
8. Ogawa, J.; Sasahara, A.; Yoshida, T.; Sira, M.M.; Futatani, T.; Kanegane, H.; Miyawaki, T. Role of transforming growth factor-beta in breast milk for initiation of IgA production in newborn infants. *Early Hum. Dev.* **2004**, *77*, 67–75. [CrossRef] [PubMed]
9. Ando, T.; Hatsushika, K.; Wako, M.; Ohba, T.; Koyama, K.; Ohnuma, Y.; Katoh, R.; Ogawa, H.; Okumura, K.; Luo, J.; et al. Orally administered TGFβ is biologically active in the intestinal mucosa and enhances oral tolerance. *J. Allergy Clin. Immunol.* **2007**, *120*, 916–923. [CrossRef] [PubMed]
10. Oddy, W.H.; Rosales, F. A systematic review of the importance of milk TGFβ on immunological outcomes in the infant and young child. *Pediatr. Allergy Immunol.* **2010**, *21*, 47–59. [CrossRef] [PubMed]
11. Garofalo, R. Cytokines in human milk. *J. Pediatr.* **2010**, *156*, S36–S40. [CrossRef] [PubMed]
12. Kobata, R.; Tsukahara, H.; Ohshima, Y.; Ohta, N.; Tokuriki, S.; Tamura, S.; Mayumi, M. High levels of growth factors in human breast milk. *Early Hum. Dev.* **2008**, *84*, 67–69. [CrossRef] [PubMed]
13. Nguyen, T.V.; Yuan, L.; Azevedo, M.S.; Jeong, K.I.; Gonzalez, A.M.; Saif, L.J. Transfer of maternal cytokines to suckling piglets: In vivo and in vitro models with implications for immunomodulation of neonatal immunity. *Vet. Immunol. Immunopathol.* **2007**, *117*, 236–248. [CrossRef] [PubMed]
14. Hasselbalch, H.; Engelmann, M.D.; Ersboll, A.K.; Jeppesen, D.L.; Fleischer-Michaelsen, K. Breast-feeding influences thymic size in late infancy. *Eur. J. Pediatr.* **1999**, *158*, 964–967. [CrossRef] [PubMed]
15. Goldman, A.S. Modulation of the gastrointestinal tract of infants by human milk. Interfaces and interactions. An evolutionary perspective. *J. Nutr.* **2000**, *130*, S426–S431.
16. Yamada, Y.; Saito, S.; Morikawa, H. Hepatocyte growth factor in human breast milk. *Am. J. Reprod. Immunol.* **1998**, *40*, 112–120. [CrossRef] [PubMed]
17. Srivastava, M.D.; Lippes, J.; Srivastava, B.I. Hepatocyte growth factor in human milk and reproductive tract fluids. *Am. J. Reprod. Immunol.* **1999**, *42*, 347–354. [CrossRef] [PubMed]
18. Ito, W.; Kanehiro, A.; Matsumoto, K.; Hirano, A.; Ono, K.; Maruyama, H.; Kataoka, M.; Nakamura, T.; Gelfand, E.W.; Tanimoto, M. Hepatocyte growth factor attenuates airway hyperresponsiveness, inflammation, and remodeling. *Am. J. Respir. Cell Mol. Biol.* **2005**, *32*, 268–280. [CrossRef] [PubMed]

19. Okunishi, K.; Sasaki, O.; Okasora, T.; Nakagome, K.; Imamura, M.; Harada, H.; Matsumoto, T.; Tanaka, R.; Yamamoto, K.; Tabata, Y.; et al. Intratracheal delivery of hepatocyte growth factor directly attenuates allergic airway inflammation in mice. *Int. Arch. Allergy Immunol.* **2009**, *149* (Suppl. S1), 14–20. [CrossRef] [PubMed]
20. Nakamura, T.; Mizuno, S. The discovery of hepatocyte growth factor (HGF) and its significance for cell biology, life sciences and clinical medicine. *Proc. Jpn. Acad. Ser. B Phys. Biol. Sci.* **2010**, *86*, 588–610. [CrossRef] [PubMed]
21. Munblit, D.; Treneva, M.; Peroni, D.G.; Colicino, S.; Chow, L.; Dissanayeke, S.; Abrol, P.; Sheth, S.; Pampura, A.; Boner, A.L.; et al. Colostrum and mature human milk of women from London, Moscow, and Verona: Determinants of immune composition. *Nutrients* **2016**, *8*, 695. [CrossRef] [PubMed]
22. Munblit, D.; Boyle, R.J.; Warner, J.O. Factors affecting breast milk composition and potential consequences for development of the allergic phenotype. *Clin. Exp. Allergy* **2015**, *45*, 583–601. [CrossRef] [PubMed]
23. Snijders, B.E.; Damoiseaux, J.G.; Penders, J.; Kummeling, I.; Stelma, F.F.; van Ree, R.; van den Brandt, P.A.; Thijs, C. Cytokines and soluble CD14 in breast milk in relation with atopic manifestations in mother and infant (KOALA study). *Clin. Exp. Allergy* **2006**, *36*, 1609–1615. [CrossRef] [PubMed]
24. Ramirez-Santana, C.; Perez-Cano, F.J.; Audi, C.; Castell, M.; Moretones, M.G.; Lopez-Sabater, M.C.; Castellote, C.; Franch, A. Effects of cooling and freezing storage on the stability of bioactive factors in human colostrum. *J. Dairy Sci.* **2012**, *95*, 2319–2325. [CrossRef] [PubMed]
25. Jones, C.A.; Holloway, J.A.; Popplewell, E.J.; Diaper, N.D.; Holloway, J.W.; Vance, G.H.; Warner, J.A.; Warner, J.O. Reduced soluble CD14 levels in amniotic fluid and breast milk are associated with the subsequent development of atopy, eczema, or both. *J. Allergy Clin. Immunol.* **2002**, *109*, 858–866. [CrossRef] [PubMed]
26. WHO. *Infant and young child feeding*; World Health Organization: Geneva, Switzerland, 2009.
27. Bottcher, M.F.; Jenmalm, M.C.; Bjorksten, B. Cytokine, chemokine and secretory IgA levels in human milk in relation to atopic disease and IgA production in infants. *Pediatr. Allergy Immunol.* **2003**, *14*, 35–41. [CrossRef] [PubMed]
28. Bottcher, M.F.; Abrahamsson, T.R.; Fredriksson, M.; Jakobsson, T.; Bjorksten, B. Low breast milk TGFβ2 is induced by lactobacillus reuteri supplementation and associates with reduced risk of sensitization during infancy. *Pediatr. Allergy Immunol.* **2008**, *19*, 497–504. [CrossRef] [PubMed]
29. Kuitunen, M.; Kukkonen, A.K.; Savilahti, E. Impact of maternal allergy and use of probiotics during pregnancy on breast milk cytokines and food antibodies and development of allergy in children until 5 years. *Int. Arch. Allergy Immunol.* **2012**, *159*, 162–170. [CrossRef] [PubMed]
30. Ismail, I.H.; Licciardi, P.V.; Oppedisano, F.; Boyle, R.J.; Tang, M.L. Relationship between breast milk sCD14, TGFβ1 and total IgA in the first month and development of eczema during infancy. *Pediatr. Allergy Immunol.* **2013**, *24*, 352–360. [CrossRef] [PubMed]
31. Orivuori, L.; Loss, G.; Roduit, C.; Dalphin, J.C.; Depner, M.; Genuneit, J.; Lauener, R.; Pekkanen, J.; Pfefferle, P.; Riedler, J.; et al. Soluble immunoglobulin a in breast milk is inversely associated with atopic dermatitis at early age: The pasture cohort study. *Clin. Exp. Allergy* **2014**, *44*, 102–112. [CrossRef] [PubMed]
32. Joseph, C.L.; Havstad, S.; Bobbitt, K.; Woodcroft, K.; Zoratti, E.M.; Nageotte, C.; Misiak, R.; Enberg, R.; Nicholas, C.; Ezell, J.M.; et al. Transforming growth factor beta (TGFβ1) in breast milk and indicators of infant atopy in a birth cohort. *Pediatr. Allergy. Immunol.* **2014**, *25*, 257–263. [CrossRef] [PubMed]
33. Ferguson, M.W.; O'Kane, S. Scar-free healing: From embryonic mechanisms to adult therapeutic intervention. *Philo. Trans. R. Soc. Lond. B Biol. Sci.* **2004**, *359*, 839–850. [CrossRef] [PubMed]
34. Whitby, D.J.; Ferguson, M.W. Immunohistochemical localization of growth factors in fetal wound healing. *Dev. Biol.* **1991**, *147*, 207–215. [CrossRef]
35. Whitby, D.J.; Ferguson, M.W. The extracellular matrix of lip wounds in fetal, neonatal and adult mice. *Development* **1991**, *112*, 651–668. [PubMed]
36. Ferguson, M.W.; Duncan, J.; Bond, J.; Bush, J.; Durani, P.; So, K.; Taylor, L.; Chantrey, J.; Mason, T.; James, G.; et al. Prophylactic administration of avotermin for improvement of skin scarring: Three double-blind, placebo-controlled, phase I/II studies. *Lancet* **2009**, *373*, 1264–1274. [CrossRef]
37. Yokobori, T.; Nishiyama, M. TGFβ signaling in gastrointestinal cancers: Progress in basic and clinical research. *J. Clin. Med.* **2017**, *6*, 11. [CrossRef] [PubMed]
38. Verhasselt, V. Neonatal tolerance under breastfeeding influence. *Curr. Opin. Immunol.* **2010**, *22*, 623–630. [CrossRef] [PubMed]

39. Munblit, D.; Verhasselt, V. Allergy prevention by breastfeeding: Possible mechanisms and evidence from human cohorts. *Curr. Opin. Allergy Clin. Immunol.* **2016**, *16*, 427–433. [CrossRef] [PubMed]
40. Dixon, D.L. The role of human milk immunomodulators in protecting against viral bronchiolitis and development of chronic wheezing illness. *Children (Basel)* **2015**, *2*, 289–304. [CrossRef] [PubMed]
41. Gdalevich, M.; Mimouni, D.; Mimouni, M. Breast-feeding and the risk of bronchial asthma in childhood: A systematic review with meta-analysis of prospective studies. *J. Pediatr.* **2001**, *139*, 261–266. [CrossRef] [PubMed]
42. Chonmaitree, T.; Alvarez-Fernandez, P.; Jennings, K.; Trujillo, R.; Marom, T.; Loeffelholz, M.J.; Miller, A.L.; McCormick, D.P.; Patel, J.A.; Pyles, R.B. Symptomatic and asymptomatic respiratory viral infections in the first year of life: Association with acute otitis media development. *Clin. Infect. Dis.* **2015**, *60*, 1–9. [CrossRef] [PubMed]
43. Dasgupta, S.; Arya, S.; Choudhary, S.; Jain, S.K. Amniotic fluid: Source of trophic factors for the developing intestine. *World J. Gastrointest Pathophysiol.* **2016**, *7*, 38–47. [CrossRef] [PubMed]
44. Silverberg, J.I.; Patel, N.; Immaneni, S.; Rusniak, B.; Silverberg, N.B.; Debashis, R.; Fewkes, N.; Simpson, E.L. Assessment of atopic dermatitis using self- and caregiver- report: A multicenter validation study. *Br. J. Dermatol.* **2015**, *135*, S53. [CrossRef] [PubMed]
45. Odhiambo, J.A.; Williams, H.C.; Clayton, T.O.; Robertson, C.F.; Asher, M.I.; Group, I.P.T.S. Global variations in prevalence of eczema symptoms in children from ISAAC phase three. *J. Allergy Clin. Immunol.* **2009**, *124*, 1251–1258. [CrossRef] [PubMed]
46. Schafer, T.; Heinrich, J.; Wjst, M.; Krause, C.; Adam, H.; Ring, J.; Wichmann, H.E. Indoor risk factors for atopic eczema in school children from east germany. *Environ. Res.* **1999**, *81*, 151–158. [CrossRef] [PubMed]

9

Food Processing: The Influence of the Maillard Reaction on Immunogenicity and Allergenicity of Food Proteins

Malgorzata Teodorowicz [1,2,*], Joost van Neerven [1,3] and Huub Savelkoul [1,2]

[1] Cell Biology and Immunology Group, Wageningen University & Research, 6708 WD Wageningen, The Netherlands; joost.vanneerven@frieslandcampina.com (J.v.N.); huub.savelkoul@wur.nl (H.S.)

[2] Allergy Consortium Wageningen, Wageningen University & Research, 6708 WD Wageningen, The Netherlands

[3] FrieslandCampina, 3818 LE Amersfoort, The Netherlands

* Correspondence: gosia.teodorowicz@wur.nl

Abstract: The majority of foods that are consumed in our developed society have been processed. Processing promotes a non-enzymatic reaction between proteins and sugars, the Maillard reaction (MR). Maillard reaction products (MRPs) contribute to the taste, smell and color of many food products, and thus influence consumers' choices. However, in recent years, MRPs have been linked to the increasing prevalence of diet- and inflammation-related non-communicable diseases including food allergy. Although during the last years a better understanding of immunogenicity of MRPs has been achieved, still only little is known about the structural/chemical characteristics predisposing MRPs to interact with antigen presenting cells (APCs). This report provides a comprehensive review of recent studies on the influence of the Maillard reaction on the immunogenicity and allergenicity of food proteins.

Keywords: Maillard reaction; advanced glycation end products (AGEs); Maillard reaction products (MRPs); immunogenicity of AGEs; allergenicity of AGEs; Maillard reaction in food

1. Food Processing

Most of the food consumed nowadays by developed societies is processed. The diversity of processed food products increased exponentially during the last century, along with the need for more safe, convenient and varied food products. Methods used for food processing can be categorized into two processing types: conventional thermal methods, including pasteurization, sterilization, drying and roasting [4,5] and non-thermal, novel methods such as high pressure treatment [6], electric field treatment [7,8], irradiation [9] or applications of cold plasma [10]. Foods are subjected to thermal processing mainly to preserve them by inactivating microbes (high temperature treatment), to improve their sensory qualities (e.g., flavor, texture, taste, and smell) or to obtain another food product or ingredient from a food source (e.g., protein isolates, cheese, oils). From a biochemical perspective, thermal processing promotes chemical and physical changes of food proteins, and affects protein conformation—and therefore also immunogenicity and allergenicity—by promoting interactions of food proteins with other components present in the food matrix.

2. Thermal Processing Induces Conformational Changes in Food Proteins

Native proteins are folded into specific and compact 3D structures. This is determined by primary structure (sequence of amino acids), secondary structure (formation of α-helixes and β-sheets) and tertiary structure. The formation of α-helixes and β-sheets is driven by interactions between polypeptide chains linked together by hydrophobic and hydrophilic interactions, electrostatic interactions and disulfide bonds [11]. All these chemical interactions create a unique protein conformation that is reorganized at all structural levels during heat treatment. Changes in α-helix and β-sheet structures start to occur at heating temperatures above 55 °C, and almost complete loss of secondary and tertiary structure as well as cleavage of disulfide bonds occurs at temperatures above 70–80 °C [12,13]. At the same time, because of protein denaturation, irreversible intermolecular interactions may result in protein aggregation and cross-linking reactions between amino acids, e.g., through formation of lysinoalanine (LAL) [14]. These heat-induced conformational changes of food proteins may further affect digestion and absorption of proteins/peptides by the intestinal epithelium, as well as their recognition by immune cells. Moreover, if sugars are present during the heat treatment, the free amino groups of side chains of amino acids can be blocked due to the Maillard reaction [11,13].

3. The Maillard Reaction in Food Processing

One of the best-known interactions between proteins and sugars occurring during heat processing of food is the Maillard reaction (MR), also known as glycation. During the MR, sugars are linked to proteins by a covalent bond between free amino groups of amino acids (mostly lysine and arginine) and the carbonyl groups of a reducing sugar (simplified scheme on Figure 1).

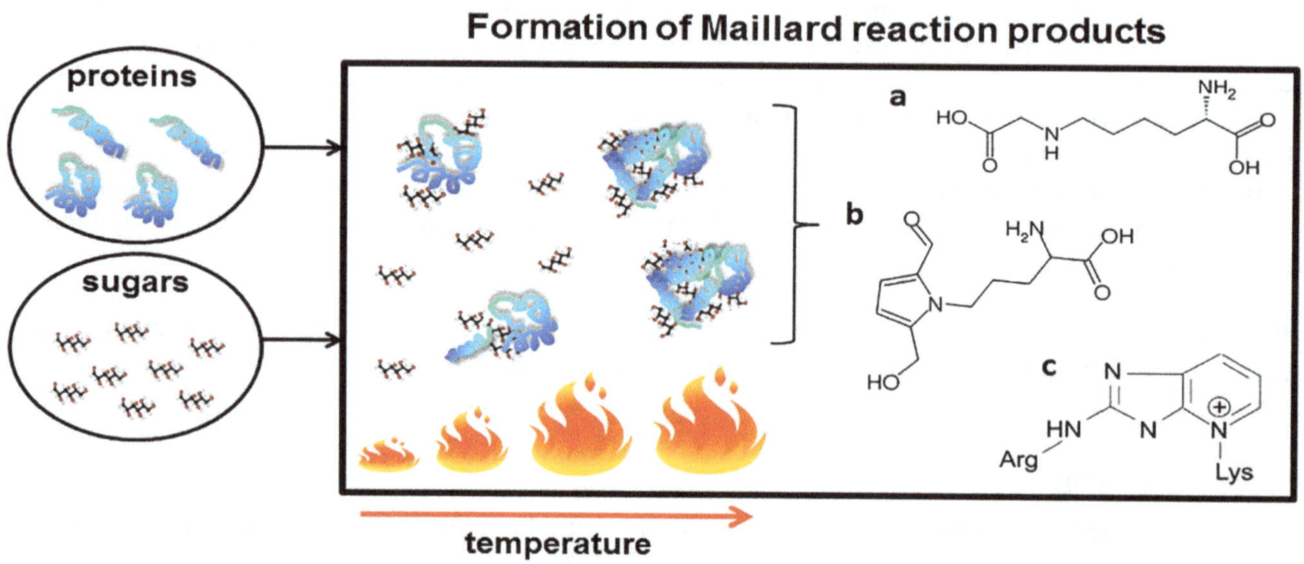

Figure 1. Simplified scheme of the formation of Maillard reaction product during food processing. Amadori rearrangement leads to the formation of a number of advanced glycation end products, among others: (a) Nε-(carboxymethyl)lysine; (b) pyrraline and (c) pentosidine.

The MR occurs naturally during regular food processing and meal preparation (cooking, frying, and baking) [15–17]. However, the chemistry of the reaction is extremely complex. A cascade of chemical rearrangements including condensation, oxidation and hydration, leads to formation of numerous Maillard reaction products (MRPs). The Schiff bases formed as the first products of the reaction are followed by their Amadori rearrangement and subsequent oxidative modifications (glycoxidations) resulting in the formation of advanced glycation end products (AGEs). The chemical nature of many of the AGEs is unknown due to their heterogeneous and unstable nature. However, a growing number of structurally defined AGEs such as pyrraline, pentosidine and Nε-carboxymethyllysine (CML) have been found in processed food [18,19].

Moreover, the type and amounts of MRPs formed are under the control of factors such as the structural diversity of (poly)saccharides and proteins, reaction temperature and time, ratio of amino group and reducing sugar, pH and water activity [15,20]. MRPs are known to confer functional characteristics to food proteins such as appearance, smell, taste and texture. For this reason, the MR is a relevant reaction for consumers therefore also for the food industry [17,21]. In addition to functional changes of proteins, many studies in the last decade have revealed that the MR also affects biological properties of food proteins such as their digestibility, bioavailability, immunogenicity and consequently their allergenicity. Biochemical and conformational changes of proteins caused by MR may result in masking of existing antibody binding epitopes, but also in creating new structures that are more immunogenic and are thus able to promote the initiation of IgE-mediated allergies [22–25].

4. Influence of Maillard Reaction of Digestibility of Proteins

In order to elicit an allergic immune response, food proteins (or peptides thereof) must survive digestion and remain in the gastrointestinal tract for a period of time that is sufficient to induce sensitization. From that perspective, the susceptibility of food proteins to enzymatic hydrolysis seems to be an important factor determining their allergenicity [26–28]. Even so, not all food allergens are resistant to digestion [29,30]. As described above, both heating and the MR can alter the susceptibility of proteins to gastrointestinal digestion due to unfolding, heat-induced disulfide bond interchanges, aggregation, the formation of lactulosyllysine, and formation of AGEs, thereby affecting the availability of enzymatic cleavage sites on the protein backbone.

Heating itself causes unfolding of protein and exposure of linear epitopes and may result in enhanced susceptibility to enzymatic proteolysis as described for β-lactoglobulin heated at the temperature of 90 °C [31]. However, Corzo-Martínez and colleagues demonstrated that denaturation and aggregation of heated β-lactoglobulin caused by MR led to decreased β-LG proteolysis [32]. A band corresponding to intact β-LG was observed on SDS-PAGE picture after trypsin/chymotrypsin digestion of β-LG glycated with galactose and tagatose at 40 °C for one day, even after 1 h of digestion. Resistance to gastrointestinal digestion was more evident in β-LG glycated with galactose than tagatose which was shown previously to be a less efficient sugar in formation of MRPs [33]. Therefore, the results of that study revealed that higher degrees of glycation of bovine β-LG lead to a higher resistance to proteolysis. This could be explained by lower susceptibility of glycated lysine and arginine residues to trypsin/chymotrypsin proteolysis by masking the sites of cleavage [18]. In addition, Maillard reaction-induced protein aggregates may protect proteins during in vitro gastrointestinal digestion, which was shown by inhibition of aggregation of β-LG in the presence of pyridoxamine [32], an effective inhibitor of formation of MRPs on all stages [34]. Those results are in line with a number of other studies that demonstrated impaired enzymatic hydrolysis in vitro due to the MR observed together with decreased protein solubility caused by denaturation, structural rearrangements and aggregation of proteins heated with sugar [25,35–37]. In contrast, glycation has also been reported to increase protein solubility [38,39] as well as protein digestibility as it has been shown for lysozyme [40] and codfish parvalbumin [41], suggesting that an effect of MR on protein digestibility may be connected with structural characteristic of the protein that is studied. Moreover, the diversity of conditions used for glycation in the different experiments as pH, time of heating, temperature of heating, ionic strength of the medium, water activity and type of sugar may also explain the disparity often observed in the literature on the influence of MR on protein digestibility. Liu and colleagues showed that the glycation of whey proteins at different conditions of water activity and pH alternates the peptide profiles observed on HPLC chromatograms [42]. The local environment of lysine changes in differently unfolded proteins at pH 5, 7 or 9, which affected the susceptibility for glycation, the type of formed MRPs (e.g., formation of agglomerates), and subsequently modified the protease action, resulting in a different peptide composition after enzymatic hydrolysis [42].

The number of studies involving in vivo experiments investigating an effect of MR on digestibility of food proteins is limited to date. A recently published study performed on humans compared the effects of diets with different MRP contents on dietary protein utilization in adolescent males. The study revealed that a diet high in the MRPs limits the digestibility of proteins since 47% higher fecal nitrogen excretion, 12% lower apparent nitrogen absorption and 6% lower nitrogen digestibility was observed in the group consuming diet high in MRPs [43]. Hellwig and colleagues [44] have shown that the human colonic microbiota are able to degrade the following MRPs: Nε-fructosyllysine, CML and pyrraline. This suggests that the released glycated peptides and amino acids may be used by microbes as the source of energy or can be transported via intestinal barrier as it was proposed for small pyrraline peptides [45]. This shows the relevance of microbiota in the degradation process of Maillard reaction-modified proteins and therefore also their absorption in the intestine.

5. Absorption of MRPs in Intestine

The question if the glycated protein/peptide can have immunological effect in vivo depends on whether these molecules are available in the gastrointestinal mucosa to be absorbed into the circulation and subsequently to get in contact with the immune system. Dietary MPRs were shown to appear in the circulation and/or urine of human subjects after consumption of MRPs rich diet [18,46–52]. The study performed by Hellwig and colleagues on glycated casein samples revealed that fructoselysine and (CML) are released after digestion bound to peptides smaller than 1000 Da, which makes them available for absorption [52]. This was confirmed in the studies performed in the rat model showing that advanced MRP such as CML, pyrraline and pentosidine may be absorbed by the gut. Ingested dietary CML in rats appeared to be approximately 26.0–29.0% excreted in the urine, and 15.0–22.0% excreted in feces [14,53]. Approximately 1.7% of dietary CML accumulated in the circulation, kidney and liver and approximately 50.0% of the ingested CML was not recovered. This was later confirmed in a human study where 31.2% of ingested dietary CML was excreted in the feces, 14.4% in the urine, and 54.4% left unrecovered [48]. More than 60% of dietary pyrraline and approximately 2.0% of dietary pentosidine were excreted in urine in humans [49,50]. Different percentage of recovery of total diet amount of AGEs found in urine suggest different resorption and metabolic pathways of individual Maillard products [50]. In addition, LAL, a compound formed by cross-linking of protein, was found in the urine, plasma, liver and kidneys of rats fed with the diet with low and high LAL-content [14] although it has been reported to be released during digestion process into larger peptides of at least 30–40 amino acids [52].

Cross-linking of proteins seems to reduce an epithelial uptake of proteins although promote an uptake through Peyer's patches as was shown for crossed-linked β-lactoglobulin and α-lactalbumin [54,55]. In addition, the larger agglomerates, as well as other MRPs can be further metabolised by intestinal microbes [44,56,57] resulting in formation of new bioactive compounds but also modulating the intestinal microbiota composition in humans [58,59]. The fact that the dietary protein-bond AGEs, such as CML, pentosidine and pyrraline, are available in the gastrointestinal tract and circulation means that they can also interact with the immune cells.

6. Influence of Maillard Reaction on Immunogenicity of Proteins

6.1. MR-Modified Proteins and Allergic Sensitization

Even though the role of AGEs in chronic inflammatory diseases is more well-known and studied [47,60,61], evidence is emerging that AGEs also play a role in allergy. As this paper focuses on allergy, the role of AGEs in chronic inflammation will not be discussed in details.

Allergy is commonly divided in two phases. An initial phase of allergic sensitization represents principally a particular immune reaction leading to the formation of allergen-specific IgE antibodies. IgE antibodies can crosslink adjacent cell-bound IgE molecules on basophils and mast cells upon repeated exposure to allergens, leading to degranulation and the release of mediators, including histamine, prostaglandins, leukotriens and tromboxanes. These mediators cause the typical symptoms of a type 1 (within 20 min) IgE-mediated allergy, including rhinitis, atopic dermatitis, allergic asthma, and occasionally even anaphylaxis [62].

Immunogenicity of proteins is thus dependent on their ability to eventually induce adaptive T-and B-lymphocyte responses during the allergic sensitization phase (see Figure 2). This is strongly influenced by the efficiency of antigen uptake and processing, as well as by the activation status and production of cytokines by myeloid antigen presenting cells (APC: monocytes, macrophages, and dendritic cells). Receptor-mediated endocytosis—as opposed to pinocytosis—is an efficient way of antigen uptake that facilitates adaptive immune responses at low antigen exposure and also induces activation and cytokine production by antigen presenting cells. APCs such as dendritic cells (DC) can use Fc receptors [63], RAGE (receptor for advanced glycation end products) [64,65], dectin-1, 2 and 3 [66,67], DC-SIGN [68], galectin-3 [69] and mannose receptors [70] for efficient antigen uptake. For example, it is known that IgG-immune complexes are more immunogenic because they are targeted to CD32/FcγRII receptors on APCs [71]. This was also shown for an uptake of allergen-IgE complexes via CD23/FcεRII, resulting in efficient T cell activation at 100-fold lower antigen concentrations [72]. These findings suggest that interaction with specific receptors on APC may be of importance to understand an immunogenic character of dietary AGEs (see Figure 2).

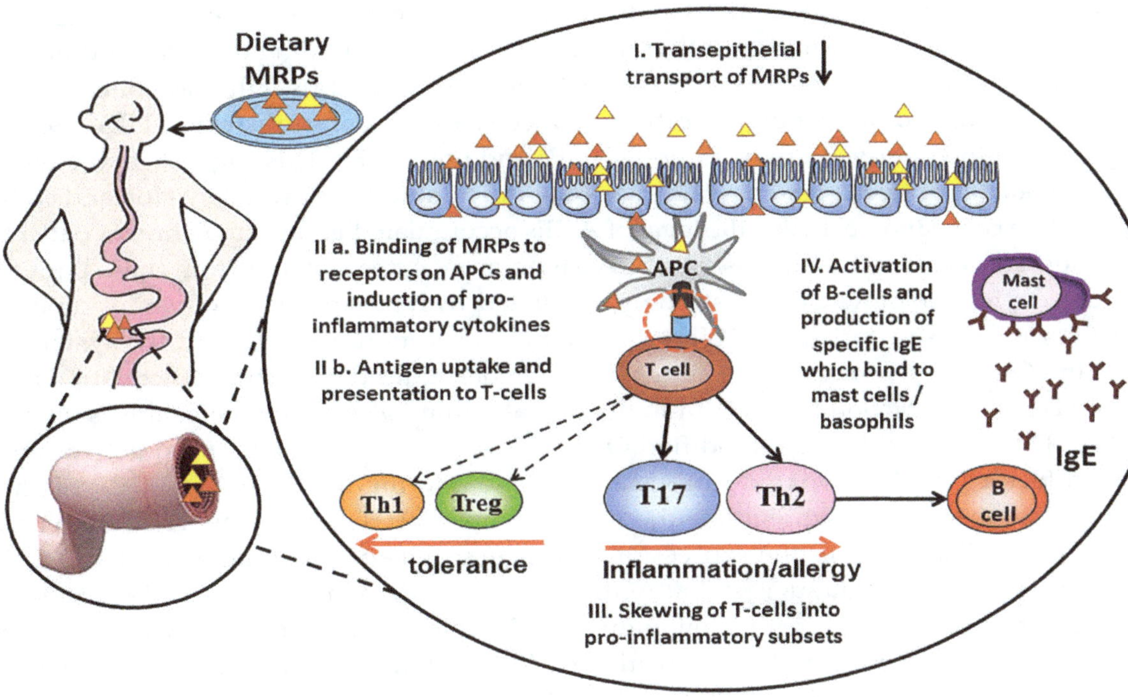

Figure 2. Schematic contribution of dietary Advanced glycation end products in the allergic sensitization process. Dietary Maillard reaction products (MRP) are taken up in the gut by crossing the epithelial barrier (I), leading to antigen uptake by mucosal dendritic cells and presentation of peptides to specific T-cells (II). Activated antigen-specific helper Th cells differentiate into pro-inflammatory and allergy-inducing Th17 and Th2 subsets (III). Allergen-specific B-cells become activated upon ligand binding and start the production of allergen-specific IgE antibodies (IV) that bind to mast cells and basophils and become detectable in the circulation.

6.2. Interaction of MR-Modified Proteins with Receptors Present on APCs

To induce an allergic immune response the MR-modified protein need to be recognized and taken up by antigen presenting cells (APCs) and subsequently presented to T-cells [24]. Recently more evidence has been found that some MRPs may function as activators of dendritic cells (DCs) via targeting AGE receptors [23,73–75]. Several receptors mediating antigen uptake, activation and maturation in DCs were identified as potential receptors for dietary MRPs, including AGE-receptor complex (AGE-R1/OST-48, AGE-R2/80K-H, AGE-R3/galectin-3) [76–78], members of the scavenger receptor family A (SR-A) and B (SR-B) [23,24,75,79–81] as well as mannose receptor [82–84]. Dry roasted Ara h1 was bound to the scavenger receptor, CD36 and the receptor for advanced glycation end products (RAGE) [24,85].

RAGE is the most studied receptor that can recognize and bind dietary AGEs [24,42,85–88]. Cellular signaling due to AGE–RAGE interactions seem to be a key component in pro-oxidative and pro-inflammatory condition [89] and this may be involved in enhanced allergic sensitization [85]. Soluble RAGE (sRAGE), the extracellular ligand-binding domains of RAGE present in the circulation, competes with membrane RAGE in binding AGEs acting as a decoy domain receptor [90,91]. Binding of AGEs to sRAGE, in contrast to interactions with membrane form of RAGE, does not result in inflammatory signal transduction therefore sRAGE acts as inhibitor of RAGE-AGE signaling and is potentially applicable for the treatment of various AGE-related diseases including diabetic cardiovascular complications [92,93], diabetic kidney disease [94] and a number of aging-related diseases including atherosclerosis, cataracts, Alzheimer's disease and Parkinson's disease [95,96].

The recent study of Liu and colleagues revealed that whey proteins glycated by dry heating (at 130 °C) interacts with sRAGE. The strength of binding was positively correlated with the time of heating and the formation of agglomerates and was more prominent in the samples with lower water activity [86]. These findings are in line with other studies showing binding of AGE-modified peanut allergens to recombinant form of RAGE [24]. The study performed by Zill and colleagues [85,97] revealed RAGE-mediated activation of both Caco-2 cells and RAGE-transfected HEK-293 cells by chemically defined food-derived products, both, AGEs and non-AGEs. This suggests that diet-derived AGEs may activate the antigen presenting cells via RAGE. The study performed by Hou and colleagues suggest a positive correlation between the level of AGEs accumulated in the circulation of patients with chronic kidney disease and the expression of RAGE on monocytes isolated from these patients [98]. The enhanced expression of RAGE was strongly correlated with plasma levels of pentosidine, plasma levels of tumor necrosis factor alpha (TNF-α), monocyte activation markers, and the systemic acute phase reactant, C-reactive protein [98]. Hilmenyuk and colleagues demonstrated activation of RAGE on immature DC via interaction with AGE-modified ovalbumin (OVA). Increased expression of RAGE on immature DCs exposed to AGE-modified OVA was seen as well as enhanced activation of the transcription factor NF-κB compared to DCs exposed to non-modified OVA [83]. The ligation of RAGE by CML was shown to upregulate the RAGE expression in human neuroblastoma cell line SH-SY5Y [87] as well as enhance the expression of vascular cell adhesion molecule-1 (VCAM-1) on endothelial cells [99]. These data suggest that AGE-RAGE interaction may result in NF-κB activation as well as upregulation of RAGE expression on immune cells what in consequence may result in secretion of pro-inflammatory cytokines and thus activation of APCs. In opposite to these results other studies show that CML-modified proteins [100] as well as Maillard-reaction modified β-lactoglobulin [101] and coffee [102] are not able to stimulate inflammatory signaling pathways in RAGE-expressing human cell lines [100,101]. Interestingly, ovalbumin modified by pyrraline, the other AGE, was also not shown to interact with RAGE [23]. Thus, the discussion on the ligation of RAGE with food-derived AGEs and its physiological consequences remains open and more data on activation of RAGE by AGEs are needed to prove the role of RAGE in the activation of APCs during the allergic sensitization process.

6.3. Influence of MR-Modified Proteins on T-Cell Activation and Polarization

Interaction of AGEs with receptors present on APCs may result in internalization and therefore presentation of antigen to T-cells. Ilchman and colleagues demonstrated that AGE-modified OVA was taken up much more efficiently by bone marrow-derived murine myeloid dendritic cells (mDCs) than native OVA, and enhanced activation of OVA-specific CD4+ T cells [75]. Scavenger receptor class A type I and II (SR-AI/II) were identified as receptors mediating the uptake of AGE-OVA [75]. These results are in line with a study using human DCs as a model for an uptake of FITC-labeled AGE-modified OVA. Enhanced uptake of AGE-modified OVA was mediated by mannose receptor, scavenger receptor and macropinocytosis. Co-culturing of CD4+ T cells with AGE-OVA-loaded mature

DCs induced greater Th2 cytokine production (IL-5, IL-4, and IL-6), while OVA-loaded DCs induced a significant Th1 or regulatory cytokine profile [83]. The study of Moghaddam and colleagues performed on dry roasted peanut proteins confirm the ability of dietary AGEs to target antigen presenting cells via RAGE and CD36. Moreover, mice sensitized with dry-roasted peanut extract showed higher IL-4, IL-5 and IL-13 secretion by mesenteric lymph node cells showing skewing of T cell response into Th2 when compared with mice sensitized with non-treated peanut extract. High reactivity of mice primed with dry roasted peanut to raw peanut antigens suggest that roasting enhances immunogenicity of peanut extract having an important impact on the priming step of sensitization [24].

Heilmann and colleagues aimed to identify glycation structures enhancing T-cell immunogenicity of a food allergen by modification of OVA with different AGEs such as CML, CEL and pyrraline. To assess the T-cell immunogenicity of glycated OVAs, murine OVA-specific CD4+ T-cells were co-cultured with bone marrow-derived DCs in the presence of differently processed OVA samples. Pyrraline modified OVA enhanced CD4+ T-cell immunogenicity, as evidenced by increased IL-2 production, higher production of IFN-γ and IL-17A when compared with native OVA. Moreover, pyrraline-OVA and AGE-OVA were efficiently taken up by BMDCs via SR-A. In addition to antigen uptake, cell maturation is required for DCs to gain their full T-cell stimulatory capacity. However, no differences in expression of co-stimulatory molecules CD40, CD80, CD86, and MHC class II on the cell surface of DC were seen suggesting that pyrraline modification does not induce BMDC maturation. This is in line with observations of Moghaddam and colleagues [24], who suggested enhanced targeting and presentation via AGE receptors rather than conventional DC maturation may be implicated in the increased immunogenicity of DR peanut antigens in vivo. However, this is in contrast with the work of Buttari and colleagues who showed that AGEs of plasma β2 glycoprotein I (β2 GPI) triggered the maturation of monocyte-derived human DCs and polarized allogenic naive CD4+ T-cells into Th2 cells in a co-culture with matured DCs [73]. These different observations could be explained by heterogeneity of the structures MRPs and the expression profiles of receptors in these human and murine DCs.

6.4. Role of Agglomeration in Immunogenicity of MR-Modified Proteins

These results raise the question which structural changes triggered by MRPs can explain the immunogenicity of AGEs and capabilities to initiate the polarization of allogenic naive CD4+ T-cells into Th2 cells. Maillard reaction caused agglomeration of proteins was excluded as a major contributor to increased immunogenicity of proteins in the studies of Moghaddam and colleagues [24] and Heilmann and colleagues [23] since the samples underwent multiple rounds of filtration and centrifugation that depleted cross-linked species. However, the agglomeration of MR-modified proteins and level of cross-linking were not measured in these studies. Moreover, food processing of proteins promotes the formation of β-sheet-rich, fibrillar structures [103] known to possess high affinity binding to RAGE [104] and CD36 [105]. Pasteurization caused aggregation of beta-lactoglobulin and alpha-lactalbumin enhanced uptake of cross-linked proteins via Peyer's patches, which promoted significantly higher Th2-associated antibody and cytokine production in mice than their native counterparts [54,55]. These results suggest that not only Maillard reaction but also protein cross-linking can enhance immunogenicity of proteins and their sensitizing capacity.

The research outcomes discussed above provide strong evidence that some dietary AGEs can bind to receptors on antigen presenting cells and thus modify T-cell immunogenicity (the schematic contribution of dietary AGEs in the allergic sensitization process is presented on Figure 2). However, information about selectivity of AGEs structures binding to AGEs receptors is very limited. The heterogeneity of AGEs and the diversity of their receptors indicate that more study is required to elucidate the precise receptors and pathways implicated in enhanced DC-mediated uptake and presentation of antigens to T cells.

6.5. *Influence of MR-Modified Proteins on B-Cells Switching and the Production of Antigen Specific IgG and IgE*

When membrane-bound immunoglobulin (Ig) of naïve B cells come in contact with specific dietary antigens, and are activated by ligation of the surface molecule CD40 to CD40L on activated Th2 cells that produce IL-4 and IL-13 , the B cells are induced to switch to produce IgE. Naïve B cells further differentiate and proliferate into activated plasma cells synthesizing and secreting antigen-specific IgE (see Box 2). Lymphocytes activated in the GALT leave through the draining lymphatics and reach the MLN, where they stay for a period for further differentiation, before migration into the bloodstream [62,106]. Moghaddam and colleagues demonstrated that BALB/c mice primed subcutaneously with soluble fractions of peanut protein extract from raw or dry roasted (DR) peanuts show enhanced peanut-specific IgG titers in DR-primed groups. These results were confirmed in intra-gastric gavages of DR and raw peanut extracts showing 100-fold higher IgG titers, enhanced titers of anti-peanut IgE as well as functional basophil degranulation in DR group. Moreover, mesenteric lymph node cells from DR but not raw peanut protein-primed mice proliferated robustly in response to raw and DR peanut extract with the dominance of IL-4 and IL-5 over IFN-γ and TNF-α. The authors suggested that the observed increased immunogenicity of DR peanut antigens can be explained by selective targeting, activation and presentation of antigen via binding to AGE receptors on DCs [24].

7. Influence of Maillard Reaction on Recognition of Food Allergens by Specific IgE

MR induced during food processing may also modulate binding potential of specific IgE to food allergens. This can be induced by: (a) disruption of the conformational and linear epitopes accompanied with the changes of the tertiary and secondary structure that impair the IgE binding potential of the protein [12,106,107]; (b) formation of agglomerates carrying high number of epitopes that cause enhanced degranulation capacity of basophils [108]; or (c) formation of new epitopes due to aggregation and/or Maillard reaction [24] (Figure 3). These new epitopes called neo-allergens are able to target APCs resulting in antigen presentation and subsequently modulating T-cell differentiation as well as a production of antigen-specific IgE. Production of specific IgE is therefore a consequence of sensitization phase by interaction of immunogenic MRPs with APCs (see Boxes 1 and 2). Moghaddam and colleagues observed that enhanced anti-raw peanut IgE titers in mice sensitized with dried peanut extract versus those sensitized with raw peanut extract was also reflected in enhanced degranulation of basophils [24].

The MR was shown to either reduce or enhance IgG and/or IgE binding capacities of some food allergens [25,109–113]. For instance, the proteins that belong to pathogenesis-related (PR) protein family and being the homologous to birch pollen allergen Bet v 1 show reduced IgE binding capacity after processing with sugar as it was shown for Pru av 1 [109] and Cor a 1 [114]. This can be explained by a masking effect of carbohydrates reducing an accessibility of epitopes for IgE binding (Figure 3). In contrast to (PR) protein family MR was shown to enhance IgE binding capacity to peanut proteins and scallop tropomyosin [115–117]. Thus, the influence of MR on IgE binding seems to depend on physicochemical properties of proteins (hydrophobicity, size, amino acid composition, charge) as well as on conditions of MR (type of sugar, time, water activity, pH, temperature, presence of salts) [118,119].

The study of Vissers and colleagues showed reduced allergenicity of MR-modified peanut allergen Ara h 1 in IgE binding test while enhanced β-hexosaminidase release from basophils upon incubation with the same MR-modified allergen [113]. The authors suggest that MR-induced agglomeration of Ara h 1 may be responsible for the observed increased capacity of antigen to cross-link the IgE and initiate the mediator release from RBL-2H3 cells (see Box 1). That indicates a need to include the functional assays, next to the IgE binding tests, in the studies on allergenicity of MRPs to be able to link the results to development of acute complaints of a clinically observable allergic response (see Box 3). Based on the functional basophil activation test (BAT) Cucu et al. showed that two out of six hazelnut allergic patients showed enhanced basophil activation after exposition to MR-modified hazelnut extract [114]. Other study revealed that 70% of the patients (out of 15) sensitized to soy showed enhanced basophil activation in BAT assay upon incubation of basophils with MR-modified soy proteins when compared with soy proteins modified only by heating (without sugars) [22]. Moreover study of Vojdani and colleagues revealed increased levels (3–8-fold) of specific IgE against processed food antigens in 31% of the patients when compared to raw food antigens [120]. These results suggest that some of the patients are sensitized against processed food rather than raw and the MR may play a crucial role in the enhancing of immunogenic potential of food allergens as it was already showed by Moghaddam and colleagues [24]. Therefore, the diagnosis of food allergy could be improved by incorporation of processed and MR-modified food allergens next to the raw ones into the diagnostic tests.

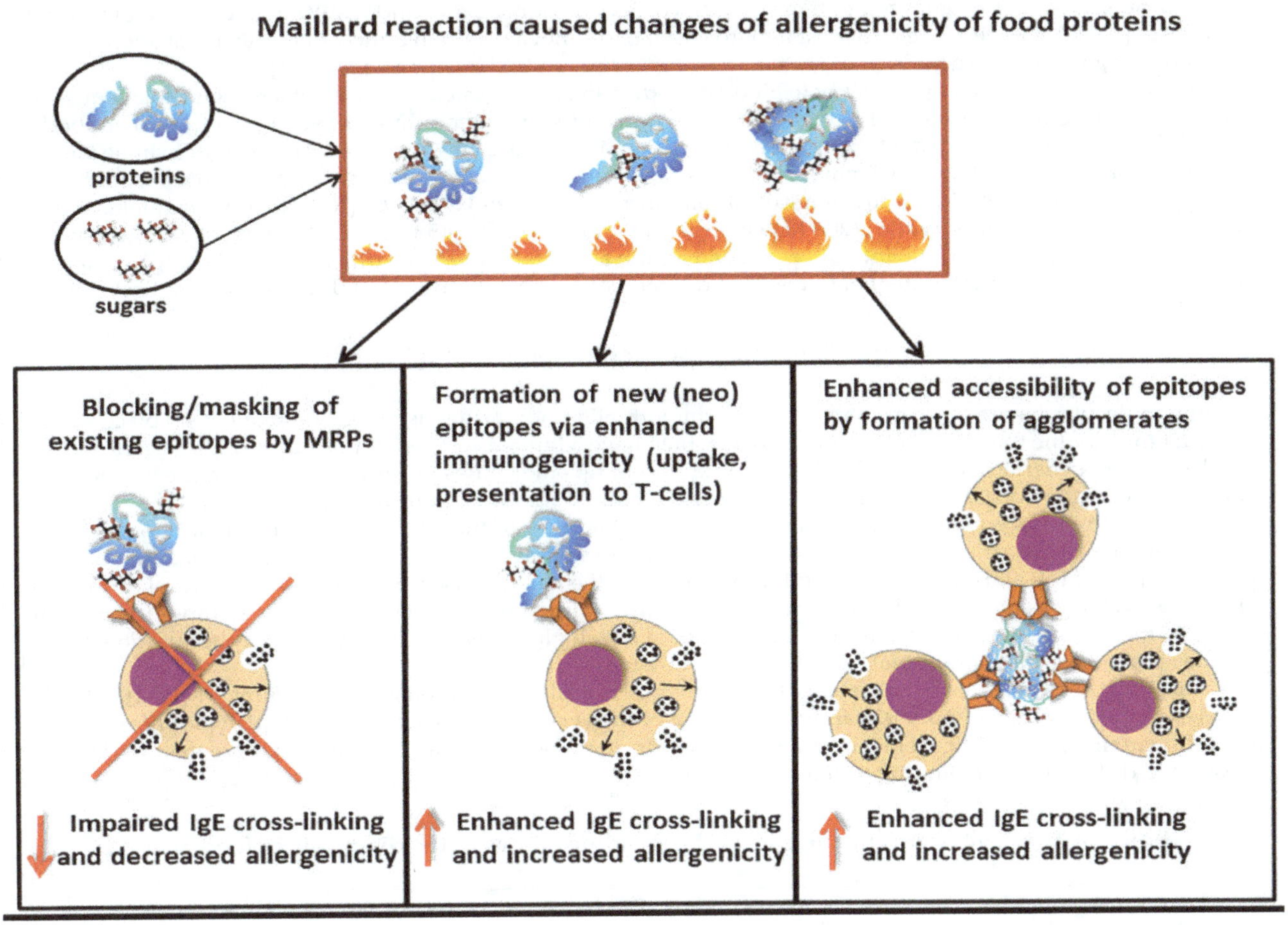

Figure 3. Modulation of allergenicity of food proteins by the Maillard reaction. Upon food processing using heating, reducing sugars will react with primary amino groups on amino acids from allergen proteins to result in Maillard reaction products (MRP). Consequently, these MRP may block epitopes thereby preventing IgE binding and crosslinking, and subsequent mediator release. This results in reduced allergenicity of the altered food allergens. Alternatively, MRP may lead to the exposure of neo-epitopes leading to enhanced uptake by antigen-presenting cells and exposure to specific T-cells and this enhanced possibility for IgE cross-linking may lead to enhanced allergenicity. Lastly, MRP may lead to the formation of agglomerates of allergen molecules resulting into enhanced IgE cross-linking and increased allergenicity. The ratio between these several possibilities determines the final outcome of the mediator release capacity of the MRP altered food allergens.

Box 1. Immunochemical properties of allergens.

Allergens are generally proteins that, when exposing genetically susceptible individuals frequently and in low doses (<1 μg) on a mucosal surface are able to induce a Th2 response associated with the production of IL-4, IL-5, and IL-13 leading to the synthesis of allergen-specific IgE antibodies.

At present, no identified antibody characteristics and no identified structural features of IgE binding epitopes seem to be associated with the phenotype of the food allergic disease. Potential allergens must necessarily contain B-cell epitopes to which IgE can bind, and T-cell epitopes capable of inducing a Th2 type response. Peptide sequences of T-cell epitopes (10–15 amino acid residues long) show no general homology across allergen families and thus it has been proven impossible to identify a consensus sequence for an allergenic epitope [121].

IgE binding allergen epitopes generally comprise conformational and more hydrophobic patches present on the allergen. A significant proportion of the IgE is directed against the glycosylated B-cell epitopes [122]. This might be a consequence of the hundred-fold increased cellular uptake of glycosylated proteins and peptides by antigen-presenting cells compared to their non-glycoslyated counterparts and resulting in enhanced immune responses [123]. However, others suggest that glycosylation is not a common critical determinant of allergenicity as food allergens comprise both glycoproteins as well as non-glycosylated proteins [124].

An epitope is identified by its ability to bind antibodies and is suggested to consist of a recognizable sequence of 6–15 amino acids (covering a 11–13 nm distance) contributing to the binding between epitope and antibody molecule [125]. Two of these identical epitopes need to span a distance between 8 and 24 nm, with a single amino acid being in the order of about 0.5 nm [126,127]. A linear unit potentially leading to degranulation would then comprise a distance of 20–54 nm equaling 40–108 amino acids (4.400 to 11.880 Da) [128]. In a 20 kDa allergen this would represent 2–5 units, while a 200 kDa allergen would harbor 16–45 units. Indeed, most allergens have only one to five immunodominant epitopes. A 40 amino acid unit would be sufficient to induce IgE antibody formation and combine the potential to result in degranulation upon binding to IgE on sensitized mast cells.

Box 2. Immunochemical properties of IgE.

IgE molecules have a 12% carbohydrate content with oligosaccharides asparagine-linked at six places all in the first three of the four constant region domains, they have a limited segmental flexibility [129]. Therefore, IgE molecules are generally considered to be more rigid than IgG molecules putting emphasis on the importance of the inter-epitope distance resulting in proper IgE binding. This way a binding stoichiometry of two can be reached as closely as possible resulting in a high binding affinity of the allergen-specific IgE antibodies [130]. The relevance of IgE affinity is illustrated in studies showing that in allergic individuals, the peanut allergen Ara h 2-specific IgE affinity correlated with the severity of the allergic disease, but not with the level of specific IgE [129,131]. In allergic individuals, IgE concentrations in the circulation may reach over 10 times the normal level ($\approx$150 ng/mL), and who have an increased risk of developing allergies. However, the concentration of IgE in the serum of healthy individuals is 10^4 times less than that of IgG.

These IgE antibodies have the capacity to bind to IgE Fc epsilon receptors with high affinity ($K_a \approx 10^{10}$ M^{-1}). This exceptionally high affinity is mainly a reflection of the very slow dissociation rate with a half-life of about 20 h for circulating IgE. The residence time on mast cells in tissues is further extended to more than 14 days by restricted diffusion and rebinding to cell receptors [130].

Box 3. Advantage of functional tests on IgE binding assays in the diagnosis of food allergy.

Diagnosis of allergy is routinely based on binding of IgE antibodies to the relevant allergen in a serological test. Principally, this binding of one Fab fragment to a single epitope results in a positive reading representing immunogenicity. This mostly conformational monovalent binding interaction is not related to the capacity to induce an allergic response resulting into mediator release. For this reaction it is essential to achieve cross-linking of several specific IgE molecules bound to adjacent FcεRI on mast cells and basophils (hence allergenicity). Principally, this elicitation phase requires a multivalent interaction between (mostly linear) allergen multi-epitopes and multiple Fab fragments on IgE antibodies. This allergen capacity can be analyzed ex vivo with blood-derived basophils or in vitro by using e.g., the rat basophilic leukemia (RBL)-HE3 cell line and is generally called allergenicity of the allergen. To analyze the basophil degranulation capacity sensitive assays are required as these cells comprise only 0–2% of leukocytes equaling 1–8 $\times$ 10^4 cells/mL [130]. This different capacity of allergens should be taken into account when relating the functional activity of allergens to the clinical symptoms of allergy. High affinity Fcε receptors are abundantly expressed (6000–600,000 receptors per cell) on mast cells in tissues and basophils in the blood. The number of FcεRI per basophil varies between different donors (range 29,000–680,000) and is also related to the IgE concentration in the serum [131]. Upon IgE binding to their specific receptors, these cells are sensitized and therefore the individual is called sensitized. Minimally, 2000 of these FcεRI bound specific IgE molecules need to be cross-linked by the relevant epitopes on the allergen in order to cause degranulation of the mast cell and/or basophil resulting in the release of the mediators and the development of acute complaints of a clinically observable allergic response. Therefore, functional assays such as histamine, β-hexosaminidase release assays or basophil activation tests should be included next to the conventional IgE binding tests to study the influence of Maillard reaction on allergenicity of proteins.

8. Conclusions

In conclusion, the MR can alter immunoreactivity towards food proteins, and MR-modified proteins may enhance the immune response by selective interaction with APCs carrying receptors for AGE. In addition, it has become clear that the presentation of MR-modified allergens to T-cells may skew the subsequent T-cell differentiation into Th2 cells producing IL-4, IL-5 and IL-13, which are responsible for the initiation of IgE antibody production. Some studies also observed enhanced mediator release from basophils incubated with MR-modified proteins that may be resulting from: (a) the immunogenic potential of MRPs enhancing the sensitization; and/or (b) agglomeration leading to more efficient cross-linking and therefore mediator release. These findings reveal a need for better understanding of the influence of MR on both the sensitization phase as well as the development of the symptoms of the allergy. Understanding the mechanisms involved in immunoreactivity of AGEs would help to improve the diagnostics of food allergy as well as develop optimized conditions for food processing to control the rate of MR.

Acknowledgments: MT was partially supported by European Seventh Framework Program FP7-PEOPLE-2011-IEF, grant number PIEF-GA-2011-302295.

Author Contributions: MT, RJJvN and HFJS equally contributed to the writing process.

References

1. Pereira, R.N.; Vicente, A.A. Environmental impact of novel thermal and non-thermal technologies in food processing. *Food Res. Int.* **2010**, *43*, 1936–1943. [CrossRef]
2. Ling, B.; Tang, J.; Kong, F.; Mitcham, E.J.; Wang, S. Kinetics of food quality changes during thermal processing: A review. *Food Bioprocess Technol.* **2015**, *8*, 343–358. [CrossRef]
3. Sevenich, R.; Bark, F.; Kleinstueck, E.; Crews, C.; Pye, C.; Hradecky, J.; Reineke, K.; Lavilla, M.; Martinez-de-Maranon, I.; Briand, J.C.; et al. The impact of high pressure thermal sterilization on the microbiological stability and formation of food processing contaminants in selected fish systems and baby food puree at pilot scale. *Food Control* **2015**, *50*, 539–547. [CrossRef]
4. Peng, P.; Song, H.; Zhang, T.; Addy, M.; Zhang, Y.; Cheng, Y.; Hatzenbeller, R.; Zhu, X.; Liu, S.; Liu, Y.; et al. Concentrated high intensity electric field (chief) system for non-thermal pasteurization of liquid foods: Modeling and simulation of fluid mechanics, electric analysis, and heat transfer. *Comput. Chem. Eng.* **2017**, *97*, 183–193. [CrossRef]
5. Halpin, R.M.; Duffy, L.; Cregenzán-Alberti, O.; Lyng, J.G.; Noci, F. The effect of non-thermal processing technologies on microbial inactivation: An investigation into sub-lethal injury of *Escherichia coli* and *Pseudomonas fluorescens*. *Food Control* **2014**, *41*, 106–115. [CrossRef]
6. Roberts, P.B. Food irradiation is safe: Half a century of studies. *Radiat. Phys. Chem.* **2014**, *105*, 78–82. [CrossRef]
7. Thirumdas, R.; Sarangapani, C.; Annapure, U.S. Cold plasma: A novel non-thermal technology for food processing. *Food Biophys.* **2015**, *10*, 1–11. [CrossRef]
8. Davis, P.J.; Williams, S.C. Protein modification by thermal processing. *Allergy* **1998**, *53*, 102–105. [CrossRef] [PubMed]
9. Tong, P.; Gao, J.; Chen, H.; Li, X.; Zhang, Y.; Jian, S.; Wichers, H.; Wu, Z.; Yang, A.; Liu, F. Effect of heat treatment on the potential allergenicity and conformational structure of egg allergen ovotransferrin. *Food Chem.* **2012**, *131*, 603–610. [CrossRef]
10. Murayama, K.; Tomida, M. Heat-induced secondary structure and conformation change of bovine serum albumin investigated by fourier transform infrared spectroscopy. *Biochemistry* **2004**, *43*, 11526–11532. [CrossRef] [PubMed]
11. Somoza, V.; Wenzel, E.; Weiss, C.; Clawin-Radecker, I.; Grubel, N.; Erbersdobler, H.F. Dose-dependent utilisation of casein-linked lysinoalanine, N(epsilon)-fructoselysine and N(epsilon)-carboxymethyllysine in rats. *Mol. Nutr. Food Res.* **2006**, *50*, 833–841. [CrossRef] [PubMed]

12. Van Boekel, M.A. Kinetic aspects of the maillard reaction: A critical review. *Mol. Nutr. Food Res.* **2001**, *45*, 150–159.
13. Hellwig, M.; Henle, T. Baking, ageing, diabetes: A short history of the maillard reaction. *Angew. Chem. Int. Ed.* **2014**, *53*, 10316–10329. [CrossRef] [PubMed]
14. De Oliveira, F.C.; Coimbra, J.S.; de Oliveira, E.B.; Zuniga, A.D.; Rojas, E.E. Food protein-polysaccharide conjugates obtained via the maillard reaction: A review. *Crit. Rev. Food Sci. Nutr.* **2016**, *56*, 1108–1125. [CrossRef] [PubMed]
15. Henle, T. Protein-bound advanced glycation endproducts (ages) as bioactive amino acid derivatives in foods. *Amino Acids* **2005**, *29*, 313–322. [CrossRef] [PubMed]
16. Somoza, V. Five years of research on health risks and benefits of maillard reaction products: An update. *Mol. Nutr. Food Res.* **2005**, *49*, 663–672. [CrossRef] [PubMed]
17. Liu, J.; Ru, Q.; Ding, Y. Glycation a promising method for food protein modification: Physicochemical properties and structure, a review. *Food Res. Int.* **2012**, *49*, 170–183. [CrossRef]
18. Ames, J.M. Applications of the maillard reaction in the food industry. *Food Chem.* **1998**, *62*, 431–439. [CrossRef]
19. Teodorowicz, M.; Jansen, A.P.H.; Roovers, M.H.W.M.; Ruinemans-Koerts, J.; Wichers, H.J.; Savelkoul, H.F.J. Maillard-type neoallergens present in processed soy extract may cause an allergic reaction in soy allergic patients. *Clin. Trans. Allergy* **2015**, *5*, 21. [CrossRef]
20. Heilmann, M.; Wellner, A.; Gadermaier, G.; Ilchmann, A.; Briza, P.; Krause, M.; Nagai, R.; Burgdorf, S.; Scheurer, S.; Vieths, S.; et al. Ovalbumin modified with pyrraline, a maillard reaction product, shows enhanced T-cell immunogenicity. *J. Biol. Chem.* **2014**, *289*, 7919–7928. [CrossRef] [PubMed]
21. Moghaddam, A.E.; Hillson, W.R.; Noti, M.; Gartlan, K.H.; Johnson, S.; Thomas, B.; Artis, D.; Sattentau, Q.J. Dry roasting enhances peanut-induced allergic sensitization across mucosal and cutaneous routes in mice. *J. Allergy Clin. Immunol.* **2014**, *134*, 1453–1456. [CrossRef] [PubMed]
22. Iwan, M.; Vissers, Y.M.; Fiedorowicz, E.; Kostyra, H.; Kostyra, E.; Savelkoul, H.F.; Wichers, H.J. Impact of maillard reaction on immunoreactivity and allergenicity of the hazelnut allergen cor a 11. *J.Agric. Food Chem.* **2011**, *59*, 7163–7171. [CrossRef] [PubMed]
23. Lehmann, K.; Schweimer, K.; Reese, G.; Randow, S.; Suhr, M.; Becker, W.M.; Vieths, S.; Rosch, P. Structure and stability of 2s albumin-type peanut allergens: Implications for the severity of peanut allergic reactions. *Biochem. J.* **2006**, *395*, 463–472. [CrossRef] [PubMed]
24. Suhr, M.; Wicklein, D.; Lepp, U.; Becker, W.M. Isolation and characterization of natural ara h 6: Evidence for a further peanut allergen with putative clinical relevance based on resistance to pepsin digestion and heat. *Mol. Nutr. Food Res.* **2004**, *48*, 390–399. [CrossRef] [PubMed]
25. Apostolovic, D.; Stanic-Vucinic, D.; de Jongh, H.H.; de Jong, G.A.; Mihailovic, J.; Radosavljevic, J.; Radibratovic, M.; Nordlee, J.A.; Baumert, J.L.; Milcic, M.; et al. Conformational stability of digestion-resistant peptides of peanut conglutins reveals the molecular basis of their allergenicity. *Sci. Rep.* **2016**, *6*, 29249. [CrossRef] [PubMed]
26. Bogh, K.L.; Madsen, C.B. Food allergens: Is there a correlation between stability to digestion and allergenicity? *Crit. Rev. Food Sci. Nutr.* **2016**, *56*, 1545–1567. [CrossRef] [PubMed]
27. Bannon, G.; Fu, T.J.; Kimber, I.; Hinton, D.M. Protein digestibility and relevance to allergenicity. *Environ. Health Perspect.* **2003**, *111*, 1122–1124. [CrossRef] [PubMed]
28. Peram, M.R.; Loveday, S.M.; Ye, A.; Singh, H. In vitro gastric digestion of heat-induced aggregates of β-lactoglobulin. *J. Dairy Sci.* **2013**, *96*, 63–74. [CrossRef] [PubMed]
29. Corzo-Martínez, M.; Soria, A.C.; Belloque, J.; Villamiel, M.; Moreno, F.J. Effect of glycation on the gastrointestinal digestibility and immunoreactivity of bovine β-lactoglobulin. *Int. Dairy J.* **2010**, *20*, 742–752. [CrossRef]
30. Corzo-Martinez, M.; Moreno, F.J.; Olano, A.; Villamiel, M. Role of pyridoxamine in the formation of the amadori/heyns compounds and aggregates during the glycation of beta-lactoglobulin with galactose and tagatose. *J. Agric. Food Chem.* **2010**, *58*, 500–506. [CrossRef] [PubMed]
31. Ahmad, S.; Shahab, U.; Baig, M.H.; Khan, M.S.; Khan, M.S.; Srivastava, A.K.; Saeed, M.; Moinuddin. Inhibitory effect of metformin and pyridoxamine in the formation of early, intermediate and advanced glycation end-products. *PLoS ONE* **2013**, *8*, e72128. [CrossRef] [PubMed]

32. Dominika, Ś.; Arjan, N.; Karyn, R.P.; Henryk, K. The study on the impact of glycated pea proteins on human intestinal bacteria. *Int. J. Food Microbiol.* **2011**, *145*, 267–272. [CrossRef] [PubMed]
33. Teodorowicz, M.; Fiedorowicz, E.; Kostyra, H.; Wichers, H.; Kostyra, E. Effect of maillard reaction on biochemical properties of peanut 7s globulin (ara h 1) and its interaction with a human colon cancer cell line (caco-2). *Eur. J. Nutr.* **2013**, *52*, 1927–1938. [CrossRef] [PubMed]
34. Luz Sanz, M.; Corzo-Martinez, M.; Rastall, R.A.; Olano, A.; Moreno, F.J. Characterization and in vitro digestibility of bovine beta-lactoglobulin glycated with galactooligosaccharides. *J. Agric. Food Chem.* **2007**, *55*, 7916–7925. [CrossRef] [PubMed]
35. Katayama, S.; Shima, J.; Saeki, H. Solubility improvement of shellfish muscle proteins by reaction with glucose and its soluble state in low-ionic-strength medium. *J. Agric. Food Chem.* **2002**, *50*, 4327–4332. [CrossRef] [PubMed]
36. Sato, R.; Sawabe, T.; Kishimura, H.; Hayashi, K.; Saeki, H. Preparation of neoglycoprotein from carp myofibrillar protein and alginate oligosaccharide: Improved solubility in low ionic strength medium. *J. Agric. Food Chem.* **2000**, *48*, 17–21. [CrossRef] [PubMed]
37. Yeboah, F.K.; Alli, I.; Yaylayan, V.A.; Yasuo, K.; Chowdhury, S.F.; Purisima, E.O. Effect of limited solid-state glycation on the conformation of lysozyme by esi-msms peptide mapping and molecular modeling. *Bioconj. Chem.* **2004**, *15*, 27–34. [CrossRef] [PubMed]
38. De Jongh, H.H.J.; Taylor, S.L.; Koppelman, S.J. Controlling the aggregation propensity and thereby digestibility of allergens by maillardation as illustrated for cod fish parvalbumin. *J. Biosci. Bioeng.* **2011**, *111*, 204–211. [CrossRef] [PubMed]
39. Liu, F.; Teodorowicz, M.; Wichers, H.J.; van Boekel, M.A.; Hettinga, K.A. Generation of soluble advanced glycation end products receptor (srage)-binding ligands during extensive heat treatment of whey protein/lactose mixtures is dependent on glycation and aggregation. *J Agric. Food Chem.* **2016**, *64*, 6477–6486. [CrossRef] [PubMed]
40. Seiquer, I.; Diaz-Alguacil, J.; Delgado-Andrade, C.; Lopez-Frias, M.; Munoz Hoyos, A.; Galdo, G.; Navarro, M.P. Diets rich in maillard reaction products affect protein digestibility in adolescent males aged 11–14 y. *Am. J. Clin. Nutr.* **2006**, *83*, 1082–1088. [PubMed]
41. Hellwig, M.; Bunzel, D.; Huch, M.; Franz, C.M.; Kulling, S.E.; Henle, T. Stability of individual maillard reaction products in the presence of the human colonic microbiota. *J. Agric. Food Chem.* **2015**, *63*, 6723–6730. [CrossRef] [PubMed]
42. Hellwig, M.; Henle, T. Release of pyrraline in absorbable peptides during simulated digestion of casein glycated by 3-deoxyglucosone. *Eur. Food Res. Technol.* **2013**, *237*, 47–55. [CrossRef]
43. Koschinsky, T.; He, C.-J.; Mitsuhashi, T.; Bucala, R.; Liu, C.; Buenting, C.; Heitmann, K.; Vlassara, H. Orally absorbed reactive glycation products (glycotoxins): An environmental risk factor in diabetic nephropathy. *Proc. Natl. Acad. Sci. USA* **1997**, *94*, 6474–6479. [CrossRef] [PubMed]
44. Uribarri, J.; Cai, W.; Sandu, O.; Peppa, M.; Goldberg, T.; Vlassara, H. Diet-derived advanced glycation end products are major contributors to the body's age pool and induce inflammation in healthy subjects. *Ann. N. Y. Acad. Sci.* **2005**, *1043*, 461–466. [CrossRef] [PubMed]
45. Delgado-Andrade, C.; Tessier, F.J.; Niquet-Leridon, C.; Seiquer, I.; Pilar Navarro, M. Study of the urinary and faecal excretion of nepsilon-carboxymethyllysine in young human volunteers. *Amino Acids* **2012**, *43*, 595–602. [CrossRef] [PubMed]
46. Foerster, A.; Henle, T. Glycation in food and metabolic transit of dietary ages (advanced glycation end-products): Studies on the urinary excretion of pyrraline. *Biochem. Soc. Trans.* **2003**, *31*, 1383–1385. [CrossRef] [PubMed]
47. Forster, A.; Kuhne, Y.; Henle, T. Studies on absorption and elimination of dietary maillard reaction products. *Ann. N. Y. Acad. Sci.* **2005**, *1043*, 474–481. [CrossRef] [PubMed]
48. Semba, R.D.; Ang, A.; Talegawkar, S.; Crasto, C.; Dalal, M.; Jardack, P.; Traber, M.G.; Ferrucci, L.; Arab, L. Dietary intake associated with serum versus urinary carboxymethyl-lysine, a major advanced glycation end product, in adults: The energetics study. *Eur. J. Clin. Nutr.* **2012**, *66*, 3–9. [CrossRef] [PubMed]
49. Hellwig, M.; Matthes, R.; Peto, A.; Löbner, J.; Henle, T. N-ε-fructosyllysine and n-ε-carboxymethyllysine, but not lysinoalanine, are available for absorption after simulated gastrointestinal digestion. *Amino Acids* **2014**, *46*, 289–299. [CrossRef] [PubMed]

50. Ames, J.M. Evidence against dietary advanced glycation endproducts being a risk to human health. *Mol. Nutr. Food Res.* **2007**, *51*, 1085–1090. [CrossRef] [PubMed]
51. Roth-Walter, F.; Berin, M.C.; Arnaboldi, P.; Escalante, C.R.; Dahan, S.; Rauch, J.; Jensen-Jarolim, E.; Mayer, L. Pasteurization of milk proteins promotes allergic sensitization by enhancing uptake through peyer's patches. *Allergy* **2008**, *63*, 882–890. [CrossRef] [PubMed]
52. Stojadinovic, M.; Pieters, R.; Smit, J.; Velickovic, T.C. Cross-linking of beta-lactoglobulin enhances allergic sensitization through changes in cellular uptake and processing. *Toxicol. Sci.* **2014**, *140*, 224–235. [CrossRef] [PubMed]
53. Tuohy, K.M.; Hinton, D.J.; Davies, S.J.; Crabbe, M.J.; Gibson, G.R.; Ames, J.M. Metabolism of maillard reaction products by the human gut microbiota—implications for health. *Mol. Nutr. Food Res.* **2006**, *50*, 847–857. [CrossRef] [PubMed]
54. Helou, C.; Marier, D.; Jacolot, P.; Abdennebi-Najar, L.; Niquet-Leridon, C.; Tessier, F.J.; Gadonna-Widehem, P. Microorganisms and maillard reaction products: A review of the literature and recent findings. *Amino Acids* **2014**, *46*, 267–277. [CrossRef] [PubMed]
55. Seiquer, I.; Rubio, L.A.; Peinado, M.J.; Delgado-Andrade, C.; Navarro, M.P. Maillard reaction products modulate gut microbiota composition in adolescents. *Mol. Nutr. Food Res.* **2014**, *58*, 1552–1560. [CrossRef] [PubMed]
56. Teodorowicz, M.; Świątecka, D.; Savelkoul, H.; Wichers, H.; Kostyra, E.C. Hydrolysates of glycated and heat-treated peanut 7s globulin (ara h 1) modulate human gut microbial proliferation, survival and adhesion. *J. Appl. Microbiol.* **2014**, *116*, 424–434. [CrossRef] [PubMed]
57. Yan, S.F.; Ramasamy, R.; Schmidt, A.M. Mechanisms of disease: Advanced glycation end-products and their receptor in inflammation and diabetes complications. *Nat. Rev. Endocrinol.* **2008**, *4*, 285–293. [CrossRef] [PubMed]
58. Davis, K.E.; Prasad, C.; Vijayagopal, P.; Juma, S.; Imrhan, V. Advanced glycation end products, inflammation, and chronic metabolic diseases: Links in a chain? *Crit. Rev. Food Sci. Nutr.* **2016**, *56*, 989–998. [CrossRef] [PubMed]
59. Wu, L.C.; Zarrin, A.A. The production and regulation of ige by the immune system. *Nat. Rev. Immunol.* **2014**, *14*, 247–259. [CrossRef] [PubMed]
60. Guilliams, M.; Bruhns, P.; Saeys, Y.; Hammad, H.; Lambrecht, B.N. The function of Fc[gamma] receptors in dendritic cells and macrophages. *Nat. Rev. Immunol.* **2014**, *14*, 94–108. [CrossRef] [PubMed]
61. Bertheloot, D.; Naumovski, A.L.; Langhoff, P.; Horvath, G.L.; Jin, T.; Xiao, T.S.; Garbi, N.; Agrawal, S.; Kolbeck, R.; Latz, E. Rage enhances tlr responses through binding and internalization of rna. *J. Immunol.* **2016**, *197*, 4118–4126. [CrossRef] [PubMed]
62. Schmidt, A.M.; Vianna, M.; Gerlach, M.; Brett, J.; Ryan, J.; Kao, J.; Esposito, C.; Hegarty, H.; Hurley, W.; Clauss, M.; et al. Isolation and characterization of two binding proteins for advanced glycosylation end products from bovine lung which are present on the endothelial cell surface. *J. Biol. Chem.* **1992**, *267*, 14987–14997. [PubMed]
63. Maldonado, S.; Dai, J.; Singh, S.; Mwangi, D.; Rivera, A.; Fitzgerald-Bocarsly, P. Human pdcs express the c-type lectin receptor dectin-1 and uptake and kill *Aspergillus fumigatus* spores in vitro (mpf4p.734). *J. Immunol.* **2015**, *194*, 136.10.
64. Zhu, L.L.; Zhao, X.Q.; Jiang, C.; You, Y.; Chen, X.P.; Jiang, Y.Y.; Jia, X.M.; Lin, X. C-type lectin receptors dectin-3 and dectin-2 form a heterodimeric pattern-recognition receptor for host defense against fungal infection. *Immunity* **2013**, *39*, 324–334. [CrossRef] [PubMed]
65. Sprokholt, J.K.; Overmars, R.J.; Geijtenbeek, T.B.H. Dc-sign in infection and immunity. In *C-type Lectin Receptors in Immunity*; Yamasaki, S., Ed.; Springer: Tokyo, Japan, 2016; pp. 129–150.
66. Lakshminarayan, R.; Wunder, C.; Becken, U.; Howes, M.T.; Benzing, C.; Arumugam, S.; Sales, S.; Ariotti, N.; Chambon, V.; Lamaze, C.; et al. Galectin-3 drives glycosphingolipid-dependent biogenesis of clathrin-independent carriers. *Nat. Cell Biol.* **2014**, *16*, 592–603. [CrossRef] [PubMed]
67. Azad, A.K.; Rajaram, M.V.S.; Schlesinger, L.S. Exploitation of the macrophage mannose receptor (cd206) in infectious disease diagnostics and therapeutics. *J. Cytol. Mol. Biol.* **2014**, *1*, 1000003. [PubMed]
68. Gosselin, E.J.; Wardwell, K.; Gosselin, D.R.; Alter, N.; Fisher, J.L.; Guyre, P.M. Enhanced antigen presentation using human fc gamma receptor (monocyte/macrophage)-specific immunogens. *J. Immunol.* **1992**, *149*, 3477–3481. [PubMed]

69. Van der Heijden, F.L.; Joost van Neerven, R.J.; van Katwijk, M.; Bos, J.D.; Kapsenberg, M.L. Serum-ige-facilitated allergen presentation in atopic disease. *J. Immunol.* **1993**, *150*, 3643. [PubMed]
70. Buttari, B.; Profumo, E.; Capozzi, A.; Facchiano, F.; Saso, L.; Sorice, M.; Rigano, R. Advanced glycation end products of human beta(2) glycoprotein i modulate the maturation and function of dcs. *Blood* **2011**, *117*, 6152–6161. [CrossRef] [PubMed]
71. Ge, J.; Jia, Q.; Liang, C.; Luo, Y.; Huang, D.; Sun, A.; Wang, K.; Zou, Y.; Chen, H. Advanced glycosylation end products might promote atherosclerosis through inducing the immune maturation of dendritic cells. *Arterioscler. Thromb. Vasc. Biol.* **2005**, *25*, 2157–2163. [CrossRef] [PubMed]
72. Ilchmann, A.; Burgdorf, S.; Scheurer, S.; Waibler, Z.; Nagai, R.; Wellner, A.; Yamamoto, Y.; Yamamoto, H.; Henle, T.; Kurts, C.; et al. Glycation of a food allergen by the maillard reaction enhances its t-cell immunogenicity: Role of macrophage scavenger receptor class a type i and ii. *J. Allergy Clin. Immunol.* **2010**, *125*, 175–183.e111. [CrossRef] [PubMed]
73. Ott, C.; Jacobs, K.; Haucke, E.; Navarrete Santos, A.; Grune, T.; Simm, A. Role of advanced glycation end products in cellular signaling. *Redox Biol.* **2014**, *2*, 411–429. [CrossRef] [PubMed]
74. Li, Y.M.; Mitsuhashi, T.; Wojciechowicz, D.; Shimizu, N.; Li, J.; Stitt, A.; He, C.; Banerjee, D.; Vlassara, H. Molecular identity and cellular distribution of advanced glycation endproduct receptors: Relationship of p60 to ost-48 and p90 to 80k-h membrane proteins. *Proc. Natl. Acad. Sci. USA* **1996**, *93*, 11047–11052. [CrossRef] [PubMed]
75. Vlassara, H.; Li, Y.M.; Imani, F.; Wojciechowicz, D.; Yang, Z.; Liu, F.T.; Cerami, A. Identification of galectin-3 as a high-affinity binding protein for advanced glycation end products (age): A new member of the age-receptor complex. *Mol. Med.* **1995**, *1*, 634–646. [PubMed]
76. Ohgami, N.; Nagai, R.; Ikemoto, M.; Arai, H.; Kuniyasu, A.; Horiuchi, S.; Nakayama, H. Cd36, a member of the class b scavenger receptor family, as a receptor for advanced glycation end products. *J. Biol. Chem.* **2001**, *276*, 3195–3202. [CrossRef] [PubMed]
77. Chatzigeorgiou, A.; Kandaraki, E.; Piperi, C.; Livadas, S.; Papavassiliou, A.G.; Koutsilieris, M.; Papalois, A.; Diamanti-Kandarakis, E. Dietary glycotoxins affect scavenger receptor expression and the hormonal profile of female rats. *J. Endocrinol.* **2013**, *218*, 331–337. [CrossRef] [PubMed]
78. Araki, N.; Higashi, T.; Mori, T.; Shibayama, R.; Kawabe, Y.; Kodama, T.; Takahashi, K.; Shichiri, M.; Horiuchi, S. Macrophage scavenger receptor mediates the endocytic uptake and degradation of advanced glycation end products of the maillard reaction. *Eur. J. Biochem.* **1995**, *230*, 408–415. [CrossRef] [PubMed]
79. Chakraborty, P.; Ghosh, D.; Basu, M.K. Modulation of macrophage mannose receptor affects the uptake of virulent and avirulent leishmania donovani promastigotes. *J. Parasitol.* **2001**, *87*, 1023–1027. [CrossRef]
80. Hilmenyuk, T.; Bellinghausen, I.; Heydenreich, B.; Ilchmann, A.; Toda, M.; Grabbe, S.; Saloga, J. Effects of glycation of the model food allergen ovalbumin on antigen uptake and presentation by human dendritic cells. *Immunology* **2010**, *129*, 437–445. [CrossRef] [PubMed]
81. Royer, P.J.; Emara, M.; Yang, C.; Al-Ghouleh, A.; Tighe, P.; Jones, N.; Sewell, H.F.; Shakib, F.; Martinez-Pomares, L.; Ghaemmaghami, A.M. The mannose receptor mediates the uptake of diverse native allergens by dendritic cells and determines allergen-induced t cell polarization through modulation of ido activity. *J. Immunol.* **2010**, *185*, 1522–1531. [CrossRef] [PubMed]
82. Mueller, G.A.; Maleki, S.J.; Johnson, K.; Hurlburt, B.K.; Cheng, H.; Ruan, S.; Nesbit, J.B.; Pomés, A.; Edwards, L.L.; Schorzman, A.; et al. Identification of maillard reaction products on peanut allergens that influence binding to the receptor for advanced glycation end products. *Allergy* **2013**, *68*, 1546–1554. [CrossRef] [PubMed]
83. Liu, F.; Teodorowicz, M.; van Boekel, M.A.; Wichers, H.J.; Hettinga, K.A. The decrease in the igg-binding capacity of intensively dry heated whey proteins is associated with intense maillard reaction, structural changes of the proteins and formation of rage-ligands. *Food Funct.* **2016**, *7*, 239–249. [CrossRef] [PubMed]
84. Holik, A.K.; Rohm, B.; Somoza, M.M.; Somoza, V. N(epsilon)-carboxymethyllysine (cml), a maillard reaction product, stimulates serotonin release and activates the receptor for advanced glycation end products (rage) in sh-sy5y cells. *Food Funct.* **2013**, *4*, 1111–1120. [CrossRef] [PubMed]
85. Neeper, M.; Schmidt, A.M.; Brett, J.; Yan, S.D.; Wang, F.; Pan, Y.C.; Elliston, K.; Stern, D.; Shaw, A. Cloning and expression of a cell surface receptor for advanced glycosylation end products of proteins. *J. Biol. Chem.* **1992**, *267*, 14998–15004. [PubMed]

86. Bastos, D.H.M.; Gugliucci, A. Contemporary and controversial aspects of the maillard reaction products. *Curr. Opin. Food Sci.* **2015**, *1*, 13–20. [CrossRef]
87. Devangelio, E.; Santilli, F.; Formoso, G.; Ferroni, P.; Bucciarelli, L.; Michetti, N.; Clissa, C.; Ciabattoni, G.; Consoli, A.; Davì, G. Soluble rage in type 2 diabetes: Association with oxidative stress. *Free. Radic. Biol. Med.* **2007**, *43*, 511–518. [CrossRef] [PubMed]
88. Raucci, A.; Cugusi, S.; Antonelli, A.; Barabino, S.M.; Monti, L.; Bierhaus, A.; Reiss, K.; Saftig, P.; Bianchi, M.E. A soluble form of the receptor for advanced glycation endproducts (rage) is produced by proteolytic cleavage of the membrane-bound form by the sheddase a disintegrin and metalloprotease 10 (adam10). *FASEB J.* **2008**, *22*, 3716–3727. [CrossRef] [PubMed]
89. Yamagishi, S.-I.; Nakamura, N.; Suematsu, M.; Kaseda, K.; Matsui, T. Advanced glycation end products: A molecular target for vascular complications in diabetes. *Mol. Med.* **2015**, *21*, S32–S40. [CrossRef] [PubMed]
90. Yamagishi, S.; Nakamura, K.; Matsui, T.; Ueda, S.; Fukami, K.; Okuda, S. Agents that block advanced glycation end product (age)-rage (receptor for ages)-oxidative stress system: A novel therapeutic strategy for diabetic vascular complications. *Exp. Opin. Investig. Drugs* **2008**, *17*, 983–996. [CrossRef] [PubMed]
91. Gugliucci, A.; Menini, T. The axis age-rage-soluble rage and oxidative stress in chronic kidney disease. In *Oxidative Stress and Inflammation in Non-Communicable Diseases—Molecular Mechanisms and Perspectives in Therapeutics*; Camps, J., Ed.; Springer International Publishing: Cham, Germany, 2014; pp. 191–208.
92. Reddy, V.P.; Beyaz, A. Inhibitors of the maillard reaction and age breakers as therapeutics for multiple diseases. *Drug Discov. Today* **2006**, *11*, 646–654. [CrossRef] [PubMed]
93. Maillard-Lefebvre, H.; Boulanger, E.; Daroux, M.; Gaxatte, C.; Hudson, B.I.; Lambert, M. Soluble receptor for advanced glycation end products: A new biomarker in diagnosis and prognosis of chronic inflammatory diseases. *Rheumatology* **2009**, *48*, 1190–1196. [CrossRef] [PubMed]
94. Zill, H.; Bek, S.; Hofmann, T.; Huber, J.; Frank, O.; Lindenmeier, M.; Weigle, B.; Erbersdobler, H.F.; Scheidler, S.; Busch, A.E.; et al. Rage-mediated mapk activation by food-derived age and non-age products. *Biochem. Biophys. Res. Commun.* **2003**, *300*, 311–315. [CrossRef]
95. Hou, F.F.; Ren, H.; Owen, W.F., Jr.; Guo, Z.J.; Chen, P.Y.; Schmidt, A.M.; Miyata, T.; Zhang, X. Enhanced expression of receptor for advanced glycation end products in chronic kidney disease. *J. Am. Soc. Nephrol. JASN* **2004**, *15*, 1889–1896. [CrossRef] [PubMed]
96. Kislinger, T.; Fu, C.; Huber, B.; Qu, W.; Taguchi, A.; Du Yan, S.; Hofmann, M.; Yan, S.F.; Pischetsrieder, M.; Stern, D.; et al. N(epsilon)-(carboxymethyl)lysine adducts of proteins are ligands for receptor for advanced glycation end products that activate cell signaling pathways and modulate gene expression. *J. Biol. Chem.* **1999**, *274*, 31740–31749. [CrossRef] [PubMed]
97. Buetler, T.M.; Leclerc, E.; Baumeyer, A.; Latado, H.; Newell, J.; Adolfsson, O.; Parisod, V.; Richoz, J.; Maurer, S.; Foata, F.; et al. Nε-carboxymethyllysine-modified proteins are unable to bind to rage and activate an inflammatory response. *Mol. Nutr. Food Res.* **2008**, *52*, 370–378. [CrossRef] [PubMed]
98. Buetler, T.M.; Latado, H.; Leclerc, E.; Weigle, B.; Baumeyer, A.; Heizmann, C.W.; Scholz, G. Glycolaldehyde-modified β-lactoglobulin ages are unable to stimulate inflammatory signaling pathways in rage-expressing human cell lines. *Mol. Nutr. Food Res.* **2011**, *55*, 291–299. [CrossRef] [PubMed]
99. Muscat, S.; Pelka, J.; Hegele, J.; Weigle, B.; Münch, G.; Pischetsrieder, M. Coffee and maillard products activate nf-κb in macrophages via H_2O_2 production. *Mol. Nutr. Food Res.* **2007**, *51*, 525–535. [CrossRef] [PubMed]
100. Cellmer, T.; Bratko, D.; Prausnitz, J.M.; Blanch, H.W. Protein aggregation in silico. *Trends Biotechnol.* **2007**, *25*, 254–261. [CrossRef] [PubMed]
101. Lee, J.-J.; Wang, P.-W.; Yang, I.H.; Wu, C.-L.; Chuang, J.-H. Amyloid-beta mediates the receptor of advanced glycation end product-induced pro-inflammatory response via toll-like receptor 4 signaling pathway in retinal ganglion cell line rgc-5. *Int. J. Biochem. Cell Biol.* **2015**, *64*, 1–10. [CrossRef] [PubMed]
102. Sadigh-Eteghad, S.; Sabermarouf, B.; Majdi, A.; Talebi, M.; Farhoudi, M.; Mahmoudi, J. Amyloid-beta: A crucial factor in Alzheimer's disease. *Med. Princ. Pract.* **2015**, *24*, 1–10. [CrossRef] [PubMed]
103. Cianferoni, A.; Spergel, J.M. Food allergy: Review, classification and diagnosis. *Allergol. Int.* **2009**, *58*, 457–466. [CrossRef] [PubMed]
104. Rahaman, T.; Vasiljevic, T.; Ramchandran, L. Conformational changes of beta-lactoglobulin induced by shear, heat, and ph-effects on antigenicity. *J. Dairy Sci.* **2015**, *98*, 4255–4265. [CrossRef] [PubMed]

105. Scheurer, S.; Lauer, I.; Foetisch, K.; San Miguel Moncin, M.; Retzek, M.; Hartz, C.; Enrique, E.; Lidholm, J.; Cistero-Bahima, A.; Vieths, S. Strong allergenicity of pru av 3, the lipid transfer protein from cherry, is related to high stability against thermal processing and digestion. *J. Allergy Clin. Immunol.* **2004**, *114*, 900–907. [CrossRef] [PubMed]
106. Gruber, P.; Vieths, S.; Wangorsch, A.; Nerkamp, J.; Hofmann, T. Maillard reaction and enzymatic browning Aaffect the allergenicity of pru av 1, the major allergen from cherry (*Prunus avium*). *J. Agric. Food Chem.* **2004**, *52*, 4002–4007. [CrossRef] [PubMed]
107. Jimenez-Saiz, R.; Belloque, J.; Molina, E.; Lopez-Fandino, R. Human immunoglobulin e (ige) binding to heated and glycated ovalbumin and ovomucoid before and after in vitro digestion. *J. Agric. Food Chem.* **2011**, *59*, 10044–10051. [CrossRef] [PubMed]
108. Taheri-Kafrani, A.; Gaudin, J.C.; Rabesona, H.; Nioi, C.; Agarwal, D.; Drouet, M.; Chobert, J.M.; Bordbar, A.K.; Haertle, T. Effects of heating and glycation of beta-lactoglobulin on its recognition by ige of sera from cow milk allergy patients. *J. Agric. Food Chem.* **2009**, *57*, 4974–4982. [CrossRef] [PubMed]
109. Vissers, Y.M.; Blanc, F.; Skov, P.S.; Johnson, P.E.; Rigby, N.M.; Przybylski-Nicaise, L.; Bernard, H.; Wal, J.-M.; Ballmer-Weber, B.; Zuidmeer-Jongejan, L.; et al. Effect of heating and glycation on the allergenicity of 2s albumins (ara h 2/6) from peanut. *PLoS ONE* **2011**, *6*, e23998. [CrossRef] [PubMed]
110. Vissers, Y.M.; Iwan, M.; Adel-Patient, K.; Stahl Skov, P.; Rigby, N.M.; Johnson, P.E.; Mandrup Muller, P.; Przybylski-Nicaise, L.; Schaap, M.; Ruinemans-Koerts, J.; et al. Effect of roasting on the allergenicity of major peanut allergens ara h 1 and ara h 2/6: The necessity of degranulation assays. *Clin. Exp. Allergy J. Br. Soc. Allergy Clin. Immunol.* **2011**, *41*, 1631–1642. [CrossRef] [PubMed]
111. Cucu, T.; De Meulenaer, B.; Bridts, C.; Devreese, B.; Ebo, D. Impact of thermal processing and the maillard reaction on the basophil activation of hazelnut allergic patients. *Food Chem. Toxicol. Int. J. Publ. Br. Ind. Biol. Res. Assoc.* **2012**, *50*, 1722–1728. [CrossRef] [PubMed]
112. Maleki, S.J.; Chung, S.-Y.; Champagne, E.T.; Raufman, J.-P. The effects of roasting on the allergenic properties of peanut proteins. *J. Allergy Clin. Immunol.* **2000**, *106*, 763–768. [CrossRef] [PubMed]
113. Gruber, P.; Becker, W.M.; Hofmann, T. Influence of the maillard reaction on the allergenicity of rara h 2, a recombinant major allergen from peanut (*Arachis hypogaea*), its major epitopes, and peanut agglutinin. *J. Agric. Food Chem.* **2005**, *53*, 2289–2296. [CrossRef] [PubMed]
114. Nakamura, A.; Watanabe, K.; Ojima, T.; Ahn, D.H.; Saeki, H. Effect of maillard reaction on allergenicity of scallop tropomyosin. *J. Agric. Food Chem.* **2005**, *53*, 7559–7564. [CrossRef] [PubMed]
115. Toda, M.; Heilmann, M.; Ilchmann, A.; Vieths, S. The maillard reaction and food allergies: Is there a link? *Clin. Chem. Lab. Med. CCLM/FESCC* **2014**, *52*, 61–67. [CrossRef] [PubMed]
116. Gupta, R.K.; Gupta, K.; Sharma, A.; Das, M.; Ansari, I.A.; Dwivedi, P.D. Maillard reaction in food allergy: Pros and cons. *Crit. Rev. Food Sci. Nutr.* **2016**, 1–19. [CrossRef] [PubMed]
117. Vojdani, A. Detection of ige, igg, iga and igm antibodies against raw and processed food antigens. *Nutr. Metab.* **2009**, *6*, 22. [CrossRef] [PubMed]
118. Sampson, H.A.; Ho, D.G. Relationship between food-specific ige concentrations and the risk of positive food challenges in children and adolescents. *J. Allergy Clin. Immunol.* **1997**, *100*, 444–451. [CrossRef]
119. Huby, R.D.; Dearman, R.J.; Kimber, I. Why are some proteins allergens? *Toxicol. Sci.* **2000**, *55*, 235–246. [CrossRef] [PubMed]
120. Aalberse, R.C. Structural biology of allergens. *J. Allergy Clin. Immunol.* **2000**, *106*, 228–238. [CrossRef] [PubMed]
121. Bredehorst, R.; David, K. What establishes a protein as an allergen? *J. Chromatogr. B Biomed. Sci. Appl.* **2001**, *756*, 33–40. [CrossRef]
122. James, J.A.; Harley, J.B. B-cell epitope spreading in autoimmunity. *Immunol. Rev.* **1998**, *164*, 185–200. [CrossRef] [PubMed]
123. Dall'Antonia, F.; Pavkov-Keller, T.; Zangger, K.; Keller, W. Structure of allergens and structure based epitope predictions. *Methods* **2014**, *66*, 3–21. [CrossRef] [PubMed]
124. Pomes, A.; Chruszcz, M.; Gustchina, A.; Wlodawer, A. Interfaces between allergen structure and diagnosis: Know your epitopes. *Curr. Allergy Asthma Rep.* **2015**, *15*, 506. [CrossRef] [PubMed]
125. Handlogten, M.W.; Kiziltepe, T.; Serezani, A.P.; Kaplan, M.H.; Bilgicer, B. Inhibition of weak-affinity epitope-ige interactions prevents mast cell degranulation. *Nat. Chem. Biol.* **2013**, *9*, 789–795. [CrossRef] [PubMed]

126. Baenziger, J.; Kornfeld, S.; Kochwa, S. Structure of the carbohydrate units of ige immunoglobulin. I. Over-all composition, glycopeptide isolation, and structure of the high mannose oligosaccharide unit. *J. Biol. Chem.* **1974**, *249*, 1889–1896. [PubMed]
127. Gould, H.J.; Sutton, B.J. Ige in allergy and asthma today. *Nat. Rev. Immunol.* **2008**, *8*, 205–217. [CrossRef] [PubMed]
128. El-Khouly, F.; Lewis, S.A.; Pons, L.; Burks, A.W.; Hourihane, J.O.B. Igg and ige avidity characteristics of peanut allergic individuals. *Pediatr. Allergy Immunol.* **2007**, *18*, 607–613. [CrossRef] [PubMed]
129. Wang, J.; Lin, J.; Bardina, L.; Goldis, M.; Nowak-Węgrzyn, A.; Shreffler, W.G.; Sampson, H.A. Correlation of ige/igg4 milk epitopes and affinity of milk-specific ige antibodies with different phenotypes of clinical milk allergy. *J. Allergy Clin. Immunol.* **2010**, *125*, 695–702.e6. [CrossRef] [PubMed]
130. Gould, H.J.; Sutton, B.J.; Beavil, A.J.; Beavil, R.L.; McCloskey, N.; Coker, H.A.; Fear, D.; Smurthwaite, L. The biology of ige and the basis of allergic disease. *Ann. Rev. Immunol.* **2003**, *21*, 579–628. [CrossRef] [PubMed]
131. Knol, E.F. Requirements for effective ige cross-linking on mast cells and basophils. *Mol. Nutr. Food Res.* **2006**, *50*, 620–624. [CrossRef] [PubMed]

10

Role of Microbial Modulation in Management of Atopic Dermatitis in Children

Lies Hulshof [1,†], Belinda van't Land [2,3,†], Aline B. Sprikkelman [4] and Johan Garssen [3,5,*]

1 Department of Paediatric Respiratory Medicine and Allergy, Emma Children's Hospital Academic Medical Center, 1105 AZ Amsterdam, The Netherlands; l.hulshof@amc.uva.nl
2 Department of Paediatric Immunology, University Medical Center Utrecht/Wilhelmina Children's Hospital, 3584 EA Utrecht, The Netherlands; b.vantland@umcutrecht.nl
3 Nutricia Research, 3584 CT Utrecht, The Netherlands
4 Department of Paediatric Pulmonology and Paediatric Allergology, University Medical Center Groningen, 9713 GZ Groningen, The Netherlands; a.b.sprikkelman@umcg.nl
5 Utrecht Institute for Pharmaceutical Sciences, Faculty of Science, Utrecht University, 3584 CG Utrecht, The Netherlands
* Correspondence: J.Garssen@uu.nl
† These authors contributed equally to this paper.

Abstract: The pathophysiology of atopic dermatitis (AD) is multifactorial and is a complex interrelationship between skin barrier, genetic predisposition, immunologic development, skin microbiome, environmental, nutritional, pharmacological, and psychological factors. Several microbial modulations of the intestinal microbiome with pre- and/or probiotics have been used in AD management, with different clinical out-come (both positive, as well as null findings). This review provides an overview of the clinical evidence from trials in children from 2008 to 2017, aiming to evaluate the effect of dietary interventions with pre- and/or pro-biotics for the treatment of AD. By searching the PUBMED/MEDLINE, EMBADE, and COCHRANE databases 14 clinical studies were selected and included within this review. Data extraction was independently conducted by two authors. The primary outcome was an improvement in the clinical score of AD severity. Changes of serum immunological markers and/or gastrointestinal symptoms were explored if available. In these studies some dietary interventions with pre- and/or pro-biotics were beneficial compared to control diets in the management of AD in children, next to treatment with emollients, and/or local corticosteroids. However, heterogeneity between studies was high, making it clear that focused clinical randomized controlled trials are needed to understand the potential role and underlying mechanism of dietary interventions in children with AD.

Keywords: atopic dermatitis; children; mucosal immune development

---

1. Introduction

Worldwide, the most common inflammatory skin disease is atopic dermatitis (AD) with a prevalence of 10–20% in children [1]. In 60% of these children, the onset of AD occurs early in life, before one year of age [2]. Pediatric AD can be characterized by its relapsing-remitting nature and the overall severity is mild in most of these young children [3]. The pathophysiology is multifactorial with a complex interrelationship between skin barrier development, genetic predisposition, immunological development, skin microbiome composition, and environmental, nutritional, pharmacological, and psychological factors. Whether or not AD is a primarily driven barrier dysfunction or a primarily inflammatory skin disease remains open for debate. Taking into account the recent understanding of the complex role of host microbial development in early life, new insights on regarding the role of microbial modulation in AD development during infancy may be hypothesized.

1.1. Host–Microbiome Development and Nutrition

The first contact of mucosal tissues to external microbiota is crucial in the establishment and maturation of the mucosal, as well as systemic, immune systems [4,5]. In particular, the first year of life is essential for programming the immune system. The development of barrier function and the immune system are influenced by environmental factors, such as feeding patterns, antibiotic use by the mother during delivery, or postnatal use of antibiotics by the neonate [6]. Proper understanding of the protective and programming effects of a healthy immune and microbiome development may provide opportunities to reduce the risk of development of AD. Any discordance between the early developmental requirements of the infant's immune system may contribute to the development of allergic diseases [7]. A recent COCHRANE systematic review of five clinical trials (952 participants) concluded that avoiding major allergens in the maternal diet (during gestation/lactation) does not protect against development of AD in the infant during the first 18 months of life [8]. This study also concluded that there was insufficient evidence that prolonged exclusive breast feeding was protective against AD. Early sensitization to food allergens through breast milk, skin contact, and/or inhalation occurs and may explain why some infants show an allergic response to specific proteins despite having never ingested it [7]. An additional influencing factor in allergy development is the timing of solid food introduction. For instance, infants starting with solid food introduction at four or five months of age had a lower risk for AD development (Odds ratio = 0.41, 95% Confidence interval, 0.20–0.87) compared to infants which were exclusively breastfed [9]. However, except maybe for peanut allergy, strong evidence is lacking to decide whether the age of complementary food introduction should be four or six months in order to prevent the development of allergy [5]. Although scientific evidence is limited, it has been suggested that timing of the start and type of nutrition (i.e., breastfeeding/infant formula) during solid food introduction influences the development of allergic diseases [10]. The question, however, remains whether observed effects are derived from direct interaction with immune cells, or indirectly through alterations in the microbiome composition and change in derivatives thereof, followed by immune changes [11]. The microbial composition is involved in the development of the regulatory T cell response and thereby plays a key role in immune development [12]. Within in vitro assays it has been shown that the addition of specific oligosaccharides during dendritic cell development induces a regulatory T cell response potentially of benefit in an allergic setting [13]. Moreover, dietary supplementation with specific prebiotic oligosaccharides has been shown to reduce the risk of developing allergies in infants [14]. Therefore, during early life it seems likely that specific components can contribute to the normal immune development via multiple direct and indirect pathways, thereby reducing the risk of allergic manifestations.

1.2. Development of Skin and Microbiome in Early Life

The composition and diversity of the skin microbiome shows a unique habitat per location, especially within children. The skin microbiome composition may be affected by different factors including age, sex, and microbial antigen exposure. Skin microbiota of neonates varies by the mode of delivery, but the differences become less apparent with age in early childhood [15,16]. The composition is also dependent on pH, temperature, Ultraviolet (UV) exposure, natural moisturizing factors (NMFs), and can easily change over time [17]. Specific changes in the skin microbiome have been associated with AD and other allergic manifestations [18]. AD has been associated with early life colonization of *Staphylococcus aureus* (*S. aureus*). A reduced bacterial diversity in the skin microbiome is of major importance in AD pathogenesis [19]. Only 5% of the skin microbiome in non-atopic individuals is colonized with *S. aureus*, compared to 39% in non-lesional skin and 70% in lesional skin of AD patients [20,21]. Although within a birth cohort it was shown that 10 infants with AD at the age of 12 months were not colonized with *S. aureus* before their first AD manifestation [22], colonization and infection with *S. aureus* has been associated with increased IgE responses, food allergy, and severity of AD skin disease [23,24]. In addition to the bacterial composition, the fungal and viral community differences are also associated with allergic manifestations such as rhinitis and asthma, as well [25,26].

This underscores the complexity of the host-microbe balance induction, as well as the sensitivity towards modulations herein [27].

Although whether or not AD is primarily driven by microbial dysbiosis leading to barrier dysfunction remains a key question, the skin barrier is hampered in AD. Within infants the skin has a higher ability to restore itself as a barrier. This adaptive flexibility results in unique properties of infant skin [28]. In a recent meta-analysis of genome-wide association studies of more than 15 million genetic variants in 21,399 cases and 95,464 controls, 10 new loci associated with AD risk were identified, bringing the total susceptibility loci until to 31 at the time of this publication [28–30]. Children with AD have changes in their skin barrier due to filaggrin deficiency or tight-junction dysfunction, which allows the penetration of irritants, allergens, and bacteria, leading to inflammation [31,32].

1.3. Immune Deregulation within AD

In AD, the skin barrier function is compromised, allowing penetration of environmental factors, such as irritants, allergens, and bacteria, leading to inflammation and/or allergic sensitization [33,34]. Skin barrier dysfunction induces the release of several inflammatory factors, including thymic stromal lymphopoietin (TSLP) and other cytokines and chemokines, which trigger inflammation in the skin [35]. These pro-inflammatory mediators (including chemokines) are released by the affected keratinocytes to attract leukocytes to the site of inflammation [36,37]. The characteristic leukocyte migration into the skin is driven by excessive chemokine production at the site of inflammation. Several chemokines (classically characterized within the Th1-type of response: CXCL9, CXCL10, and CXCL11; the Th2-type response: CCL-17, CCL22; and for inflammation: CCL-20) have been associated with an AD phenotype comprising complex pathology [38]. Studies on the pathology of early paediatric AD are limited and correlation of disease activity has been shown with only a few serum biomarkers (i.e., CCL17, CCL22, CCL27, and IgE) in infants [38,39]. Recently, profound immune activation in non-lesional skin in paediatric patients with AD has also been detected [38]. While little is known about the alterations in skin-derived immunity and skin barrier function that occur during the early-onset phase of AD, Th2 (IL-13, IL-31, and CCL17), Th22 (IL-22 and S100As), and some Th1-skewing (IFN-γ and CXCL10) have been detected in the skin, which is also observed in adults [38]. An increase in recruited Th2 cell populations classically leads to the increased production of interleukins IL-4, IL-5, and IL-13, which may be locally involved in the induction of IgE and eosinophil activation [39]. However, the identification of the trigger in AD development is still very complex.

1.4. Current Understanding in the Specific Microbial Modulations in AD

Due to the potential role of the microbiome in children with AD and development in early childhood, this seems a promising time frame for effective nutritional interventions including those with pre- and/or probiotics. In 2008 a comprehensive COCHRANE review (analysing 10 clinical trials (up to April 2008 (781 children)) concluded that overall probiotics in general seem not to be effective as a treatment of AD [40]. On the contrary, a modest role for probiotic interventions in paediatric dermatitis was suggested [41,42], as well as within later studies regarding pre- and/or probiotic interventions [43]. As stated by the recent meta-analysis by Kim et al. [44], the difference between age and severity of AD as measured by scoring of childhood atopic dermatitis (SCORAD) should be taken into account when analysing the impact of microbial modulations. Collectively, there was a large heterogeneity between trials complicating the comparison between specific species, strains, dosage, duration, time or age, and clinical outcomes. The aim of this review is to give an overview of the results of recently performed clinical intervention studies published after the COCHRANE review in 2008 until June 2017, studying the effect of microbial modulations for treatment of AD in children.

2. Methods

2.1. Search Strategy

To identify clinical dietary intervention studies with prebiotics/probiotics and/or synbiotics in children with AD, from birth up to 18 years of age, the PUBMED/MEDLINE, EMBASE, and COCHRANE databases have been searched. Since the COCHRANE review included all clinical trials up to April 2008, the literature search started from 2008 to June 2017. The following keywords were used: (probiotics OR prebiotics OR synbiotics) AND (atopic dermatitis OR eczema).

2.2. Study Selection

Published clinical intervention studies were included within this review meeting the following criteria: clinical studies with a dietary intervention with prebiotic(s) and/or probiotic(s), all participants were human, more specifically children from birth up to 18 years of age, all children with AD before the start of intervention, only studies with a clinical outcome for AD severity, studies published in the last 10 years, written in English, and presenting original data. A total of 75 abstracts have been retrieved through the database searches. Two authors independently checked the fulfilment of the inclusion criteria for this review by screening titles and abstracts and excluded studies that obviously did not fulfil the inclusion criteria. Seventy-three were published between April 2008 and 2017. A total of 59 from the 73 studies were excluded for this review, due to different outcomes than the inclusion criteria for this overview. The majority of these clinical studies had prevention of AD or other allergic manifestations as the primary outcome (N = 31). Other reasons to exclude studies were: no clinical AD outcome value, only gastrointestinal outcomes, safety studies, or genetic outcomes. In addition, three long-term follow-up studies were excluded. Finally the reference lists of the positively identified articles were checked for additional clinical studies and led to one additional study.

2.3. Data Extraction

Data extraction was independently conducted by two authors and cross-checked to avoid errors. Disagreements were resolved through consensus and, when needed, using the opinion of a third author. Details of the study were recorded: methods, objectives, study population, age of children with AD, inclusion and exclusion criteria, mild-to moderate-to severe AD, mean SCORAD scores, specific dietary intervention, strain and dosage of prebiotics and or probiotics, control diet, duration of intervention, number of randomized children in each group, clinical outcome of AD severity and change in AD severity (using primarily the AD scoring system SCORAD [45]). In addition, if available, the immunological outcomes, as well as the gastrointestinal outcomes, were included.

3. Results

3.1. Study Characteristics

The literature search resulted in 75 clinical intervention studies and, after inclusion, 13 studies could be used. One publication included two different types of interventions; open label versus randomized control using the same probiotic strain. Therefore, those two clinical studies will be mentioned separately in this overview. The study characteristics of the 14 selected clinical trials (N = 1008 children with AD) are summarized in Table 1 [43,46–57].

Table 1. Effects of microbial modulation in children with AD.

Subjects (Age, N, Treatment vs. Control)	Inclusion Criteria	Dietary Intervention	Treatment Period and Dose of Pre/Probiotics	Primary Parameter	Clinical Outcome, AD Severity and IgE	Immunological Outcomes	Gastro Intestinal Outcomes	Reference
Term infants 6–8 weeks N = 120 60 vs. 60	Positive history of allergy in one parent or sibling No breastfeeding at inclusion	Hydrolysed formula (HA) with GOS Control diet Only HA formula	For six months; Per 100 mL GOS 0.5 g	Differences in SCORAD score	After dietary intervention decrease of SCORAD in both groups (ns)	No serum data was available	Significant softer stool consistency in prebiotic group ($p < 0.05$)	Bozensky, et al. 2015 [46]
Term infants 0–7 months N = 89 42/47	SCORAD > 15 No more breastfeeding at inclusion No antibiotics four weeks before inclusion	Extensively hydrolysed formula with *Bifidobacterium Breve* M-16V and GOS/FOS Control diet Only extensively hydrolysed formula	For 12 weeks; Per 100 mL *BB.* 1.3×10^9 CFU GOS 0.72 g (90%) FOS 0.08 g (10%)	Change in severity of AD	After dietary intervention significant reduction of SCORAD in both groups. In subgroup of 50 infants, with elevated IgE levels, improvement in SCORAD after 12 weeks was greater in synbiotic group compared to control diet ($p = 0.04$)	No differences in spec IgE after 12 weeks between groups, No significant differences on IL-5, IgG1, IgG4, CCL17 and CCL27 after 12 weeks between groups. Significant increase of total IgE levels in both groups	Faecal pH was significantly lower in synbiotic group ($p = 0.001$) Significant softer stool consistency in synbiotic group ($p = 0.05$). Diaper dermatitis less prevalent in synbiotic group ($p = 0.008$)	Van der Aa, et al. 2010 [43]
Infants 1–36 months N = 36 18/18	Moderate to severe AD (SCORAD > 25)	Daily sachet with 7 strains of probiotics and FOS Control diet Daily sachet 1000 mg sucrose	For eight weeks; 10 mg probiotic mixture of 1×10^9 CFU 990 mg FOS	Clinical effect	After dietary intervention the mean total SCORAD in both groups decreased by 56% of all children. No differences between groups. In IgE + subgroup, similar decrease of AD severity in both groups	No serum data was available	No gastro intestinal data was available	Shafiei, et al. 2011 [47]
>34 weeks gestation 3–6 months N = 137 90 vs. 47	SCORAD>10 >200 mL standard formula daily	Extensively hydrolysed formula with a sachet *Lactobacillus paracasei CNCM I-2116* or with a sachet *Bifidobacterium lactis CNCM I-3446* Control diet; Extensively hydrolysed formula with maltodextrin sachet	For 12 weeks; *LP.* 10^{10} CFU *BL.* 10^{10} CFU *LP.* N = 45 *BL.* N = 45 C. N = 47	Change in SCORAD	After dietary intervention SCORAD reduction decreased significantly over time in all groups	No significant effect of probiotic treatments on the prevalence of allergen sensitization post-intervention	No differences in infants administered the L/M-permeability test between the groups	Gore, et al. 2012 [48]
Infants 3–72 months N = 40 19 vs. 21	Mild to severe AD No prior exposure to antibiotics or probiotics	1 g sachet with a mixture of 7 probiotic strains and FOS Control diet; 1 g sachet with placebo powder	For eight weeks; Twice daily mixture of 1×10^9 CFU and FOS	Change in AD severity	After dietary intervention greater reduction in SCORAD in synbiotic group compared to control diet ($p = 0.005$)	No significant differences on cytokine production of IFN-γ or IL-4 between groups	No gastro intestinal data was available	Farid, et al. 2011 [49]

Table 1. *Cont.*

Subjects (Age, N, Treatment vs. Control)	Inclusion Criteria	Dietary Intervention	Treatment Period and Dose of Pre/Probiotics	Primary Parameter	Clinical Outcome, AD Severity and IgE	Immunological Outcomes	Gastro Intestinal Outcomes	Reference
Infants 12–36 months N = 90 43 vs. 47	Moderate to severe AD (8 vs. 9 children with proven DBPCFC milk or egg allergy two months before inclusion on a milk or egg diet)	*Lactobacillus achidophilus DDS-1* and *Bifidobacterium lactis UABLA-12* and FOS in a rice maltodextrin powder Control diet; Pure powder of rice maltodextrin	For eight weeks; Twice daily Mixture of *LA.* and *BL2.* 5 × 10^9 CFU and 50mg FOS	Percentage change in SCORAD	After dietary intervention greater decrease in mean SCORAD in synbiotic group compared to control diet ($p = 0.001$)	Absolut count of CD4 and CD25 lymphocyte subsets were decreased whereas CD8 count increased in synbiotic group after dietary intervention compared to control diet.	No gastro intestinal data was available	Gerasimov, et al. 2010 [50]
Children 0–11 years N = 43	AD symptoms	Sachet *Lactobacillus salivarius LS01 DSM22775* No control diet	For eight weeks; Twice daily *LS.* 1 × 10^9 CFU	Change in AD severity	After dietary intervention significant reduction SCORAD in N = 28 ($p = 0.001$)	No serum data was available	No gastro intestinal data was available	Niccoli A, et al. 2014 [51]
Children 1–13 years N = 83 44 vs. 39	SCORAD ranged from 20 to 50	*Lactobacillus plantarum CJLP133* Control diet; placebo preparation No fermented food products containing live microorganisms were allowed	For 12 weeks; Twice daily *LP2.* 0.5 × 10^{10} CFU	Improvement of clinical and immunological parameters in children with AD	After dietary intervention greater decrease in SCORAD compared to control ($p = 0.004$)	Total eosinophil counts, Logarithmic IFN-y and IL-4 were significantly lower after dietary intervention in probiotic group compared to control ($p = 0.023$) ($p < 0.001$) ($p = 0.049$)	No gastro intestinal data was available	Han, et al. 2012 [52]
Children 1–18 years N = 220 165 vs. 55	AD symptoms > 6 months before inclusion SCORAD >15 At least 1 positive SPT or spec. IgE antibodies to common allergens	Capsule with *Lactobacillus para-casei GMNL-133* or capsule with *Lactobacillus fermentum GM090* or capsule with both probiotics Control diet; Placebo capsule	For three months; *LP3.* 2 × 10^9 CFU *LF.* 2 × 10^9 CFU *LP3* + *LF* 4 × 10^9 CFU *LP3.* N = 55 *LF.* N = 53 *LP3* + *LF* N = 51 C. N = 53	Change in AD severity	After dietary intervention (three groups LP, LF, and LP + LF mixture) lower SCORAD compared to control ($p < 0.001$) Difference remained at four months after discontinuing the probiotics	Total IgE levels were reduced within the *LP* and *LP* + *LF* group, but no significant differences compared to control. Significant change in IL-4 compared to control ($p = 0.04$)	The probiotics groups had significant higher fecal colony counts of *Bifidobacterium* ($p = 0.004$) and lower counts of *Clostridium* ($p = 0.03$) compared to control	Wang IJ, et al. 2015 [53]
Children 2–10 years N = 75 41 vs. 34	AEDS for six months prior to study Total SCORAD > 25	Microcrystalline cellulose with *Lactobacillus sakei KCTC 10755BP* Control diet; only microcrystalline cellulose	For 12 weeks; Twice daily *LS2.* 5 × 10^9 CFU	Evaluation of clinical outcome of AD	After dietary intervention mean change in Total SCORAD was significantly greater in probiotic group compared to the control group ($p = 0.008$)	Serum CCL17 and CCL27 levels were significantly decreased in probiotic group compared to control (both $p < 0.001$)	No gastro intestinal data was available	Woo, et al. 2010 [54]

Table 1. *Cont.*

Subjects (Age, N, Treatment vs. Control)	Inclusion Criteria	Dietary Intervention	Treatment Period and Dose of Pre/Probiotics	Primary Parameter	Clinical Outcome, AD Severity and IgE	Immunological Outcomes	Gastro Intestinal Outcomes	Reference
Children 2–14 years N = 54 27 vs. 27	AD symptoms for at least four days SCORAD > 25	Capsule with *Lactobacillus salivarius PM-A0006* and FOS Control diet; Capsule with corn starch and FOS	For eight weeks; Twice daily 25 mg *LS3.* (2×10^9 CFU), 475 mg FOS Control; 25 mg corn starch 475 mg FOS	SCORAD changes	After dietary intervention SCORAD significant lower in synbiotic group compared to prebiotic group ($p = 0.022$), differences remained at week 10	The median serum eosinophil cationic protein decreased significant within the groups but not significant different between the groups	No gastro intestinal data was available	Wu, et al. 2012 [55]
Children 4–10 years N = 51 26 vs. 25	AD symptoms No antibiotics for eight weeks No local corticosteroid use for eight weeks prior to study	Chewable tablet with *Lactobacillus reuteri ATCC55730* Control diet; chewable placebo tablet	For eight weeks; Once daily *LR.* 1×10^8 CFU	Effects on exhaled breath condensate (EBC) cytokine expression	After dietary intervention, no significant changes SCORAD mean values in probiotic group compared to control group	EBC IFN-y increased and IL4 decreased significantly in 16 IgE positive AD children in probiotic group compared to 14 IgE positive AD children in the control group (both $p = 0.001$)	No gastro intestinal data was available	Miniello, et al. 2010 [56]
Children 4–15 years N = 20	AD No cow's milk spec IgE	Fermented milk with *Lactobacillus acidophilus L-92* No control diet	For eight weeks; once daily 150 mL milk + *LA2*. 3×10^{10} CFU	Symptom-medication score (SMS), which is calculated as sum ADASI and calculated medication score of less topical steroid use.	Changes in ADASI, in SMS, and itch (all three; $p < 0.001$)	No changes in blood biochemical parameters, including the total plasma IgE concentration.	Significant decrease in the total faecal Bacteroidaceae count ($p = 0.034$), Significant increase in the faecal Lactobacillus count ($p = 0.007$)	Torii S, et al. 2010 [57]
Children 1–12 years N = 50	AD No cow's milk spec IgE	Fermented milk with dried and heat-killed *Lactobacillus acidophilus 92* and dextrin. Control diet; Fermented milk with dextrin	For eight weeks; once daily 150 mL milk + heat-killed *LA2* 1.5×10^{11} CFU + 900 mg dextrin	Symptom-medication score (SMS).	Significantly decreased of SMS in probiotic group compared to control group ($p = 0.0127$)	Changes in CCL17 levels were significantly different between probiotic group compared to control group ($p < 0.01$)	No gastro intestinal data was available	Torii S, et al. 2010 [57]

The clinical dietary intervention studies have been ordered according to the age of the children at inclusion. Abbreviations Table 1: AD, atopic dermatitis; IgE, Immunoglobulin E; HA, hydrolysed infant formula; GOS, galacto-oligosaccharides; SCORAD, scoring atopic dermatitis score; FOS, Fructo-oligosaccharides; BB, *Bifidobacterium breve M-16V*; CFU, colony-forming units; LP, *Lactobacillus paracasei CNCMI-2116*; BL *Bifidobacterium lactis CNCMI-3446*; C, control group; DBPCFC, double blind placebo controlled food challenge; LA, *Lactobacillus achidophilus DDS-1*, BL2 *Bifidobacterium lactis UABLA-12*; LS *Lactobacillus salivarius LS01 DSM22775*; LP2, *Lactobacillus plantarum CJLP133*; LP3, *Lactobacillus para-casei GMNL-133*; LF, *Lactobacillus fermentum GM090*; LS2 *Lactobacillus sakei KCTC10755BP*; LS3, *Lactobacillus salivarius PM-A0006*; LR, *Lactobacillus reuteri ATCC55730*; LA2, *Lactobacillus acidophilus L-92*.

3.2. *Specific Dietary Intervention*

Since the results of clinical intervention studies in the past showed inconclusive results of prebiotics and/or probiotics in the treatment of AD, it was hypothesized that the beneficial effects of prebiotics and probiotics are strain- and dose-dependent. *Lactobacillus* and *Bifidobacterium* are the two most investigated bacterial species in allergy research. Again, a wide variety in the dietary intervention studies was found in the clinical trials between 2008 and 2017 (Table 1). In total, 12 included trials were randomized controlled trials (RCTs) which had a total of 601 AD children in the treatment groups and 444 AD children in the control groups. The two additional clinical trials provided an open label intervention and were conducted with 63 children with AD. Not one intervention study used the same strain of probiotics or the same combination with prebiotics. More specifically, five RCTs provided synbiotic mixtures [43,47,49,50,55], four RCTs provided only one probiotic as dietary intervention [52,54,56,57], two RCTs provided more than one probiotic strain within the study [48,53], one trial explored the effect of prebiotics only [46], and the two open label studies were conducted with only one probiotic strain [51,57].

3.3. *Effect of Dietary Intervention on Clinically-Detected AD Severity*

In total, 12 out of the 14 studies reported the severity in AD using SCORAD. Three of the five RCTs with synbiotic intervention showed significant AD improvement by reduction of AD severity after dietary intervention compared to control diet [49,50,55]. The remaining two synbiotic RCTs showed a significant reduction of SCORAD score in both groups [43,47]. Improvement of AD severity was shown in three out of the four RCTs with one probiotic strain [52,54,57]. In addition, the result of the two open label intervention studies with one strain of probiotics is an improvement in AD symptoms [51,57]. Additionally, the RCT with the highest enrolment of children with AD (N = 220), showed an improvement in AD severity compared to the control group [53]. The trial of Gore et al. with two strains of probiotics showed a reduction of the SCORAD score in both groups [48]. The prebiotic trial showed improvement of AD severity in both groups [46]. In addition, the RCT with synbiotic intervention showed improvement of AD severity (SCORAD score). In the trial of van der Aa et al., a subgroup analysis of AD infants with elevated IgE levels showed a greater SCORAD score reduction in the synbiotic group [43]. A previous study also showed that synbiotic interventions may have beneficial effects, especially in AD with elevated IgE [58]. Taking IgE further into account, Shafiei et al. found no differences in comparing SCORAD scores in the IgE and non-IgE AD infants [47]. In contrast to Wang et al., who included only AD children with at least one positive skin prick test or at least one elevated specific IgE level within their study, showed improvement in AD [53], suggesting an important role for IgE.

3.4. *Additional Effect of Dietary Interventions*

Knowing the complexity of development in early life, some studies provide additional exploratory markers within the different RCTs. Three RCTs showed changing levels in cytokines IL-4 and/or IFN-y, which were significantly lower after intervention or did not show any change [51–53]. Additionally, changes in serum chemokine markers were detected, showing significant changes in two [54,57] groups, and no significant differences between groups in another study [43]. Some studies showed changes in IgE levels, but no significance between treatment and control [43,48,53]. In addition to serum markers, a few studies provide additional data on the effect of dietary intervention cellular composition [50]. For instance, the eosinophil count was significantly lower between groups in one study [52], and over time in one other study [55]. In three studies no immunological data was available, which may be due to the young age of infants included in those studies [46,47,51]. Only three RCTs reported on faecal bacterial counts after dietary intervention; all, however, confirmed changes in gut microbial composition after dietary intervention. Gastrointestinal symptoms, such as stool consistency and diaper dermatitis, were also positively influenced in the treatment group compared to control after the specific dietary interventions [43,46].

3.5. Treatment Duration and Time of Intervention

Within the identified clinical intervention studies, the treatment duration was variable, ranging from eight weeks up to six months [43,46–57]. There seemed to be no association between the duration of dietary intervention and the outcome of clinical improvement of AD. The trials indicating improvement of AD in both groups had intervention periods of eight or 12 weeks [43,46,48]. The effective duration of dietary intervention remains unclear. In two trials included in this review, a positive beneficial effect on AD severity remained detectable after the intervention period [53,55].

4. Discussion

This review summarizes the clinical outcome on AD severity among children receiving dietary intervention with or without prebiotics, probiotics, or synbiotics. It presents an overview of data from 2008 to June 2017 regarding the use of the specific dietary interventions in the treatment of AD in children, from birth up to 18 years of age available to date. As in earlier studies and meta-analyses published up to 2008, overall, strong evidence to clarify insights into the role of pre-, pro-, and synbiotics in treatment of AD is lacking, which may be due to high heterogeneity among the trials. Moreover, the outcome on AD severity seems to depend of multiple factors, including age, season, UV exposure, the use of local corticosteroids, number of AD exacerbations, etc.

Within the clinical intervention studies included in this review, several confounding factors need to be considered when interpreting the results. For example, since it is unethical to withhold AD children AD treatment with emollients and/or topical steroids, most studies provided treatment simultaneously with the dietary intervention. However, not all trials reported the amount and frequency of topical steroid use and, therefore, it is not clear if children in the treatment group were using the same amount of topical steroids as in the control groups. Within future studies, the method of randomisation, as well as amount and frequency of used topical steroids, should be reported. Although in some trials a decrease of local steroid use was mentioned, the effect of nutritional intervention compared to pharmacological treatment may both influence the AD severity score. For clinical outcome comparisons, the SCORAD score is validated for AD severity, but it is known to be difficult to assess in young infants, providing possible inter-observer variability. Moreover, due to the relapsing-remitting nature of AD in these young children (which occurs randomly in time), this may complicate the evaluation of AD severity and the impact of nutritional intervention effects in time. Recently, the evaluation on AD measurements provided recommendations about scoring AD severity, providing an interesting tool for future research. These include SIS (skin intensity score) (paediatric version), POEM (patient-oriented eczema measure), SCORAD (Severity Scoring of Atopic Dermatitis index), SA-EASI (self-administered eczema area and severity index score), and adapted SA-EASI, which are currently the most appropriate instruments to assess AD and, therefore, should be recommended as core symptom instruments in future clinical trials [59].

With the knowledge that both the child's microbiome and mucosal immunity evolves from infancy into early childhood, the age of inclusion in a study of AD is of utmost importance. In infants the cheeks are a typical preferred site of AD and the nasal tip is usually spared. After one year of age, a change of AD sites is more prone to the antecubital and popliteal fossa. Possible explanation for this change is change in the diversity in the skin microbiome and changes in skin barrier function in early life. Nevertheless the age of inclusion was within the dietary intervention studies, which may explain the differing results. Hypothesizing that the first year of life is the essential period for programming the mucosal immune system, this may also be the preferred time to prevent the development of AD with microbial modulations. However, as shown within some recent meta-analyses with a specific focus on the clinical evidence from dietary intervention studies, it was concluded that dietary intervention during pregnancy, or lactation in the mothers, or in the early life of the infant led to a decreased risk of AD development, but not the development of other allergies [60–62]. It should be noted that the overall evidence is low due to the inconsistent results among studies. In order to investigate and understand the mechanisms involved in immune modulation capacities of microbiota by dietary interventions on clinical outcome severity of AD in childhood, the consistency between trials must increase. Therefore, criteria should be formulated on how to conduct future studies in this field in order to be able to compare clinical trial outcomes, so that subsequently reliable and valid advice can be given to implement dietary interventions in the management of AD.

5. Conclusions

Identifying high-risk children for atopic manifestations and AD children who can benefit from these microbial modulations seems highly relevant. Moreover, a better understanding of the contributing factors, such as the skin microbiome, faecal composition, and biomarkers of skin barrier function, leading to changes within serum biomarker profiles would be of great value for a more individualized therapeutic approach in AD management in children. In addition, to overcome the problem of heterogeneity of the studies and therefore the limitation of comparing clinical trial outcomes, an international committee of experts should focus on definitions of outcome measures, treatment duration, administration of the product, etc. Since the development and evolution of each child's microbiome starts from infancy up to childhood, an early life dietary intervention (in pregnancy and/or in infancy) seems preferable. Further standardized clinical research is, however, necessary to gain more insight into specific strains, prebiotics and timing for optimal intervention. By combining the individual factors of a child with AD, as mentioned above, it may be possible to eventually match the clinical needs with the best dietary management option available.

Author Contributions: L.H. and B.v.L. contributed equally to data extraction, analyses, and interpretation. A.B.S. and J.G. supervised the project, and all authors approved the final version of the manuscript.

Abbreviations

AD	Atopic dermatitis
CCL	CC chemokine ligand (−17, −20, −22, −27)
CXCL	CXC chemokine ligand (−9,−10,−11)
EASI	Eczema area and severity index
FLG	Filaggrin
lcFOS	long chain—Fructo-oligosaccharides
scGOS	short chain—Galacto-oligosaccharides
IgE	Immunoglobulin E (total, specific)
IL	Interleukin (−4, −5, −13, −22, −31)
IFN	Interferon ($-\gamma$)
NMF	Natural moisturizing factors
POEM	Patient-oriented eczema measure
RCT	Randomized controlled trial
SA-EASI	Self-administered eczema area and severity index score
SASSAD	Six Area, Six Sign Atopic Dermatitis severity score
SIS	Skin intensity score
SCORAD	Scoring atopic dermatitis score, clinical tool for scoring AD severity
SC	Stratum corneum
TEWL	Trans epidermal water loss
Th-	T helper cell type (1, 2, 17, 22)
TIS	Three Item Severity score
TJ	Tight junction
TSLP	Thymic stromal lymphopoietin
UV	Ultraviolet

References

1. Weidinger, S.; Novak, N. Atopic dermatitis. *Lancet* **2016**, *387*, 1109–1122. [CrossRef]
2. Illi, S.; von Mutius, E.; Lau, S.; Nickel, R.; Gruber, C.; Niggemann, B.; Wahn, U.; Multicenter Allergy Study group. The natural course of atopic dermatitis from birth to age 7 years and the association with asthma. *J. Allergy Clin. Immunol.* **2004**, *113*, 925–931. [CrossRef] [PubMed]
3. Ballardini, N.; Kull, I.; Soderhall, C.; Lilja, G.; Wickman, M.; Wahlgren, C.F. Eczema severity in preadolescent children and its relation to sex, filaggrin mutations, asthma, rhinitis, aggravating factors and topical treatment: A report from the BAMSE birth cohort. *Br. J. Dermatol.* **2013**, *168*, 588–594. [CrossRef] [PubMed]
4. Van't Land, B.; Schijf, M.A.; Martin, R.; Garssen, J.; van Bleek, G.M. Influencing mucosal homeostasis and immune responsiveness: The impact of nutrition and pharmaceuticals. *Eur. J. Pharmacol.* **2011**, *668* (Suppl. 1), S101–S107. [CrossRef] [PubMed]
5. Abrams, E.M.; Greenhawt, M.; Fleischer, D.M.; Chan, E.S. Early Solid Food Introduction: Role in Food Allergy Prevention and Implications for Breastfeeding. *J. Pediatr.* **2017**, *184*, 13–18. [CrossRef] [PubMed]
6. Ahmadizar, F.; Vijverberg, S.J.H.; Arets, H.G.M.; de Boer, A.; Turner, S.; Devereux, G.; Arabkhazaeli, A.; Soares, P.; Mukhopadhyay, S.; Garssen, J.; et al. Early life antibiotic use and the risk of asthma and asthma exacerbations in children. *Pediatr. Allergy Immunol.* **2017**, *28*, 430–437. [CrossRef] [PubMed]
7. Verhasselt, V.; Milcent, V.; Cazareth, J.; Kanda, A.; Fleury, S.; Dombrowicz, D.; Glaichenhaus, N.; Julia, V. Breast milk-mediated transfer of an antigen induces tolerance and protection from allergic asthma. *Nat. Med.* **2008**, *14*, 170–175. [CrossRef] [PubMed]
8. Kramer, M.S.; Kakuma, R. Maternal dietary antigen avoidance during pregnancy or lactation, or both, for preventing or treating atopic disease in the child. *Cochrane Database Syst. Rev.* **2012**, CD000133. [CrossRef]
9. Turati, F.; Bertuccio, P.; Galeone, C.; Pelucchi, C.; Naldi, L.; Bach, J.F.; La Vecchia, C.; Chatenoud, L.; HYGIENE Study Group. Early weaning is beneficial to prevent atopic dermatitis occurrence in young children. *Allergy* **2016**, *71*, 878–888. [CrossRef] [PubMed]
10. Snijders, B.E.; Thijs, C.; van Ree, R.; van den Brandt, P.A. Age at first introduction of cow milk products and other food products in relation to infant atopic manifestations in the first 2 years of life: The KOALA Birth Cohort Study. *Pediatrics* **2008**, *122*, e115–e122. [CrossRef] [PubMed]
11. Te Velde, A.A.; Bezema, T.; van Kampen, A.H.; Kraneveld, A.D.; t Hart, B.A.; van Middendorp, H.; Hack, E.C.; van Montfrans, J.M.; Belzer, C.; Jans-Beken, L.; et al. Embracing Complexity beyond Systems Medicine: A New Approach to Chronic Immune Disorders. *Front Immunol.* **2016**, *7*, 587. [CrossRef] [PubMed]
12. Round, J.L.; Mazmanian, S.K. Inducible Foxp3+ regulatory T-cell development by a commensal bacterium of the intestinal microbiota. *Proc. Natl. Acad. Sci. USA* **2010**, *107*, 12204–12209. [CrossRef] [PubMed]
13. Lehmann, S.; Hiller, J.; van Bergenhenegouwen, J.; Knippels, L.M.; Garssen, J.; Traidl-Hoffmann, C. In Vitro Evidence for Immune-Modulatory Properties of Non-Digestible Oligosaccharides: Direct Effect on Human Monocyte Derived Dendritic Cells. *PLoS ONE* **2015**, *10*, e0132304. [CrossRef] [PubMed]
14. Boyle, R.J.; Tang, M.L.; Chiang, W.C.; Chua, M.C.; Ismail, I.; Nauta, A.; Hourihane, J.O.; Smith, P.; Gold, M.; Ziegler, J.; et al. Prebiotic-supplemented partially hydrolysed cow's milk formula for the prevention of eczema in high-risk infants: A randomized controlled trial. *Allergy* **2016**, *71*, 701–710. [CrossRef] [PubMed]
15. Dominguez-Bello, M.G.; Costello, E.K.; Contreras, M.; Contreras, M.; Magris, M.; Hidalgo, G.; Fierer, N.; Knight, R. Delivery mode shapes the acquisition and structure of the initial microbiota across multiple body habitats in newborns. *Proc. Natl. Acad. Sci. USA* **2010**, *107*, 11971–11975. [CrossRef] [PubMed]
16. Human Microbiome Project C. Structure, function and diversity of the healthy human microbiome. *Nature* **2012**, *486*, 207–214.
17. Huang, Y.J.; Marsland, B.J.; Bunyavanich, S.; O'Mahony, L.; Leung, D.Y.; Muraro, A.; Fleisher, T.A. The microbiome in allergic disease: Current understanding and future opportunities-2017 PRACTALL document of the American Academy of Allergy, Asthma & Immunology and the European Academy of Allergy and Clinical Immunology. *J. Allergy Clin. Immunol.* **2017**, *139*, 1099–1110. [PubMed]
18. Oh, J.; Byrd, A.L.; Park, M.; Program, N.C.S.; Kong, H.H.; Segre, J.A. Temporal Stability of the Human Skin Microbiome. *Cell* **2016**, *165*, 854–866. [CrossRef] [PubMed]
19. Kong, H.H.; Oh, J.; Deming, C.; Conlan, S.; Grice, E.A.; Beatson, M.A.; Nomicos, E.; Polley, E.C.; Komarow, H.D.; NISC Comparative Sequence Program; et al. Temporal shifts in the skin microbiome associated with disease flares and treatment in children with atopic dermatitis. *Genome Res.* **2012**, *22*, 850–859. [CrossRef] [PubMed]

20. Hanifin, J.M.; Rogge, J.L. Staphylococcal infections in patients with atopic dermatitis. *Arch. Dermatol.* **1977**, *113*, 1383–1386. [CrossRef] [PubMed]
21. Zollner, T.M.; Wichelhaus, T.A.; Hartung, A.; Von Mallinckrodt, C.; Wagner, T.O.; Brade, V.; Kaufmann, R. Colonization with superantigen-producing Staphylococcus aureus is associated with increased severity of atopic dermatitis. *Clin. Exp. Allergy* **2000**, *30*, 994–1000. [CrossRef] [PubMed]
22. Kennedy, E.A.; Connolly, J.; Hourihane, J.O.; Fallon, P.G.; McLean, W.H.; Murray, D.; Jo, J.H.; Segre, J.A.; Kong, H.H.; Irvine, A.D. Skin microbiome before development of atopic dermatitis: Early colonization with commensal staphylococci at 2 months is associated with a lower risk of atopic dermatitis at 1 year. *J. Allergy Clin. Immunol.* **2017**, *139*, 166–172. [CrossRef] [PubMed]
23. Jones, A.L.; Curran-Everett, D.; Leung, D.Y. Food allergy is associated with Staphylococcus aureus colonization in children with atopic dermatitis. *J. Allergy Clin. Immunol.* **2016**, *137*, 1247–1248.e3. [CrossRef] [PubMed]
24. Tauber, M.; Balica, S.; Hsu, C.Y.; Jean-Decoster, C.; Lauze, C.; Redoules, D.; Viodé, C.; Schmitt, A.M.; Serre, G.; Simon, M.; et al. Staphylococcus aureus density on lesional and nonlesional skin is strongly associated with disease severity in atopic dermatitis. *J. Allergy Clin. Immunol.* **2016**, *137*, 1272–1274.e3. [CrossRef] [PubMed]
25. Jung, W.H.; Croll, D.; Cho, J.H.; Kim, Y.R.; Lee, Y.W. Analysis of the nasal vestibule mycobiome in patients with allergic rhinitis. *Mycoses* **2015**, *58*, 167–172. [CrossRef] [PubMed]
26. Van Woerden, H.C.; Gregory, C.; Brown, R.; Marchesi, J.R.; Hoogendoorn, B.; Matthews, I.P. Differences in fungi present in induced sputum samples from asthma patients and non-atopic controls: A community based case control study. *BMC Infect. Dis.* **2013**, *13*, 69. [CrossRef] [PubMed]
27. Williams, M.R.; Gallo, R.L. The role of the skin microbiome in atopic dermatitis. *Curr. Allergy Asthma Rep.* **2015**, *15*, 65. [CrossRef] [PubMed]
28. Kezic, S.; Novak, N.; Jakasa, I.; Jungersted, J.M.; Simon, M.; Brandner, J.M.; Middelkamp-Hup, M.A.; Weidinger, S. Skin barrier in atopic dermatitis. *Front. Biosci.* **2014**, *19*, 542–556. [CrossRef]
29. Paternoster, L.; Standl, M.; Waage, J.; Baurecht, H.; Hotze, M.; Strachan, D.P.; Curtin, J.A.; Bønnelykke, K.; Tian, C.; Takahashi, A.; et al. Multi-ancestry genome-wide association study of 21,000 cases and 95,000 controls identifies new risk loci for atopic dermatitis. *Nat. Genet.* **2015**, *47*, 1449–1456. [CrossRef] [PubMed]
30. Paternoster, L.; Standl, M.; Chen, C.M.; Ramasamy, A.; Bonnelykke, K.; Duijts, L.; Ferreira, M.A.; Alves, A.C.; Thyssen, J.P.; Albrecht, E.; et al. Meta-analysis of genome-wide association studies identifies three new risk loci for atopic dermatitis. *Nat. Genet.* **2011**, *44*, 187–192. [CrossRef] [PubMed]
31. Irvine, A.D.; McLean, W.H.; Leung, D.Y. Filaggrin mutations associated with skin and allergic diseases. *N. Engl. J. Med.* **2011**, *365*, 1315–1327. [CrossRef] [PubMed]
32. Yuki, T.; Tobiishi, M.; Kusaka-Kikushima, A.; Ota, Y.; Tokura, Y. Impaired Tight Junctions in Atopic Dermatitis Skin and in a Skin-Equivalent Model Treated with Interleukin-17. *PLoS ONE* **2016**, *11*, e0161759. [CrossRef] [PubMed]
33. Fluhr, J.W.; Darlenski, R.; Taieb, A.; Hachem, J.P.; Baudouin, C.; Msika, P.; De Belilovsky, C.; Berardesca, E. Functional skin adaptation in infancy - almost complete but not fully competent. *Exp. Dermatol.* **2010**, *19*, 483–492. [CrossRef] [PubMed]
34. Leung, D.Y. New insights into atopic dermatitis: Role of skin barrier and immune dysregulation. *Allergol. Int.* **2013**, *62*, 151–161. [CrossRef] [PubMed]
35. Albanesi, C. Keratinocytes in allergic skin diseases. *Curr. Opin. Allergy Clin. Immunol.* **2010**, *10*, 452–456. [CrossRef] [PubMed]
36. Castan, L.; Magnan, A.; Bouchaud, G. Chemokine receptors in allergic diseases. *Allergy* 2016. [CrossRef] [PubMed]
37. Homey, B.; Steinhoff, M.; Ruzicka, T.; Leung, D.Y. Cytokines and chemokines orchestrate atopic skin inflammation. *J. Allergy Clin. Immunol.* **2006**, *118*, 178–189. [CrossRef] [PubMed]
38. Esaki, H.; Brunner, P.M.; Renert-Yuval, Y.; Czarnowicki, T.; Huynh, T.; Tran, G.; Lyon, S.; Rodriguez, G.; Immaneni, S.; Johnson, D.B.; et al. Early-onset pediatric atopic dermatitis is TH2 but also TH17 polarized in skin. *J. Allergy Clin. Immunol.* **2016**, *138*, 1639–1651. [CrossRef] [PubMed]
39. Van der Velden, V.H.; Laan, M.P.; Baert, M.R.; de Waal Malefyt, R.; Neijens, H.J.; Savelkoul, H.F. Selective development of a strong Th2 cytokine profile in high-risk children who develop atopy: Risk factors and regulatory role of IFN-gamma, IL-4 and IL-10. *Clin. Exp. Allergy* **2001**, *31*, 997–1006. [CrossRef] [PubMed]

40. Boyle, R.J.; Bath-Hextall, F.J.; Leonardi-Bee, J.; Murrell, D.F.; Tang, M.L. Probiotics for treating eczema. *Cochrane Database Syst. Rev.* **2008**, CD006135. [CrossRef]
41. Lee, J.; Seto, D.; Bielory, L. Meta-analysis of clinical trials of probiotics for prevention and treatment of pediatric atopic dermatitis. *J. Allergy Clin. Immunol.* **2008**, *121*, 116–121.e11. [CrossRef] [PubMed]
42. Michail, S.K.; Stolfi, A.; Johnson, T.; Onady, G.M. Efficacy of probiotics in the treatment of pediatric atopic dermatitis: A meta-analysis of randomized controlled trials. *Ann. Allergy Asthma Immunol.* **2008**, *101*, 508–516. [CrossRef]
43. Van der Aa, L.B.; Heymans, H.S.; van Aalderen, W.M.; Sillevis Smitt, J.H.; Knol, J.; Ben Amor, K.; Goossens, D.A.; Sprikkelman, A.B.; synbad Study Group. Effect of a new synbiotic mixture on atopic dermatitis in infants: A randomized-controlled trial. *Clin. Exp. Allergy* **2010**, *40*, 795–804. [PubMed]
44. Kim, S.O.; Ah, Y.M.; Yu, Y.M.; Choi, K.H.; Shin, W.G.; Lee, J.Y. Effects of probiotics for the treatment of atopic dermatitis: A meta-analysis of randomized controlled trials. *Ann. Allergy Asthma Immunol.* **2014**, *113*, 217–226. [CrossRef] [PubMed]
45. Schmitt, J.; Langan, S.; Deckert, S.; Svensson, A.; von Kobyletzki, L.; Thomas, K.; Spuls, P.; Harmonising Outcome Measures for Atopic Dermatitis (HOME) Initiative. Assessment of clinical signs of atopic dermatitis: A systematic review and recommendation. *J. Allergy Clin. Immunol.* **2013**, *132*, 1337–1347. [PubMed]
46. Bozensky, J.; Hill, M.; Zelenka, R.; Skyba, T. Prebiotics Do Not Influence the Severity of Atopic Dermatitis in Infants: A Randomised Controlled Trial. *PLoS ONE* **2015**, *10*, e0142897. [CrossRef] [PubMed]
47. Shafiei, A.; Moin, M.; Pourpak, Z.; Gharagozlou, M.; Aghamohammadi, A.; Sajedi, V.; Soheili, H.; Sotoodeh, S.; Movahedi, M. Synbiotics could not reduce the scoring of childhood atopic dermatitis (SCORAD): A randomized double blind placebo-controlled trial. *Iran. J. Allergy Asthma Immunol.* **2011**, *10*, 21–28. [PubMed]
48. Gore, C.; Custovic, A.; Tannock, G.W.; Munro, K.; Kerry, G.; Johnson, K.; Peterson, C.; Morris, J.; Chaloner, C.; Murray, C.S.; et al. Treatment and secondary prevention effects of the probiotics Lactobacillus paracasei or Bifidobacterium lactis on early infant eczema: Randomized controlled trial with follow-up until age 3 years. *Clin. Exp. Allergy* **2012**, *42*, 112–122. [CrossRef] [PubMed]
49. Farid, R.; Ahanchian, H.; Jabbari, F.; Moghiman, T. Effect of a new synbiotic mixture on atopic dermatitis in children: A randomized-controlled trial. *Iran. J. Pediatr.* **2011**, *21*, 225–230. [PubMed]
50. Gerasimov, S.V.; Vasjuta, V.V.; Myhovych, O.O.; Bondarchuk, L.I. Probiotic supplement reduces atopic dermatitis in preschool children: A randomized, double-blind, placebo-controlled, clinical trial. *Am. J. Clin. Dermatol.* **2010**, *11*, 351–361. [CrossRef] [PubMed]
51. Niccoli, A.A. Preliminary results on clinical effects of probiotic Lactobacillus salivarius LS01 in children affected by atopic dermatitis. *J. Clin. Gastroenterol.* **2014**, *48* (Suppl. 1), S34–S36. [CrossRef] [PubMed]
52. Han, Y.; Kim, B.; Ban, J.; Lee, J.; Kim, B.J.; Choi, B.S.; Hwang, S.; Ahn, K.; Kim, J. A randomized trial of Lactobacillus plantarum CJLP133 for the treatment of atopic dermatitis. *Pediatr. Allergy Immunol.* **2012**, *23*, 667–673. [CrossRef] [PubMed]
53. Wang, I.J.; Wang, J.Y. Children with atopic dermatitis show clinical improvement after Lactobacillus exposure. *Clin. Exp. Allergy* **2015**, *45*, 779–787. [CrossRef] [PubMed]
54. Woo, S.I.; Kim, J.Y.; Lee, Y.J.; Kim, N.S.; Hahn, Y.S. Effect of Lactobacillus sakei supplementation in children with atopic eczema-dermatitis syndrome. *Ann. Allergy Asthma Immunol.* **2010**, *104*, 343–348. [CrossRef] [PubMed]
55. Wu, K.G.; Li, T.H.; Peng, H.J. Lactobacillus salivarius plus fructo-oligosaccharide is superior to fructo-oligosaccharide alone for treating children with moderate to severe atopic dermatitis: A double-blind, randomized, clinical trial of efficacy and safety. *Br. J. Dermatol.* **2012**, *166*, 129–136. [CrossRef] [PubMed]
56. Miniello, V.L.; Brunetti, L.; Tesse, R.; Natile, M.; Armenio, L.; Francavilla, R. Lactobacillus reuteri modulates cytokines production in exhaled breath condensate of children with atopic dermatitis. *J. Pediatr. Gastroenterol. Nutr.* **2010**, *50*, 573–576. [CrossRef] [PubMed]
57. Torii, S.; Torii, A.; Itoh, K.; Urisu, A.; Terada, A.; Fujisawa, T.; Yamada, K.; Suzuki, H.; Ishida, Y.; Nakamura, F.; et al. Effects of oral administration of Lactobacillus acidophilus L-92 on the symptoms and serum markers of atopic dermatitis in children. *Int. Arch. Allergy Immunol.* **2011**, *154*, 236–245. [CrossRef] [PubMed]
58. Viljanen, M.; Savilahti, E.; Haahtela, T.; Juntunen-Backman, K.; Korpela, R.; Poussa, T.; Tuure, T.; Kuitunen, M. Probiotics in the treatment of atopic eczema/dermatitis syndrome in infants: A double-blind placebo-controlled trial. *Allergy* **2005**, *60*, 494–500. [CrossRef] [PubMed]

59. Gerbens, L.A.; Prinsen, C.A.; Chalmers, J.R.; Drucker, A.M.; von Kobyletzki, L.B.; Limpens, J.; Nankervis, H.; Svensson, Å.; Terwee, C.B.; Zhang, J.; et al. Evaluation of the measurement properties of symptom measurement instruments for atopic eczema: A systematic review. *Allergy* **2017**, *72*, 146–163. [CrossRef] [PubMed]
60. Forsberg, A.; West, C.E.; Prescott, S.L.; Jenmalm, M.C. Pre- and probiotics for allergy prevention: Time to revisit recommendations? *Clin. Exp. Allergy* **2016**, *46*, 1506–1521. [CrossRef] [PubMed]
61. Cuello-Garcia, C.A.; Brozek, J.L.; Fiocchi, A.; Pawankar, R.; Yepes-Nunez, J.J.; Terracciano, L.; Gandhi, S.; Agarwal, A.; Zhang, Y.; Schünemann, H.J. Probiotics for the prevention of allergy: A systematic review and meta-analysis of randomized controlled trials. *J. Allergy Clin. Immunol.* **2015**, *136*, 952–961. [CrossRef] [PubMed]
62. Zuccotti, G.; Meneghin, F.; Aceti, A.; Barone, G.; Callegari, M.L.; Di Mauro, A.; Fantini, M.P.; Gori, D.; Indrio, F.; Maggio, L.; et al. Probiotics for prevention of atopic diseases in infants: Systematic review and meta-analysis. *Allergy* **2015**, *70*, 1356–1371. [CrossRef] [PubMed]

11

The Role of Nutritional Aspects in Food Allergy: Prevention and Management

Alessandra Mazzocchi [1,*], Carina Venter [2], Kate Maslin [3] and Carlo Agostoni [1]

1 Pediatric Intermediate Care Unit, Fondazione IRCCS Ospedale Ca' Granda-Ospedale Maggiore Policlinico, Department of Clinical Sciences and Community Health, University of Milan, 20122 Milan, Italy; carlo.agostoni@unimi.it
2 Section of Allergy and Immunology, Children's Hospital Colorado, University of Colorado, Aurora, CO 80045, USA; carina.venter@childrenscolorado.org
3 MRC Lifecourse Epidemiology Unit, University of Southampton, Southampton SO16 6YD, UK; maslinkate@gmail.com
* Correspondence: alessandra.mazzocchi@unimi.it

Abstract: The prevalence of food allergy in childhood appears to be increasing in both developed and transitional countries. The aim of this paper is to review and summarise key findings in the prevention and management of food allergy, focusing on the role of dietary components and nutritional habits in the development and optimal functioning of the immune system. Essential fatty acids, zinc and vitamin D are likely to enhance the anti-inflammatory and antioxidative barrier and promote immunologic tolerance. Additionally, nutritional components such as pre- and probiotics represent a novel research approach in the attempt to induce a tolerogenic immune environment. For all these reasons, the traditional avoidance diet has been, in recent years, completely reconsidered. New findings on the protective effect of an increased diversity of food introduced in the first year of life on allergic diseases are consistent with the hypothesis that exposure to a variety of food antigens during early life might play a role in the development of immune tolerance. Accordingly, therapeutic (and even preventive) interventions should be planned on an individual basis.

Keywords: food allergy; children; diet diversity; adequate nutrition

---

1. Introduction

Food allergy (FA) represents a substantial health problem in childhood. The prevalence appears to be increasing in both developed and transitional countries, however a true increase has been difficult to demonstrate [1]. Over 90% of food allergies are caused by eight common allergens; namely: eggs, peanuts, cow's milk, soy, nuts, shellfish, fish, or wheat [2]. On the whole, food allergy affects approximately 6% of infants younger than three years [2], and prevalence decreases over the first decade. The cumulative incidence of food hypersensitivity over a 10-year period is 6.7% (95% CI: 5.2–8.4%); 3.0% (95% CI: 1.8–4.2%) had IgE-mediated food allergy and 0.6% (95% CI: 0.07–1.3%) had non-IgE-mediated food allergy/food intolerance [3]. A systematic review from the European Academy of Allergy and Clinical Immunology concluded that food allergy prevalence in Europe ranges between 0.1 and 6.0% [4]. The Institute of Medicine report states that the prevalence of food allergies in children ranges between 1.1 and 10.4% [1]. Food-allergic infants commonly present with symptoms and signs of atopic eczema, gastrointestinal symptoms and/or recurrent wheezing [5]. Diet plays a crucial role in both the prevention and management of food allergy. A number of factors, including the maternal diet, the microbiome and early life feeding, have been investigated for the prevention of allergic diseases [6]. The aim of this paper is to review and summarise key findings in the prevention and management of food allergy, with particular reference to nutrients of concern (fats, micronutrients), gut flora (including the role of pre- and probiotics), early-life feeding and formula choice in cow's milk allergy.

2. Prevention of Food Allergy: The Role of Nutrition in the Development and Optimal Functioning of the Immune System

Allergy results when there is a breakdown in normal "tolerance" mechanisms, which leads to inappropriate and detrimental immune responses to normally harmless substances, including food allergens such as cow's milk protein, eggs, nuts, or shellfish [7]. At birth, the immune system is immature, but it develops with age, antigen stimulation, and appropriate nutrition [8]. In addition, bacterial colonisation occurs during the first weeks of life, and interactions between intestinal flora and the developing mucosa result in further development of immune responses and oral tolerance [7].

Nutrition plays a key role in the development, maintenance, and optimal functioning of immune cells. Nutrients, such as zinc and vitamin D and nutritional factors, such as pre- and probiotics, can influence the nature of an immune response and are important in ensuring appropriate functioning of the immune system, as described in the paragraphs below.

2.1. Fat

Appropriate fat intake may become seriously compromised in allergen-restricted diets and may be further influenced by the "westernized" dietary practices. The role of fat on the immune system can be divided into the role of saturated vs. unsaturated fats and the particular role of the essential fatty acids.

2.1.1. Saturated vs. Unsaturated Fats

It has been reported that typical western diets rich in protein and saturated fat and low in complex carbohydrates may negatively affect the diversity of the gut microbiome [9]. This was supported by David et al. [10], showing that an animal-based diet high in protein and fat, with very little fibre intake, resulted in increased abundance of bile-tolerant microorganisms (*Alistipes*, *Bilophila*, and *Bacteroides*) and decreased levels of Firmicutes that metabolize dietary plant polysaccharides (*Roseburia*, *Eubacterium rectale*, and *Ruminococcus bromii*) within a five-day period. A recent review also concluded that the amount, type (e.g., unsaturated vs saturated), and mixture of dietary fats can dramatically shift gut microbial community membership and function [11]. In addition, high fat, high sugar diets also affect the gut barrier function in mice, as demonstrated by high horseradish peroxidase (HRP) influx, lower portal vein endotoxin levels and decreased goblet cell numbers [12]. The gut barrier function may be permanently affected in non-IgE mediated food allergies, and temporarily affected during allergen exposure in IgE mediated food allergies [13,14].

2.1.2. Essential Fatty Acids (EFAs)

EFAs are important immune regulators. Linoleic acid (LA), the parental *n*-6 polyunsaturated fatty acid (PUFA), is converted into arachidonic acid (AA) by fatty acid elongase and desaturase, and subsequently may give origin to pro-inflammatory and pro-allergic lipid mediators, whose collective name is eicosanoids [15]. In contrast, α-linolenic acid (ALA), an *n*-3 PUFA, is converted in the mammalian body to eicosapentaenoic acid (EPA) and docosahexaenoic acid (DHA), which are subsequently converted into anti-inflammatory and/or pro-resolving lipid mediators (such as resolvins and protectins). EPA forms the precursors of the 3 series of prostaglandins and the 5 series of leukotrienes, which are biologically less powerful than the corresponding derivatives which form the *n*-6 compounds. Because *n*-3 and *n*-6 PUFAs compete for the same metabolic pathways, an increase of *n*-3 PUFA, parallel to a decrease of *n*-6 PUFA intake, might theoretically reduce the onset of human immunologic conditions, including allergies, thanks to the replacement of AA with EPA and DHA in the membranes of inflammatory cells. EFA, including long-chain PUFAs, may be consumed as part of the normal diet through breast milk, formula and food, or as supplements at any stage in the life cycle [15].

The fatty acid status is of particular concern in infants and children. Essential fatty acids (EFA) promote the renewal of the protective hydrolipidic film layer of the skin and, accordingly, an altered EFA metabolism has been associated with the pathogenesis of atopic dermatitis (AD). Moreover, the clinical spectrum of EFA deficiency may range from mild skin irritation to life-threatening conditions [16].

In spite of intensive research in the field, a recent systematic review [17] concerning the role of dietary PUFAs in the development of allergy shows that PUFA supplementation in infancy seems not to affect infant incidence, childhood incidence or childhood prevalence of food allergy (GRADE level of evidence: very low; GRADE, Grading of Recommendations Assessment, Development and Evaluation) in infants up to two years of age, even taking into account a moderate heterogeneity between studies that reported infant incidence of food allergy (3 studies; 915 infants; RR (risk ratio) 0.81, 95% CI 0.56–1.19%, I^2 (fraction of variance due to heterogeneity) = 63%; RD (risk difference) 0.02, 95% CI: 0.06–0.02%, I^2 = 74%). However, while well-documented immunomodulatory effects of *n*-3 PUFAs (both in vitro and in vivo) highlight the potential role in preventing and treating allergic disease, larger longitudinal intervention studies are clearly warranted to confirm this observation [18].

2.2. Zinc

Children with food hypersensitivity have increased amounts of mastocytes, eosinophils and neutrophils in the digestive tract. Persistent exposure to allergen can lead to chronic inflammatory changes of mucous membrane and increased production of reactive oxygen species (ROS) [19]. Excess ROS should be neutralized by components of the antioxidative barrier. Therefore, all disturbances of enzymatic and non-enzymatic mechanisms of this barrier lead to many unfavourable reactions, including oxidation of cell membrane lipids. Zinc is an essential trace element and it is needed for various cellular functions; specifically, it is a cofactor of many enzymes, including superoxide dismutase (SOD), which play an important role in maintaining the oxidative-antioxidative balance. A study performed in 134 children with food allergy, aged 1 to 36 months, showed that children with food allergy had significantly lower concentrations of zinc, and therefore a weakened antioxidative barrier [19]. To our knowledge there are no randomized controlled trials (RCTs) investigating zinc supplementation and allergic outcomes.

2.3. Vitamin D

The classical role of Vitamin D is, in fact, related to calcium homeostasis and bone health. However, over the last decade, the effects of vitamin D on the innate and adaptive immune system have been investigated and expanded [20]. The active form of the vitamin, i.e., 1,25(OH)2D (calcitriol), has effects on epithelial cells, T cells, B cells, macrophages and dendritic cells. It stimulates innate immune responses by enhancing the chemotactic and phagocytotic responses of macrophages, as well as the production of antimicrobial proteins such as cathelicidin. This action plays a role in maintaining mucosal integrity by stimulating junction genes. Nevertheless, the potential effect of vitamin D on Th1/Th2 adaptive immune response is of interest and related to food allergy [21–23]. Almost all cells of the adaptive immune system express the vitamin D receptor, making them also capable of being vitamin responsive. When specifically considering a potential role for vitamins in food allergy, vitamin D has been shown to affect several mechanisms that promote immunologic tolerance, including T regulatory cell function and the induction of tolerogenic dendritic cells. However, clinical trials on vitamin D supplementation in children and the possible role in preventing food allergy are lacking. A systematic review of vitamin D supplementation for the prevention of allergic diseases found no evidences about the protective role of this nutrient in children, but the currently available data are poor [24].

2.4. *The Role of Prebiotics, Probiotics and Microbiota in the Prevention of Food Allergy*

The innate immune system has the ability to modulate adaptive immune responses to food proteins. Therefore, the type of gastrointestinal microbiota of the newborn and the preservation of intestinal permeability is crucial for preventing the development of food allergies. The dietary modulation of nutritional factors through pre-, pro- and synbiotic preparations represent a novel research hypothesis and a challenge for dietitians and paediatric allergists. The modulation of the immune system using functional foods is a promising research hypothesis in the attempt to induce a tolerogenic immune environment [16].

2.4.1. Prebiotics

Prebiotics have been defined as "non-digestible food components that beneficially affect the host by selectively stimulating the growth and/or activity of one or a limited number of bacteria in the colon and thereby improving host health", and recently redefined as "a selectively fermented ingredient that allows specific changes, both in the composition and/or activity in the gastrointestinal microbiota that confers benefits" [25]. In December 2016, the panel of experts convened by the International Scientific Association for Probiotics and Prebiotics (ISAPP) suggested a new definition, i.e., "a substrate that is selectively utilized by host microorganisms conferring a health benefit" [26]. Based on the body of available evidence, the Guidelines for Atopic Disease Prevention (GLAD-p) panel concluded that it is likely that prebiotic supplementation in infants reduces the risk of developing recurrent wheezing and possibly also the development of food allergy. However, there is very low certainty that there is an effect of prebiotics on other outcomes, other than an indirect effect due to its effect on the microbiome. In fact, their activity can be affected by many individual factors, (e.g., host's microbiota or the genetic predisposition to diseases). Environmental factors such as diet or antibiotics can also influence the use of prebiotics [26].

2.4.2. Probiotics

Probiotics are living microorganisms that have been proposed as immune-modulators of the allergic response by affecting phagocytosis and production of pro-inflammatory cytokines, and thus have been advocated as therapeutic and preventive interventions for allergic diseases [27]. They are present in everyday food (not only in yoghurt or fermented milk, but also in cheese—either hard or soft—and also in less expected sources such as kefir, miso soup or tempeh) and they are a common exposure in almost everyone's life [27]. The probiotic effects of complex oligosaccharides in human milk promote the establishment of a bifidogenic microbiota which, in turn, induces a milieu of tolerogenic immune responses to foods. Earlier studies suggested a positive effect of probiotic interventions on atopic dermatitis, but meta-analyses have failed to confirm it.

The new World Allergy Organization (WAO) guidelines determined that it is likely that probiotic supplementation in infants reduces the risk of developing eczema and suggested that probiotics should be recommended in mothers of high-risk infants and in infants at high risk of allergic disease, where "high risk for allergy in a child" is defined as having a biological parent or sibling with an existing or history of allergic rhinitis, asthma, eczema, or food allergy [27]. The recommendations are conditional, and based on very low-quality evidence, with no specific recommendation regarding strains, dose, treatment duration etc.

In terms of tolerance development in those with established food allergy, one study from Australia performed oral immunotherapy (OIT) to peanut in combination with Lactabillus GG, showing that 89.7% of the study participants in this arm were desensitized to peanut. The authors speculate that this protective effect may be seen because of the possible effect of the probiotic on T regulatory cells [28]. Further scientific confirmation is required to include probiotics and prebiotics in the therapeutic plans. Practical implications and how this should be incorporated in advising food allergy sufferers are also unclear in terms of advising regular intake of foods high in short-chain fructo-oligo saccharides, fermented foods and yoghurts.

3. The Role of Allergen Intake and Dietary Diversity in Prevention of Food Allergy

3.1. Allergen Intake

Measures to prevent allergy and food allergy have traditionally included maternal allergen avoidance during pregnancy and/or lactation, periods of exclusive breast feeding and avoidance of potential allergens, including food and environmental antigens, during the first year of life and beyond [29]. The value and significance of food avoidance for preventive purposes has been completely reconsidered in recent years.

On the contrary, an ideal age to introduce potentially allergenic foods into an infant's diet has been debated for the past 2 decades, particularly in high-income countries where allergic disease has become highly prevalent. Initial approaches to primary prevention of food allergy largely focused on "avoidance" strategies. In 2000 [30], practice guidelines generally recommended that allergenic foods (such as egg, cow's milk, and peanut) be avoided during the first 1 to 3 years of life. As data accumulated from both observational studies and experimental models, it became apparent that avoidance practices may not be beneficial.

Given the increasing interest in the role of time of introduction of allergic food into the infant diet (the so-called "window of opportunity") and the risk of allergic diseases, intervention trials evaluating the intake of food, as milk, egg, peanuts, etc., during the first year of life have been performed.

For instance, a recent RCT found no evidence that regular egg intake from age 4 to 6.5 months substantially alters the risk of egg allergy by age 1 year in infants who are at hereditary risk of allergic disease and had no eczema symptoms at study entry [31]. These findings are generally supportive of other data in high-risk patients showing a risk-reducing benefit for early egg introduction, and risk-reducing benefit for early peanut introduction [32]. The EAT study [33] also showed a reduced risk in the general population using the per protocol analysis, but not the intention to treat analysis. For peanut, clinical practice guidelines in the US have incorporated these findings and do recommend early peanut introduction in the first year of life for high- and standard-risk children [34]. However, despite some evidence for early introduction of egg, the US guidelines only made recommendations regarding peanut intake, and concluded that there was not enough evidence to suggest early introduction of egg. Surprisingly, the UK COT report [35], published very recently, suggested that all foods should be introduced after a period of exclusive breast feeding from 6 months and that there is no need to introduce peanut or egg differently from other foods. It seems as if despite the data from recent RCTs on peanut and egg, the weaning debate will continue, as there is still no consensus about the age of introduction of these foods. The only consistent messages are: start weaning once the infant is developmentally ready; don't delay introduction of allergens: once they are introduced into the diet, continue to feed them.

3.2. Diet Diversity and Other Related Factors

3.2.1. Dietary Diversity

Recent findings on the protective effect of an increased diversity of food introduced in the first year of life on allergic diseases (asthma, atopic dermatitis, food allergy and atopic sensitisation) are consistent with the hypothesis that exposure to a variety of food antigens during early life might be important for the development of immune tolerance [36–38].

The microbiome plays an important role in ensuring the gut wall integrity and regulation of the immune system. Diet diversity has been shown to reduce allergic diseases [36,38]. It may well be that the more diverse diet leads to a more diverse microbiome [39], and that natural microbial load of food enhances this process [40]. This in turn may improve the gut wall integrity and regulation of the immune system, but human trials are needed to confirm this theory.

3.2.2. Food Production

Food production and cooking methods, inclusive of canning, putting food in pouches, producing "ready to eat" foods, may affect the natural microbioal load of food and hence the immune system as it may affect the microbiome and, possibly, the allergic response.

Lang et al. [40] reported that the microbial load of different diets (e.g., USA diet vs. vegan diet) differs due to the foods excluded and cooking methods used. Chaturvedi, et al. [41] reported that the natural microbial load of fruits and vegetables differ between groups from a different socio-economic status. In addition, Venter and Maslin reported an association between an increase in baby food sales and allergic diseases [42], underlining that commercial baby foods are sterile and that the diversity of ingredients and nutrient content is variable. All these factors highlight that the foods we eat (irrespective of their nutrient content) may affect the immune system and perhaps development and management of allergic diseases.

3.2.3. Healthy Diet

It is unclear at present what a "healthy diet" in terms of allergy prevention and management means, and if a healthy diet as we know it (20% protein, 50% carbohydrate, 30% fat) has any relevance in allergy prevention. Currently, either the healthy eating index [43] or a Mediterranean-style diet [44] is being used as a proxy measure for healthy eating. Research using the healthy eating index tool, specific to the pregnancy diet, found no association between overall healthy eating score and recurrent wheeze in infants at the age of 3 years [43], and this was confirmed in another study by Moonesinghe et al. focusing on eating patterns in pregnancy and allergic diseases [45]. In addition to these two studies, two review papers addressed the issue of the Mediterranean diet on allergy prevention. Venter et al. summarised studies during pregnancy [46]. Three observational studies have investigated the role of the Mediterranean diet on allergy outcomes. One study showed a possible increased risk for the infant to develop allergic disease [47], one showed a reduction in wheeze [48], and another study showed no effect on allergy prevention [49]. Mediterranean style eating patterns shows more promising effects with reduction in asthma/wheezing symptoms seen but no effect on other allergic symptoms [44]. More studies are therefore needed with well-defined criteria for healthy eating to study its effect on allergy prevention.

3.2.4. Other Factors

More recently, the role of advanced glycosylated end products in food and the direct effect on the Th2 immune system and the microbiome has been described [50]. One mouse model study also questioned the role of emulsifiers on the gut microbiome. This study showed that a diet high in emulsifiers destroyed the epithelial mucous layer in the gut, altered gut microbial composition and promoted inflammation [51].

4. The Role of Diet in the Management of Food Allergy

The cornerstone of the nutritional management of food allergies is an individualized allergen avoidance management plan. In children, the main goals are to prevent the occurrence of acute and chronic symptoms by avoiding the offending food(s), whilst providing an adequate, healthy and nutritionally balanced diet and maintaining optimal growth; ideally, under the guidance of a trained dietitian [52]. Complete avoidance of the allergen is still required by some, but latest developments in food allergy have indicated that some individuals with food allergies tolerate baked forms of milk and egg [53]. Additionally, complete avoidance of all nuts is not necessarily recommended anymore, and only those nuts reacted to should be eliminated from the diet [54]. In addition to nutritional consequences of food allergy, it is known that children and families with food allergies experience a decreased quality of life across a number of domains, which can create anxiety and lead to avoidance of social situations [55–58]. Hence, it is suggested that liberalisation of the diet, when appropriate and safe, will increase both quality of life and nutritional intake.

4.1. Cow's Milk Allergy

Exclusion of any food group can result in a nutritionally deficient diet, but the elimination of milk and products in infancy is particularly likely to cause nutritional deficiencies [59] and deserves special emphasis. Cow's milk proteins (CM) are among the first foods introduced into an infant's diet, and accordingly they represent one of the first and most common causes of food allergy in early childhood. Cow's milk allergy generally requires a strict exclusion diet, usually for the first year of life. This exclusion of a main food group occurs at a critical time in the development of food preferences and eating habits. The management of CMA (cow's milk allergy) in infants and young children requires individualized advice regarding avoidance of cow's milk, including advice to breastfeeding mothers and/or guidance on the most appropriate specialized formula or milk substitute [60]. In many cases, micronutrient supplements will also be required; however, their usage is not always intuitive with both under- and over-supplementation occurring [61].

Cow's milk proteins could induce an allergic reaction: in particular beta-lactoglobulin (BLG), included in the whey fraction, is not present in human milk, and is therefore is considered the principal component involved in the etiology of the disease. During the production of infant formula, only the processes of extensive hydrolysis, ultrafiltration or an enzymatic cleavage result in truly hypoallergenic formulas [16].

4.1.1. Choice of Formula in CMA

The nutritional value of a milk substitute must be taken into account at ages lower than 2 years of life, when such a type of food is needed and may represent the only source of nutrients in the first months of life [16]. As breast milk composition differs both in component ratios and structure from other milks, the composition of infant formula should serve to meet the particular nutritional requirements and to promote normal growth and development of the infants for whom they are intended [62,63]. When a replacement formula is needed, allergologists can avail themselves of different types of formula [64]. The alternative formulas considered for CMA are extensively hydrolysed whey or casein formula (eHWF or eHCF), and amino acid-based formula (AAF), which are considered to be of low antigenic potential and are therefore preferred in highly allergic children. The unpalatable taste of hydrolysed formulas has often been associated with reduced intakes and a consequent growth faltering in infants fed these types of formula, particularly in the first year of life [59].

In recent years, an alternative explanation has been proposed based on the content of free amino acids (FAAs) in hydrolysed formulas, added to complete their biologic value. Glutamic acid, in particular, has been suggested to downregulate appetite during feeding by interacting with specific receptors in the oral cavity and gastrointestinal tract. However recent studies have shown no negative effect of feeding AA formulas in infants; on the contrary, they may be beneficial for growth [65].

Other studies have demonstrated that dietary management with extensively hydrolysed casein-based formula (eHCF) supplemented with the probiotic Lactobacillus rhamnosus GG (LGG) results in a higher rate of tolerance acquisition in infants with CMA than in those treated with eHCF without supplementation or with other non-casein-based formulas. The mechanistic basis for this effect could be the possible influence of eHCF+LGG on the strain-level bacterial community structure of the infant gut [66]. However, randomised controlled trials to date have not yielded sufficient evidence to recommend probiotics for the primary prevention of allergic disorders. Indeed, the Nutrition Committee of the European Society for Paediatric Gastroenterology Hepatology and Nutrition (ESPGHAN) does not support routine supplementing with probiotics in infant formulas [67].

Soy protein-based formula may be an option in infants older than 6 months who do not accept the bitter taste of an eHCF, or in cases in which the higher cost of an eHCF is a limiting factor [68]. However, soy formulae have nutritional disadvantages. Absorption of minerals and trace elements may be lower because of their phytate content. They also contain appreciable amounts of isoflavones, with a potentially weak estrogenic action that can lead to high serum concentrations in infants. Also, the possible derivation from genetically modified soy should be considered. Hence, the European Society of Paediatric Gastroenterology, Hepatology, and Nutrition (ESPGHAN) and the American Academy of Pediatrics (AAP) recommend that cow's-milk-based formulas should be preferred over soy formulas in healthy infants, and soy protein-based formulas should not usually be used during the first 6 months of life [68].

Other mammal's milks, those of, goats, ewes, mares, donkeys, or camels, have been proposed as substitutes in the management of CMA in infants and children, but are NOT recommended, due to either nutritional issues, cross-reactions or both. The Diagnosis and Rationale for Action against Cow's Milk Allergy (DRACMA) guidelines state that milk allergens of various mammalian species cross-react [16]. The greatest homology is found between cow's, buffalo's, sheep's and goat's milk proteins. Proteins in their milks have less structural similarity with pig, horse, donkey, camel and dromedary. Goat's, buffalo's and ewe's milk are particularly not recommended by the World Allergy Organization due to cross-reactivity with cow's milk [16]. The tolerance of other mammalian milks needs to be further investigated in clinical trials, and there are some concerns about their chemical composition and sanitation. In conclusion, either amino acid-based formulas or eHCFrepresent the most available solutions for allergic infants who are no longer breast-fed. The therapeutic interventions should therefore be indicated on an individual basis.

5. Conclusions

Food allergy represents a significant health burden at either an individual and population level worldwide. Recent guidelines for the prevention of food allergies advocate that there is no need to delay the introduction of allergenic foods once weaning has commenced. In terms of food allergy management (end even prevention), individualised strategies should be implemented. These strategies will include developmental readiness to be weaned, prevalence of particular food allergies in certain countries, family eating patterns and availability of physician and dietetic care.

Care should be taken to ensure adequate intake of nutrients, particularly in relation to cow's milk allergy, when selecting a suitable hypoallergenic formula. There is emerging evidence regarding the role of fats (particularly EFAs), pre-/probiotics, commercial foods, healthy eating and micronutrients on food allergy. A better understanding of how nutrients and other aspects of food, food patterns and food preparation may affect the immune system and allergy outcomes is required to best advise those at risk of developing food allergies and those with current food allergies.

Author Contributions: All the Authors gave a significant contribution in the drafting of the paper.

References

1. Medicine, Io. Food Allergies: Global Burden, Causes, Treatment, Prevention and Public Policy Washington: National Academy of Sciences. 2016. Available online: http://www.nationalacademies.org/hmd/Activities/Nutrition/FoodAllergies.aspx (accessed on 28 March 2017).
2. Venter, C.; Pereira, B.; Voigt, K.; Grundy, J.; Clayton, C.B.; Higgins, B.; Arshad, S.H.; Dean, T. Prevalence and cumulative incidence of food hypersensitivity in the first 3 years of life. *Allergy* **2008**, *63*, 354–359. [CrossRef] [PubMed]
3. Venter, C.; Patil, V.; Grundy, J.; Glasbey, G.; Twiselton, R.; Arshad, S.H.; Dean, T. Prevalence and cumulative incidence of food hypersensitivity in the first ten years of life. *Pediatr. Allergy Immunol.* **2016**, *27*, 452–458. [CrossRef] [PubMed]

4. Nwaru, B.I.; Hickstein, L.; Panesar, S.S.; Muraro, A.; Werfel, T.; Cardona, V.; Dubois, A.E.; Halken, S.; Hoffmann-Sommergruber, K.; Poulsen, L.K.; et al. The epidemiology of food allergy in Europe: A systematic review and meta-analysis. *Allergy* **2014**, *69*, 62–75. [CrossRef] [PubMed]
5. Venter, C.; Pereira, B.; Grundy, J.; Clayton, C.B.; Roberts, G.; Higgins, B.; Dean, T. Incidence of parentally reported and clinically diagnosed food hypersensitivity in the first year of life. *J. Allergy Clin. Immunol.* **2006**, *117*, 1118–1124. [CrossRef] [PubMed]
6. Du Toit, G.; Foong, R.M.; Lack, G. Prevention of food allergy—Early dietary interventions. *Allergol. Int.* **2016**, *65*, 370–377. [CrossRef] [PubMed]
7. Caplan, M.; Calder, P.; Prescott, S. (Eds.) *Scientific Review: The Role of Nutrients in Immune Function of Infants and Young Children Emerging Evidence for Long-chain Polyunsaturated Fatty Acids*; Mead Johnson & Company: Glenview, IL, USA, 2007; p. 40.
8. Stockinger, S.; Hornef, M.W.; Chassin, C. Establishment of intestinal homeostasis during the neonatal period. *Cell. Mol. Life Sci.* **2011**, *68*, 3699–3712. [CrossRef] [PubMed]
9. Yatsunenko, T.; Rey, F.E.; Manary, M.J.; Trehan, I.; Dominguez-Bello, M.G.; Contreras, M.; Magris, M.; Hidalgo, G.; Baldassano, R.N.; Anokhin, A.P.; et al. Human gut microbiome viewed across age and geography. *Nature* **2012**, *486*, 222–227. [CrossRef] [PubMed]
10. David, L.A.; Maurice, C.F.; Carmody, R.N.; Gootenberg, D.B.; Button, J.E.; Wolfe, B.E.; Ling, A.V.; Devlin, A.S.; Varma, Y.; Fischbach, M.A.; et al. Diet rapidly and reproducibly alters the human gut microbiome. *Nature* **2014**, *505*, 559–563. [CrossRef] [PubMed]
11. Martinez, K.B.; Leone, V.; Chang, E.B. Western diets, gut dysbiosis, and metabolic diseases: Are they linked? *Gut Microbes* **2017**, *8*, 130–142. [CrossRef] [PubMed]
12. Volynets, V.; Louis, S.; Pretz, D.; Lang, L.; Ostaff, M.J.; Wehkamp, J.; Bischoff, S.C. Intestinal Barrier Function and the Gut Microbiome Are Differentially Affected in Mice Fed a Western-Style Diet or Drinking Water Supplemented with Fructose. *J. Nutr.* **2017**, *147*, 770–780. [CrossRef] [PubMed]
13. Dupont, C.; Barau, E.; Molkhou, P.; Raynaud, F.; Barbet, J.P.; Dehennin, L. Food-induced alterations of intestinal permeability in children with cow's milk-sensitive enteropathy and atopic dermatitis. *J. Pediatr. Gastroenterol. Nutr.* **1989**, *8*, 459–465. [CrossRef] [PubMed]
14. Jarvinen, K.M.; Konstantinou, G.N.; Pilapil, M.; Arrieta, M.C.; Noone, S.; Sampson, H.A.; Meddings, J.; Nowak-Węgrzyn, A. Intestinal permeability in children with food allergy on specific elimination diets. *Pediatr. Allergy Immunol.* **2013**, *24*, 589–595. [CrossRef] [PubMed]
15. Kunisawa, J.; Arita, M.; Hayasaka, T.; Harada, T.; Iwamoto, R.; Nagasawa, R.; Shikata, S.; Nagatake, T.; Suzuki, H.; Hashimoto, E.; et al. Dietary ω3 fatty acid exerts anti-allergic effect through the conversion to 17,18-epoxyeicosatetraenoic acid in the gut. *Sci. Rep.* **2015**, *5*, 9750. [CrossRef] [PubMed]
16. Fiocchi, A.; Brozek, J.; Schünemann, H.; Bahna, S.L.; von Berg, A.; Beyer, K.; Bozzola, M.; Bradsher, J.; Compalati, E.; Ebisawa, M.; et al. World Allergy Organization (WAO) Diagnosis and Rationale for Action against Cow's Milk Allergy (DRACMA) Guidelines. *Pediatr. Allergy Immunol.* **2010**, *21* (Suppl. 21), 1–125. [PubMed]
17. Schindler, T.; Sinn, J.K.; Osborn, D.A. Polyunsaturated fatty acid supplementation in infancy for the prevention of allergy. *Cochrane Database Syst. Rev.* **2016**, *10*, CD010112. [CrossRef] [PubMed]
18. Prescott, S.L.; Calder, P.C. *N*-3 polyunsaturated fatty acids and allergic disease. *Curr. Opin. Clin. Nutr. Metab. Care* **2004**, *7*, 123–129. [CrossRef] [PubMed]
19. Kamer, B.; Wąsowicz, W.; Pyziak, K.; Kamer-Bartosińska, A.; Jolanta Gromadzińska, J.; Pasowska, R. Role of selenium and zinc in the pathogenesis of food allergy in infants and young children. *Arch. Med. Sci.* **2012**, *8*, 1083–1088. [CrossRef] [PubMed]
20. Prietl, B.; Treiber, G.; Pieber, T.R.; Amrein, K. Vitamin D and Immune Function. *Nutrients* **2013**, *5*, 2502–2521. [CrossRef] [PubMed]
21. Rudders, S.A.; Camargo, C.A., Jr. Sunlight, vitamin D and food allergy. *Curr. Opin. Allergy Clin. Immunol.* **2015**, *15*, 350–357. [CrossRef] [PubMed]
22. Vassallo, M.F.; Camargo, C.A., Jr. Potential mechanisms for the hypothesized link between sunshine, vitamin D, and food allergy in children. *J. Allergy Clin. Immunol.* **2010**, *126*, 217–222. [CrossRef] [PubMed]
23. Peroni, D.G.; Boner, A.L. Food allergy: The perspectives of prevention using vitamin D. *Curr. Opin. Allergy Clin. Immunol.* **2013**, *13*, 287–292. [CrossRef] [PubMed]

24. Yepes-Nuñez, J.J.; Brożek, J.L.; Fiocchi, A.; Pawankar, R.; Cuello-García, C.; Zhang, Y.; Morgano, G.P.; Agarwal, A.; Gandhi, S.; Terracciano, L. Vitamin D supplementation in primary allergy prevention: Systematic review of randomized and non-randomized studies. *Allergy* **2017**. [CrossRef]
25. Cuello-Garcia, C.A.; Fiocchi, A.; Pawankar, R.; Yepes-Nuñez, J.J.; Morgano, G.P.; Zhang, Y.; Ahn, K.; Al-Hammadi, S.; Agarwal, A.; Gandhi, S.; et al. World Allergy Organization-McMaster University Guidelines for Allergic Disease Prevention (GLAD-P): Prebiotics. *World Allergy Organ. J.* **2016**, *9*, 10. [CrossRef] [PubMed]
26. Gibson, G.R.; Hutkins, R.; Sanders, M.E.; Prescott, S.L.; Reimer, R.A.; Salminen, S.J.; Scott, K.; Stanton, C.; Swanson, K.S.; Cani, P.D.; et al. The International Scientific Association for Probiotics and Prebiotics (ISAPP) consensus statement on the definition and scope of prebiotics. *Nat. Rev. Gastroenterol. Hepatol.* **2017**. [CrossRef] [PubMed]
27. Fiocchi, A.; Pawankar, R.; Cuello-Garcia, C.; Ahn, K.; Al-Hammadi, S.; Agarwal, A.; Beyer, K.; Burks, W.; Canonica, G.W.; Ebisawa, M.; et al. World Allergy Organization-McMaster University Guidelines for Allergic Disease Prevention (GLAD-P): Probiotics. *World Allergy Organ. J.* **2015**, *8*, 4. [CrossRef] [PubMed]
28. Tang, M.L.; Ponsonby, A.L.; Orsini, F.; Tey, D.; Robinson, M.; Su, E.L.; Licciardi, P.; Burks, W.; Donath, S. Administration of a probiotic with peanut oral immunotherapy: A randomized trial. *J. Allergy Clin. Immunol.* **2015**, *135*, 737–744. [CrossRef] [PubMed]
29. Di Mauro, G.; Bernardini, R.; Barberi, S.; Capuano, A.; Correra, A.; De' Angelis, G.L.; Iacono, I.D.; de Martino, M.; Ghiglioni, D.; Di Mauro, D.; et al. Prevention of food and airway allergy: Consensus of the Italian Society of Preventive and Social Paediatrics, the Italian Society of Paediatric Allergy and Immunology, and Italian Society of Pediatrics. *World Allergy Organ. J.* **2016**, *9*, 28. [CrossRef] [PubMed]
30. American Academy of Pediatrics. Committee on Nutrition. Hypoallergenic infant formulas. *Pediatrics* **2000**, *106*, 346–349.
31. Palmer, D.J.; Sullivan, T.R.; Gold, M.S.; Prescott, S.L.; Makrides, M. Randomized controlled trial of early regular egg intake to prevent egg allergy. *J. Allergy Clin. Immunol.* **2017**, *139*, 1600–1607. [CrossRef] [PubMed]
32. Ierodiakonou, D.; Garcia-Larsen, V.; Logan, A.; Groome, A.; Cunha, S.; Chivinge, J.; Robinson, Z.; Geoghegan, N.; Jarrold, K.; Reeves, T. Timing of Allergenic Food Introduction to the Infant Diet and Risk of Allergic or Autoimmune Disease: A Systematic Review and Meta-analysis. *JAMA* **2016**, *316*, 1181–1192. [CrossRef] [PubMed]
33. Perkin, M.R.; Logan, K.; Tseng, A.; Raji, B.; Ayis, S.; Peacock, J.; Brough, H.; Marrs, T.; Radulovic, S.; Craven, J.; et al. Randomized Trial of Introduction of Allergenic Foods in Breast-Fed Infants. *N. Engl. J. Med.* **2016**, *374*, 1733–1743. [CrossRef] [PubMed]
34. Togias, A.; Cooper, S.F.; Acebal, M.L.; Assa'ad, A.; Baker, J.R.; Beck, L.A.; Block, J.; Bredbenner, C.; Chan, E.S.; Eichenfield, L.F.; et al. Addendum guidelines for the prevention of peanut allergy in the United States: Report of the National Institute of Allergy and Infectious Diseases-sponsored expert panel. *J. Allergy Clin. Immunol.* **2017**, *139*, 29–44. [CrossRef] [PubMed]
35. Assessing the Health Benefits and Risks of the Introduction of Peanut and Hen's Egg into the Infant Diet before Six Months of Age in the UK. Available online: https://cot.food.gov.uk/sites/default/files/jointsacncotallergystatementfinal2.pdf (accessed on 31 July 2017).
36. Roduit, C.; Frei, R.; Depner, M.; Schaub, B.; Loss, G.; Genuneit, J.; Pfefferle, P.; Hyvärinen, A.; Karvonen, A.M.; Riedler, J.; et al. Increased food diversity in the first year of life is inversely associated with allergic diseases. *J. Allergy Clin. Immunol.* **2014**, *133*, 1056–1064. [CrossRef] [PubMed]
37. Roduit, C.; Frei, R.; Loss, G.; Buchele, G.; Weber, J.; Depner, M.; Loeliger, S.; Dalphin, M.L.; Roponen, M.; Hyvärinen, A.; et al. Development of atopic dermatitis according to age of onset and association with early-life exposures. *J. Allergy Clin. Immunol.* **2012**, *130*, 130–136. [CrossRef] [PubMed]
38. Nwaru, B.I.; Takkinen, H.M.; Kaila, M.; Erkkola, M.; Ahonen, S.; Pekkanen, J.; Simell, O.; Veijola, R.; Ilonen, J.; Hyöty, H.; et al. Food diversity in infancy and the risk of childhood asthma and allergies. *J. Allergy Clin. Immunol.* **2014**, *133*, 1084–1091. [CrossRef] [PubMed]
39. Claesson, M.J.; Jeffery, I.B.; Conde, S.; Power, S.E.; O'Connor, E.M.; Cusack, S.; Harris, H.M.B.; Coakley, M.; Lakshminarayanan, B.; O'Sullivan, O.; et al. Gut microbiota composition correlates with diet and health in the elderly. *Nature* **2012**, *488*, 178–184. [CrossRef] [PubMed]
40. Lang, J.M.; Eisen, J.A.; Zivkovic, A.M. The microbes we eat: Abundance and taxonomy of microbes consumed in a day's worth of meals for three diet types. *PeerJ* **2014**, *2*, e659. [CrossRef] [PubMed]

41. Chaturvedi, M.; Kumar, V.; Singh, D.; Kumar, S. Assessment of microbial load of some common vegetables among two different socioeconomic groups. *Int. Food Res. J.* **2013**, *20*, 2927–2931.
42. Venter, C.; Maslin, K. The Future of Infant and Young Children's Food: Food Supply/Manufacturing and Human Health Challenges in the 21st Century. *Nestle Nutr. Inst. Workshop Ser.* **2016**, *85*, 19–27. [PubMed]
43. Lange, N.E.; Rifas-Shiman, S.L.; Camargo, C.A., Jr.; Gold, D.R.; Gillman, M.W.; Litonjua, A.A. Maternal dietary pattern during pregnancy is not associated with recurrent wheeze in children. *J. Allergy Clin. Immunol.* **2010**, *126*, 250–255. [CrossRef] [PubMed]
44. Castro-Rodriguez, J.A.; Garcia-Marcos, L. What Are the Effects of a Mediterranean Diet on Allergies and Asthma in Children? *Front. Pediatr.* **2017**, *5*, 72. [CrossRef] [PubMed]
45. Moonesinghe, H.; Patil, V.K.; Dean, T.; Arshad, S.H.; Glasbey, G.; Grundy, J.; Venter, C. Association between healthy eating in pregnancy and allergic status of the offspring in childhood. *Ann. Allergy Asthma Immunol.* **2016**, *116*, 163–165. [CrossRef] [PubMed]
46. Venter, C.B.; Maslin, K.; Palmer, D. Maternal dietary intake in pregnancy and lactation and allergic disease outcomes in offspring. *Pediatr. Allergy Immunol.* **2016**, *28*, 135–143. [CrossRef] [PubMed]
47. Chatzi, L.; Garcia, R.; Roumeliotaki, T.; Basterrechea, M.; Begiristain, H.; Iñiguez, C.; Vioque, J.; Kogevinas, M.; Sunyer, J.; INMA Study Group; RHEA Study Group. Mediterranean diet adherence during pregnancy and risk of wheeze and eczema in the first year of life: INMA (Spain) and RHEA (Greece) mother-child cohort studies. *Br. J. Nutr.* **2013**, *110*, 2058–2068. [CrossRef] [PubMed]
48. Chatzi, L.; Torrent, M.; Romieu, I.; Garcia-Esteban, R.; Ferrer, C.; Vioque, J.; Kogevinas, M.; Sunyer, J. Mediterranean diet in pregnancy is protective for wheeze and atopy in childhood. *Thorax* **2008**, *63*, 507–513. [CrossRef] [PubMed]
49. De Batlle, J.; Garcia-Aymerich, J.; Barraza-Villarreal, A.; Anto, J.M.; Romieu, I. Mediterranean diet is associated with reduced asthma and rhinitis in Mexican children. *Allergy* **2008**, *63*, 1310–1316. [CrossRef] [PubMed]
50. Smith, P.K.; Masilamani, M.; Li, X.M.; Sampson, H.A. The false alarm hypothesis: Food allergy is associated with high dietary advanced glycation end-products and proglycating dietary sugars that mimic alarmins. *J. Allergy Clin. Immunol.* **2017**, *139*, 429–437. [CrossRef] [PubMed]
51. Chassaing, B.; Koren, O.; Goodrich, J.K.; Poole, A.C.; Srinivasan, S.; Ley, R.E.; Gewirtz, A.T. Dietary emulsifiers impact the mouse gut microbiota promoting colitis and metabolic syndrome. *Nature* **2015**, *519*, 92–96. [CrossRef] [PubMed]
52. Venter, C.; Laitinen, K.; Vlieg-Boerstra, B. Nutritional Aspects in Diagnosis and Management of Food Hypersensitivity—The Dietitians Role. *J. Allergy (Cairo)* **2012**, *2012*, 269376. [CrossRef] [PubMed]
53. Leonard, S.A.; Nowak-Wegrzyn, A.H. Baked Milk and Egg Diets for Milk and Egg Allergy Management. *Immunol. Allergy Clin. N. Am.* **2016**, *36*, 147–159. [CrossRef] [PubMed]
54. Brough, H.A.; Turner, P.J.; Wright, T.; Fox, A.T.; Taylor, S.L.; Warner, J.O.; Lack, G. Dietary management of peanut and tree nut allergy: What exactly should patients avoid? *Clin. Exp. Allergy* **2015**, *45*, 859–871. [CrossRef] [PubMed]
55. Fong, A.T.; Katelaris, C.H.; Wainstein, B. Bullying and quality of life in children and adolescents with food allergy. *J. Paediatr. Child Health* **2017**, *53*, 630–635. [CrossRef] [PubMed]
56. Meyer, R.; Godwin, H.; Dziubak, R.; Panepinto, J.A.; Foong, R.M.; Bryon, M.; Lozinsky, A.C.; Reeve, K.; Shah, N. The impact on quality of life on families of children on an elimination diet for Non-immunoglobulin E mediated gastrointestinal food allergies. *World Allergy Organ. J.* **2017**, *10*, 8. [CrossRef] [PubMed]
57. Shaker, M.S.; Schwartz, J.; Ferguson, M. An update on the impact of food allergy on anxiety and quality of life. *Curr. Opin. Pediatr.* **2017**, *29*, 497–502. [CrossRef] [PubMed]
58. Polloni, L.; Toniolo, A.; Lazzarotto, F.; Baldi, I.; Foltran, F.; Gregori, D.; Muraro, A. Nutritional behavior and attitudes in food allergic children and their mothers. *Clin. Transl. Allergy* **2013**, *3*, 41. [CrossRef] [PubMed]
59. Venter, C.; Mazzocchi, A.; Maslin, K.; Agostoni, C. Impact of elimination diets on nutrition and growth in children with multiple food allergies. *Curr. Opin. Allergy Clin. Immunol.* **2017**, *17*, 220–226. [CrossRef] [PubMed]
60. Centre for Clinical Practice at NICE. *Food Allergy in Children and Young People: Diagnosis and Assessment of Food Allergy in Children and Young People in Primary Care and Community Settings*; National Institute for Health and Clinical Excellence: London, UK, 2011.

61. Meyer, R.; De Koker, C.; Dziubak, R.; Skrapac, A.K.; Godwin, H.; Reeve, K.; Chebar-Lozinsky, A.; Shah, N. A practical approach to vitamin and mineral supplementation in food allergic children. *Clin. Transl. Allergy* **2015**, *5*, 11. [CrossRef] [PubMed]
62. Minniti, F.; Comberiati, P.; Munblit, D.; Piacentini, G.L.; Antoniazzi, E.; Zanoni, L.; Boner, A.L.; Peroni, D.G. Breast-milk characteristics protecting against allergy. *Endocr. Metab. Immune Disord. Drug Targets* **2014**, *14*, 9–15. [CrossRef] [PubMed]
63. Munblit, D.; Boyle, R.J.; Warner, J.O. Factors affecting breast milk composition and potential consequences for development of the allergic phenotype. *Clin. Exp. Allergy* **2015**, *45*, 583–601. [CrossRef] [PubMed]
64. Venter, C.; Meyer, R. Session 1: Allergic disease: The challenges of managing food hypersensitivity. *Proc. Nutr. Soc.* **2010**, *69*, 11–24. [CrossRef] [PubMed]
65. Canani, R.B.; Nocerino, R.; Frediani, T.; Lucarelli, S.; Di Scala, C.; Varin, E.; Leone, L.; Muraro, A.; Agostoni, C. Amino Acid-based Formula in Cow's Milk Allergy: Long-term Effects on Body Growth and Protein Metabolism. *J. Pediatr. Gastroenterol. Nutr.* **2017**, *64*, 632–638. [CrossRef] [PubMed]
66. Berni Canani, R.; Sangwan, N.; Stefka, A.T.; Nocerino, R.; Paparo, L.; Aitoro, R.; Calignano, A.; Khan, A.A.; Gilbert, J.A.; Nagler, C.R. Lactobacillus rhamnosus GG-supplemented formula expands butyrate-producing bacterial strains in food allergic infants. *ISME J.* **2016**, *10*, 742–750. [CrossRef] [PubMed]
67. Lis-Święty, A.; Milewska-Wróbel, D.; Janicka, I. Dietary strategies for primary prevention of atopic—What do we know? *Dev. Period Med.* **2016**, *20*, 68–74. [PubMed]
68. Koletzko, S.; Niggemann, B.; Arato, A.; Dias, J.A.; Heuschkel, R.; Husby, S.; Mearin, M.L.; Papadopoulou, A.; Ruemmele, F.M.; Staiano, A.; et al. Diagnostic approach and management of cow's-milk protein allergy in infants and children: ESPGHAN GI Committee practical guidelines. *J. Pediatr. Gastroenterol. Nutr.* **2012**, *55*, 221–229. [CrossRef] [PubMed]

12

Can Early Omega-3 Fatty Acid Exposure Reduce Risk of Childhood Allergic Disease?

Elizabeth A. Miles [1] **and Philip C. Calder** [1,2,*]

1 Human Development and Health Academic Unit, Faculty of Medicine, University of Southampton, Southampton SO16 6YD, UK; eam@soton.ac.uk
2 NIHR Southampton Biomeducal Research Centre, University Hospital Southampton NHS Foundation Trust and University of Southampton, Southampton SO16 6YD, UK
* Correspondence: pcc@soton.ac.uk

Abstract: A causal link between increased intake of omega-6 (*n*-6) polyunsaturated fatty acids (PUFAs) and increased incidence of allergic disease has been suggested. This is supported by biologically plausible mechanisms, related to the roles of eicosanoid mediators produced from the *n*-6 PUFA arachidonic acid. Fish and fish oils are sources of long chain omega-3 (*n*-3) PUFAs. These fatty acids act to oppose the actions of *n*-6 PUFAs particularly with regard to eicosanoid synthesis. Thus, *n*-3 PUFAs may protect against allergic sensitisation and allergic manifestations. Epidemiological studies investigating the association between maternal fish intake during pregnancy and allergic outcomes in infants/children of those pregnancies suggest protective associations, but the findings are inconsistent. Fish oil provision to pregnant women is associated with immunologic changes in cord blood. Studies performed to date indicate that provision of fish oil during pregnancy may reduce sensitisation to common food allergens and reduce prevalence and severity of atopic eczema in the first year of life, with a possible persistence until adolescence. A recent study reported that fish oil consumption in pregnancy reduces persistent wheeze and asthma in the offspring at ages 3 to 5 years. Eating oily fish or fish oil supplementation in pregnancy may be a strategy to prevent infant and childhood allergic disease.

Keywords: allergy; asthma; eczema; polyunsaturated fatty acid; omega-6; omega-3; inflammation; eicosanoid; resolution; early life origins

---

1. Introduction

Epidemiological studies strongly suggest that early life environmental exposures are important determinants of health and disease in later life [1,2]. Nutrition has been identified as one important exposure that influences early development and later outcomes [3,4]. Considerable development of the human immune system occurs in utero and in the weeks and months after birth [5–7], and there is evidence that early immune development can be influenced by nutritional factors [8]. Epidemiological, ecological, and case-control studies have associated differences in the patterns of exposure to omega-6 (*n*-6) and omega-3 (*n*-3) polyunsaturated fatty acids (PUFAs) with differences in the incidence and prevalence of atopic sensitisation or its clinical manifestations (allergies, atopic eczema, hayfever, allergic asthma) [9,10]. A molecular and cellular mechanism has been proposed to explain this association [9,10], thus making a causal relationship between fatty acid exposures and risk of allergic disease. In this article, the mechanisms that are proposed to underlie the causal link between early exposure to *n*-6 or *n*-3 PUFAs and altered risk of developing allergic diseases will be described, as will the literature relating early exposure to the different PUFAs to allergic diseases or to relevant immune outcomes. This is an update of an earlier discussion of this topic [11].

2. Polyunsaturated Fatty Acids: Metabolic Relationships, Dietary Sources, and Typical Intakes

There are two main families of PUFAs, the *n*-6 and the *n*-3 families. The simplest members of these families are linoleic acid (18:2*n*-6; LA) and α-linolenic acid (18:3*n*-3; ALA), respectively. LA and ALA cannot be synthesized by mammals, including humans, and so they are described as essential fatty acids. Both are synthesised by plants and are therefore found in plant tissues, like leaves, nuts, seeds, and seed oils. LA is found in significant quantities in many commonly consumed vegetable oils, like corn, sunflower, and soybean oils, and in products made from such oils, like margarines. ALA is found in green plant tissues, in some common vegetable oils, including soybean and rapeseed (canola) oils, in some nuts (e.g., walnuts), and in flaxseeds (also known as linseeds), and flaxseed oil. LA and ALA together contribute over 95% of PUFAs in most Western diets, with LA intake most often being in considerable excess of ALA intake. The intake of LA in Western countries increased greatly over the second half of the 20th century, following the introduction and marketing of cooking oils and margarines as an alternative to animal based fats and spreads [12]. The changed pattern of consumption of LA during the 20th century resulted in a marked increase in the ratio of *n*-6 to *n*-3 PUFAs in the Western diet, with this ratio currently being between 5 and 20 in most Western populations.

Although they are not synthesized by humans, LA and ALA can be metabolized to other fatty acids by humans (Figure 1). This metabolic conversion, which mainly occurs in the liver, involves the insertion of new double bonds into the hydrocarbon chain, called desaturation, and the elongation of this chain (Figure 1). This pathway enables the conversion of LA to γ-linolenic acid (18:3*n*-6), di-homo-γ-linolenic acid (20:3*n*-6) and arachidonic acid (20:4*n*-6; AA) (Figure 1). The same pathway and the same enzymes enable the conversion of ALA to eicosapentaenoic acid (20:5*n*-3; EPA). Both AA and EPA can be further metabolised. EPA can be converted to docosapentaenoic acid (22:5*n*-3) and on to docosahexaenoic acid (22:6*n*-3; DHA) (Figure 1). Dietary intakes of AA, EPA, and DHA are much lower than intakes of LA and ALA [13].

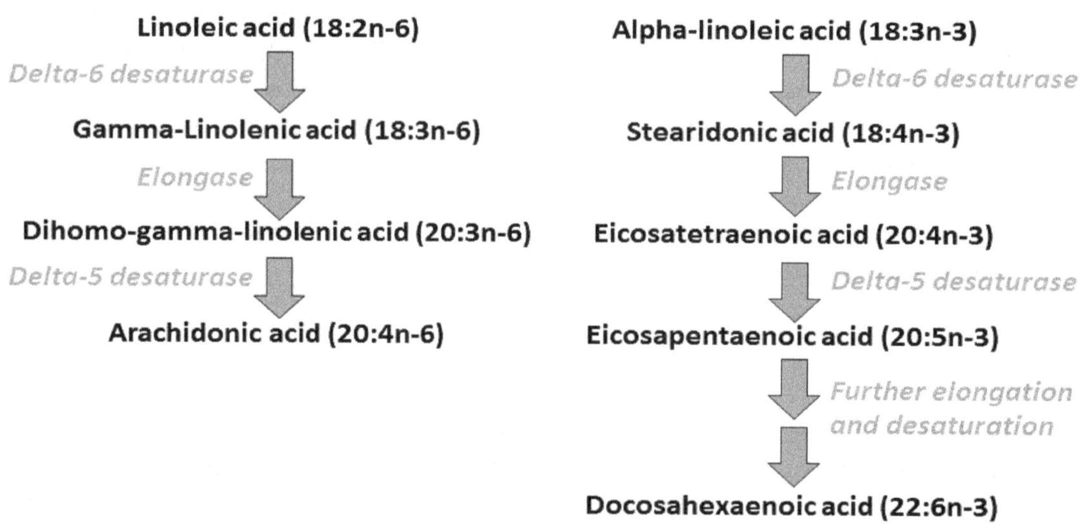

Figure 1. Overview of the pathway of conversion of linoleic and α-linolenic acids to longer chain more unsaturated *n*-6 and *n*-3 polyunsaturated fatty acids (PUFAs).

In contrast to their precursors, AA, EPA, and DHA are not found in high amounts in plant tissues. Instead, they are found in animal tissues. The most important sources of AA are eggs, meat, and organ meats (offal). The daily intake of AA is estimated to be between 50 and 500 mg among adults in Western countries, with higher intake in people who eat alot of red meat compared to those who do not. EPA and DHA are found in most seafoods, and in the highest amounts in so-called "oily" or "fatty" fish like tuna, salmon, mackerel, herring, and sardines. One serving of oily fish can provide between 1.5 and 3.5 g of EPA plus DHA [13]. A lean fish serving (e.g., of cod) can provide about one tenth of this amount. Fish oil supplements also contain EPA and DHA. A standard fish oil supplement contains about 30% EPA plus DHA; thus, a one gram capsule of such a supplement would contain about 300 mg of EPA plus DHA. In the absence of oily fish consumption or use of fish oil supplements, the dietary intake of EPA and DHA together is likely to be <100 mg/day [13].

3. Arachidonic Acid, Lipid Mediators, Inflammation, and Allergic Disease

PUFAs are important components of the phospholipids found in all cell membranes. Phospholipids and their constituent PUFAs play roles in providing the environment that enables membrane proteins to function, by influencing membrane order ("fluidity") and by promoting specific protein–lipid and protein–protein interactions. As a result of these actions, PUFAs regulate cell signaling, gene expression, and cellular function. Through such membrane-mediated actions, PUFAs can modulate immune cell function [14–16], including the inflammatory component [17], and may influence the development and manifestations of allergic diseases [18,19]. However, the key link between PUFAs and the immunological processes related to allergic diseases are the eicosanoids. Eicosanoids are a family of lipid mediators synthesised from 20-carbon PUFAs released from membrane phospholipids upon cell stimulation. Eicosanoids include prostaglandins (PGs), thromboxanes (TXs), and leukotrienes (LTs) (Figure 2). Immune cell membranes usually contain a high proportion of the *n*-6 PUFA AA and low proportions of other 20-carbon PUFAs like EPA. Therefore, the major substrate for synthesis of eicosanoids is usually AA. PGs and TXs are synthesised from the precursor PUFA by the cyclooxygenase (COX) pathway while LTs are synthesised by lipoxygenase (LOX) pathways (Figure 2). The precise mixture of eicosanoids that is produced is determined by the nature, timing, and duration of the initiating stimulus and by the particular cell involved [20–23]. Some eicosanoids, including PGE_2, play a role in promoting sensitisation to allergens as a result of their actions on dendritic cells, on T cell differentiation and on immunoglobulin (Ig) class switching in B cells [9,10,18,24]. Other eicosanoids, like the 4-series LTs, are involved in the immunologic features and clinical manifestations of allergic diseases, as a result of their actions on inflammatory, smooth muscle and epithelial cells [9,10,18]. Animal models of allergic inflammation involve increased production of PGs and LTs from AA, suggesting a role of these eicosanoids in the pathology of allergy. However, individual PGs might have different effects, with some enhancing, and others suppressing, allergic inflammation. For example, while PGD_2, $PGF_{2\alpha}$, and TXA_2 appear to increase allergic inflammation, PGE_2 and PGI_2 appear to inhibit it [25–27]. Mast cells and activated macrophages are important sources of PGD_2. PGD_2 is a potent bronchoconstrictor, promotes vascular permeability, and activates eosinophils and a pro-allergic Th2-type response [27]. TXA_2 is a bronchoconstrictor and stimulates acetylcholine release. PGE_2 is a vasodilator, promotes vascular permeability, inhibits the production of Th1-type cytokines, and primes naïve T cells to produce pro-allergic interleukin (IL)-4 and IL-5 [24]. PGE_2 also promotes Ig class switching in uncommitted B cells towards the production of pro-allergic IgE [24]. Despite these effects, which are suggestive that PGE_2 would promote allergic responses, it seems to be protective towards inflammation of the airways [25,26]. It is possible that PGE_2 has opposing roles, promoting sensitisation via its effects on T cell phenotype and B cells, but protecting against the subsequent manifestations of inflammation upon re-exposure to allergen. PGI_2 can suppress the activity of Th2 lymphocytes and recruitment of eosinophils, explaining its "anti-allergy" effects. LTB_4 is chemotactic for leukocytes, increases vascular permeability, induces the release of lysosomal enzymes and reactive oxygen species by neutrophils and of inflammatory cytokines (e.g., tumour necrosis factor-α) by macrophages, and promotes IgE production by B cells. The cysteinyl-LTs (LTC_4, D_4 and E_4) may be either vasoconstrictors or vasodilators depending upon the situation and the location of their synthesis. They cause smooth muscle contraction and bronchoconstriction, and promote vascular permeability, eosinophil recruitment, and mucus secretion. The central role of these eicosanoids in allergic inflammation is indicated by the effective treatment of asthma by LT antagonists. The complex nature of the role of eicosanoids in allergic disease is further illustrated by the interactions that exist amongst these mediators. For example, PGE_2 inhibits 5-LOX activity so down-regulating LT production [28]. This may be one mechanism by which PGE_2 is protective towards established allergic disease. Furthermore, PGE_2 induces 15-LOX, leading to production of lipoxin A_4 which is anti-inflammatory [29–31].

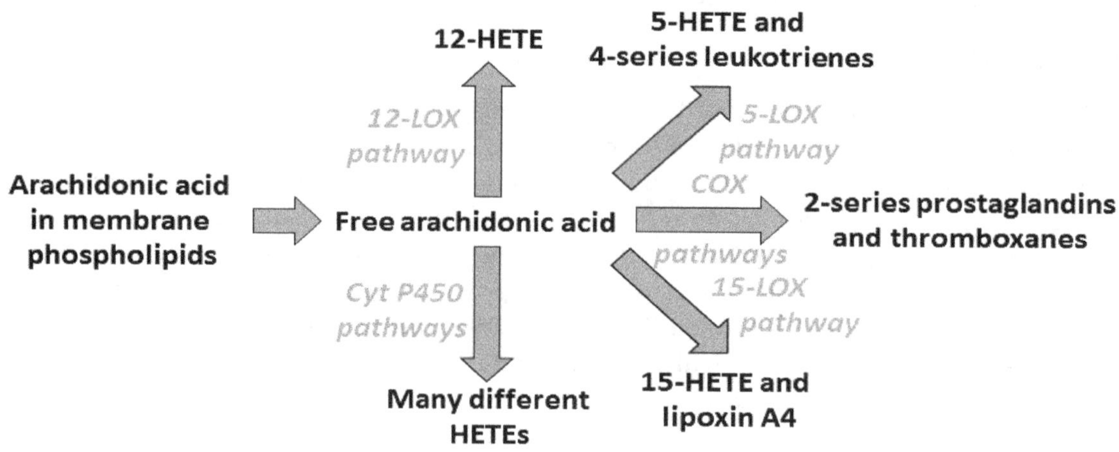

Figure 2. Outline of the pathway of conversion of arachidonic acid to eicosanoids. Abbreviations used: COX, cyclooxygenase; Cyt P450, cytochrome P450; HETE, hydroxyeicosatetraenoic acid; LOX, lipoxygenase.

The role of AA as the main substrate for the synthesis of eicosanoids and the link between these eicosanoids and inflammation, have lead to suggestions of a causal association between the increased dietary intake of *n*-6 PUFA (mainly as the AA precursor LA) during the second half of the 20th century [12], and the increased incidence and prevalence of allergic diseases over that period [9,10]. The proposed link between dietary *n*-6 PUFA, cell membrane AA, and pro-atopic and pro-allergic eicosanoids is summarised in Figure 3.

In support of the proposed biological mechanism (Figure 3), a high dietary intake of LA has been linked with increased risk of allergic diseases in several studies. Differences in the prevalence of asthma and allergic rhinitis and differences in blood concentrations of allergen-specific IgE in former East and West Germany were related to differences in consumption of LA-poor butter and LA-rich margarine in the two countries [32]. Differences in the prevalence of bronchial asthma, allergic rhinitis, and atopic dermatitis among Finnish schoolchildren were related to levels of LA in plasma cholesteryl esters, an indicator of dietary LA intake [33]. Margarine consumption among German schoolchildren was associated with higher hayfever risk compared with not consuming margarine [34]. Margarine consumption was higher among Australian schoolchildren with atopic dermatitis or with other manifestations of allergic disease compared with controls [35] and high PUFA consumption was associated with increased risk of recent asthma compared with low PUFA consumption [36]. In another study, boys with high margarine consumption were at increased risk of allergic sensitization and of allergic rhinitis compared with those who did not consume margarine [37]. For reasons that are not clear, this relationship was not seen in girls [37]. Swedish children with high consumption of PUFA-rich oils had increased risk of wheeze than those with low consumption [38], while a high dietary *n*-6 to *n*-3 PUFA ratio was associated with increased risk of asthma in Australian schoolchildren [39]. Each of these studies has associated dietary intake and disease at the same point in time. Few studies have attempted to associate early LA exposure to later allergic disease, although there are some studies reporting that LA is higher in breast milk consumed by infants who go on to develop allergic disease in infancy, although not all such studies have found this reviewed in Ref [40]. Furthermore, umbilical cord lipids from neonates who go on to develop allergic disease in early childhood contain a higher amount of LA than normally seen [40], suggesting an early programming effect of higher, compared with lower, LA exposure. A more recent Finnish study reported that a higher ratio of *n*-6 to *n*-3 PUFAs in the diet of pregnant women was associated with higher risk of rhino-conjunctivitis in the offspring at 5 years of age [41].

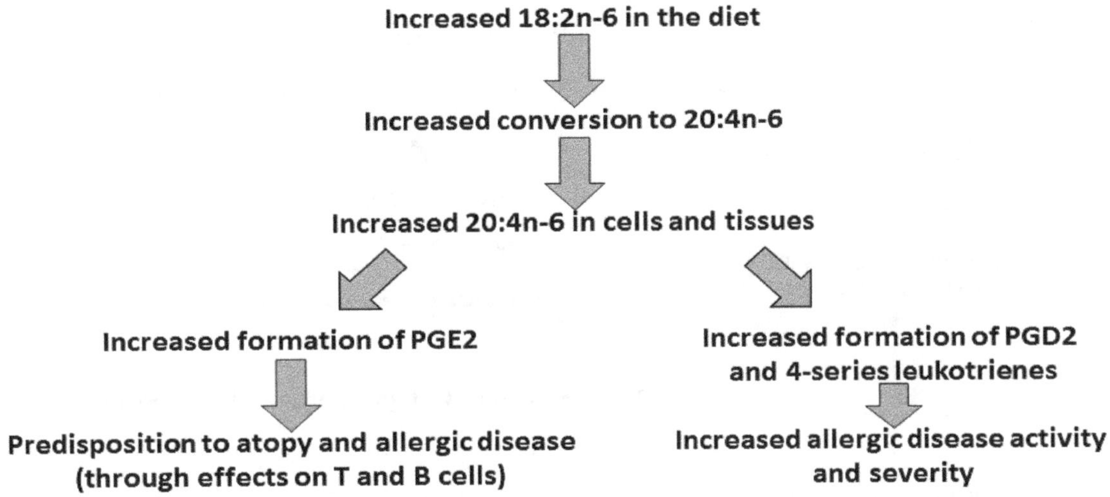

Figure 3. Proposed relationship between increased linoleic acid exposure and increased allergic disease. Abbreviation used: PG, prostaglandin.

4. Omega-3 Fatty Acids, Lipid Mediators, and Inflammatory Processes

Increased consumption of EPA and DHA (in studies this is usually through use of fish oil supplements) results in enhanced incorporation of EPA and DHA into the phospholipids of immune cell membranes resulting in an elevated proportion of these fatty acids [42–45]. The incorporation of EPA and DHA into human immune cells is partly at the expense of *n*-6 PUFAs, including AA [42–44,46]. This decreases the amount of substrate available for synthesis of 2-series PGs and TXs and 4-series LTs [17,47]. In addition to the reduced production of eicosanoids from AA, EPA is a substrate for COX and LOX enzymes, producing eicosanoids with a slightly different structure to those formed from AA, and the EPA-derived eicosanoids are frequently much less potent than the AA-derived ones [17,47,48]. As an example, LTB_5 is 10- to 100-fold less potent as a neutrophil chemotactic agent than LTB_4. In addition to *n*-3 PUFAs decreasing the metabolism of AA to eicosanoids and to EPA acting as substrate for the generation of alternative eicosanoids, another family of lipid mediators is produced from EPA and DHA (Figure 4). This family, termed specialised pro-resolving mediators, includes the D- and E-series resolvins, produced from DHA and EPA, respectively, as well as protectins and maresins produced from DHA. All of these compounds have potent anti-inflammatory and inflammation resolving properties [49–51].

The role of some resolvins in allergic inflammation has been examined in animal models. Transgenic fat-1 mice can endogenously synthesise *n*-3 PUFAs from *n*-6 PUFAs, a process that is not usually possible in animals [52]. Compared with wild-type mice, fat-1 mice that had been sensitized to ovalbumin had lower infiltration of leukocytes into the airways, lower concentrations of a range of pro-allergic cytokines including IL-5 and IL-13 in lung lavage fluid, increased resolvin E1 and D1 in lung tissue, and showed resistance of the airways to methacholine challenge [53]. These observations suggest that *n*-3 PUFAs might be protective towards allergic inflammation as a result of the synthesis and actions of resolvins. Some other studies have assessed the therapeutic role of resolvins in ovalbumin-sensitised Balb/C mice. In one study resolvin E1 decreased infiltration of eosinophils and lymphocytes into the airways, decreased production of the Th2 cytokine IL-13, lowered circulating ovalbumin-specific IgE concentrations, and reduced airway hyperresponsiveness to inhaled methacholine [54]. In another study, resolvin E1 promoted the resolution of inflammatory airway responses by directly suppressing the production of IL-23 and IL-6 in the lung [55]. More recently resolvin D1 and its epimer aspirin-triggered resolvin D1 were both shown to decrease eosinophil recruitment to the airways, to reduce the production of pro-allergic cytokines and to improve airway hyperresponsiveness to methacholine challenge [56]. These observations suggest that, in contrast to the effects of high intake of *n*-6 PUFAs, a high intake of EPA and DHA will be protective against allergic diseases perhaps acting in part through pro-resolving mediators.

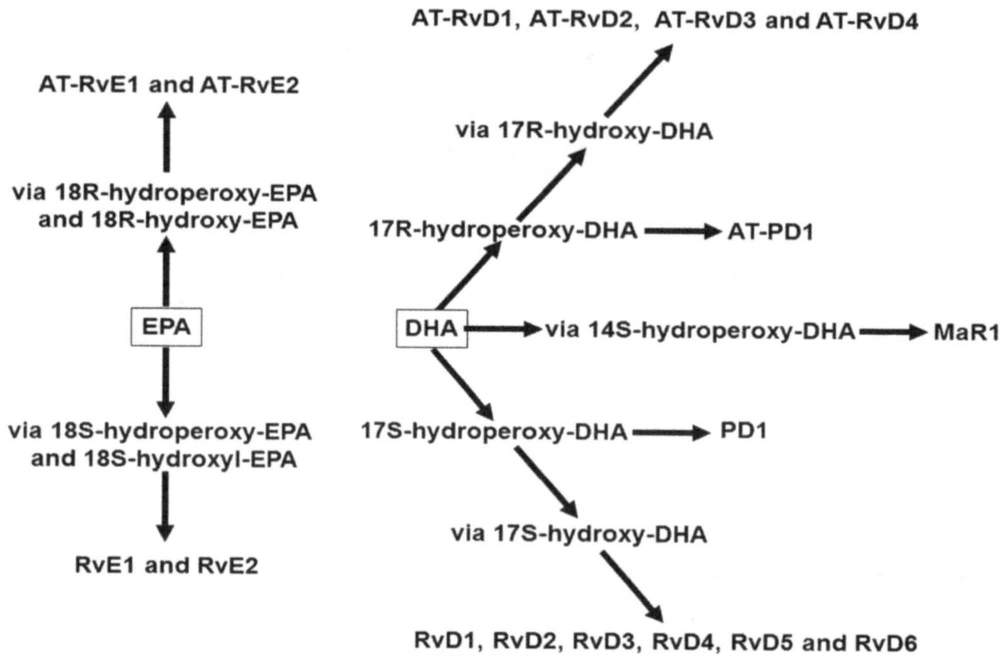

Figure 4. Overview of the pathways of synthesis of specialised pro-resolving mediators from eicosapentaenoic acid (EPA) and docosahexaenoic acid (DHA). Abbreviations used: AT, aspirin-triggered; MaR, maresin; PD, protectin D; Rv, resolvin.

5. Omega-3 Fatty Acids and Allergic Disease in Infants and Children

There is some evidence that higher intake of fish, especially fatty fish, in pregnant women is associated with lower risk of allergic disease in the offspring during infancy and childhood [57], but not all studies show this [58]. A Finnish study reported that a low intake of ALA or of total *n*-3 PUFAs in pregnancy was associated with an increased risk of asthma in the offspring at the age of 5 years [59]. Likewise, Miyake et al. [60] found that high maternal ALA intake was associated with reduced risk of wheeze in 16 to 24 months old Japanese children. Pike et al. [61] reported that higher EPA, DHA, and total *n*-3 PUFAs in blood plasma of women in late pregnancy was associated with reduced risk of non-atopic persistent/late wheeze in the offspring. A small number of studies found that infants who go on to develop allergic diseases in infancy consume breast milk with lower EPA and DHA than those who remain healthy, but this finding is not consistent across all studies [40]. Furthermore, umbilical cord blood lipids from neonates who went on to develop allergic disease in early childhood often had lower than normal amounts of EPA and DHA [40].

A small number of studies of maternal fish oil supplementation during pregnancy have been conducted in the context of early immune responses and allergic outcomes in the offspring (studies reporting clinical outcomes [62–70] are summarised in Table 1). Several studies have reported that maternal fish oil modifies immune markers in umbilical cord blood [62,71–74]. These immunologic effects might modify allergic sensitization and the risk of allergic diseases. Indeed, Dunstan et al. [62] reported less severe atopic dermatitis and lower risk of sensitisation to egg in one year old infants whose mothers had consumed fish oil supplements during pregnancy. Some other clinical outcomes were numerically lower in the infants whose mothers had taken fish oil, but the differences were not statistically significant. Olsen et al. [63] reported that fish oil supplementation in late pregnancy was associated with a marked reduction in asthma-related diagnoses in the offspring at age 16 years, suggesting a long term effect of any immunologic changes that occurred in pregnancy and early life. Furthermore, follow-up at age 24 years showed a reduced likelihood of having been prescribed anti-asthma medication in the fish oil group [64], suggesting a long term effect of any immunologic changes that occurred in pregnancy and early life. Fish oil supplementation during both pregnancy and lactation resulted in lower PGE_2 production by stimulated maternal blood [75], which might influence Th2 polarization in the fetus. In the same study, infants whose mothers had taken fish oil had a lower risk of developing allergic sensitization to egg, less IgE-associated eczema and less food allergy during the first year of life [65]. Over the period of 0 to 24 months there was a lower risk of developing any IgE-mediated disease or IgE-associated eczema or being sensitised to egg or to any allergen that was tested [66]. Palmer et al. [67] found less sensitisation to hens' egg at age 12 months in offspring of mothers who consumed a DHA-rich oil during pregnancy. There was also a strong trend to less IgE-associated eczema, but there was no difference in "any IgE-mediated disease". Over the period to age 3 years there was no effect of the DHA-rich oil on any clinical outcome including asthma [68]. However, sensitization to one species of house dust mite was lower at age 6 years [69]. In 2016 Best et al. [76] reported a meta-analysis of offspring clinical outcomes from trials of maternal fish oil supplementation in pregnancy. The results are summarised in Table 2. They identified that maternal fish oil supplementation results in a lower risk of atopic eczema, and less likelihood of having a positive skin prick test to any allergen tested, to hens' egg, or to any food extract, all in the first 12 months of life. Recently, Bisgaard et al. [70] reported significantly reduced incidence of persistent wheeze or asthma at ages 3 to 5 years in children whose mothers took fish oil during pregnancy (Figure 5). The higher dose of EPA + DHA used, especially of EPA, may explain why these recent findings [70] differ from those of Palmer et al. [67,68] and Best et al. [69]. Furthermore, the studies of Palmer et al. [67,68] and Best et al. [69] reported disease with sensitization (i.e., atopic disease), as opposed the study of Bisgaard et al. [70] which reported wheeze irrespective of sensitization as skin prick testing was only conducted at 6 and 18 months of age. One interesting finding from Bisgaard et al. [70] is that the beneficial effect of maternal EPA + DHA on offspring persistent wheeze or asthma (Figure 5) was seen mainly in the subset of children whose mothers had the lowest EPA + DHA status at study entry, but was less apparent in the subset of children whose mothers had the highest EPA + DHA status at study entry. This observation suggests that n-3 PUFAs will be of most benefit to those with the lowest status and may be less effective in those who already have a high status.

Table 1. Summary of randomized controlled trials of n-3 PUFAs in pregnancy reporting on allergic outcomes in the offspring.

Publication	Particpants	Intervention Details	Outcomes	Differences from Control in n-3 PUFA Group
Dunstan et al. [62]	atopic, non-smoking pregnant women ($n = 98$)	fish oil providing 3.7 g n-3 PUFAs daily including 1.02 g EPA and 2.07 g DHA; control group received olive oil; from 20 weeks of gestation until delivery	skin prick test positivity (hens' egg; cows' milk; peanut; house dust mite; cat), asthma, atopic eczema, food allergy all at 12 months of life	less sensitisation to hens' egg (odds ratio 0.34; $p = 0.05$); less severe atopic eczema (odds ratio 0.09; $p = 0.045$); less recurrent wheeze, persistant cough and diagnosed asthma but these were not significant
Olsen et al. [63]	pregnant women; $n = 553$	fish oil providing 2.7 g n-3 PUFAs daily including 0.86 g EPA and 0.62 g DHA; control group received olive oil; a third group received no intervention; from 30 weeks of gestation until delivery	asthma-related diagnoses at 16 years of life	less incidence of "any asthma" (3.04% vs 8.08%; $p = 0.03$) and "allegic asthma" (0.76% vs. 5.88%; $p = 0.01$)
Hansen et al. [64]	as above	as above	prescription of asthma or allergic rhinitis medication at age 24 years	less prescription of asthma medication (hazard ratio 0.54; $p = 0.02$); trend to less prescription of allerfgic rhinitis medication (hazard ratio 0.70; $p = 0.10$)

Table 1. *Cont.*

Publication	Particpants	Intervention Details	Outcomes	Differences from Control in *n*-3 PUFA Group
Furuhjelm et al. [65]	pregnant women with fetus at high allergic risk; $n = 145$	fish oil providing 2.7 g *n*-3 PUFAs daily including 1.6 g EPA and 1.1 g DHA; control group received soybean oil; from 25 weeks of gestation until 3.5 months post-natally	skin prick test positivity (hens' egg; cows' milk; wheat), IgE-antibodies (hens' egg; cows' milk; wheat), food allergy, eczema at 3, 6 and 12 months of life	less IgE-associated eczema up to 6 months of life (8% vs. 20%; $p = 0.06$); less IgE-associated eczema (7.7% vs. 20.8%; $p = 0.02$), sensitisation to hens' egg (11.5% vs. 25.4%; $p = 0.02$), any positive skin prick test (15,4% vs. 31.7%; $p = 0.04$) up to 12 months of life
Furuhjelm et al. [66]	as above	as above	skin prick test positivity (hens' egg; cows' milk; wheat; cat; tomothy; birch), food allergy, eczema at 24 months of life	less IgE-mediated disease (11.1% vs. 30.6%; $p = 0.01$), IgE-mediated food reactions (5.6% vs. 21.5%; $p = 0.01$), sensitisation to hens' egg (13.4% vs. 29.5%; $p = 0.04$), any positive skin prick test (19.2% vs. 36.1%; $p = 0.048$), IgE-associated eczema (9.3% vs. 23.8%; $p = 0.04$) up to 24 months of life
Palmer et al. [67]	pregnant women with fetus at high atopy risk; $n = 706$	fish oil providing 0.9 g *n*-3 PUFAs daily including 0.1 g EPA and 0.8 g DHA; control group received mixed vegetable oils; from 21 weeks of gestation until delivery	skin prick test positivity (hens' egg; cows' milk; peanut; wheat; tuna; grass pollen; perennial ryegrass; olive tree pollen; *Alternaria tenuis*; cat; house dust mite), asthma, food allergy, eczema at 12 months of life	less sensitisation to hens' egg (9% vs. 15%; $p = 0.02$); less IgE-associated eczema (7% vs. 12%; $p = 0.06$)
Palmer et al. [68]	as above	as above	skin prick test positivity (hens' egg; cows' milk; peanut; wheat; tuna; cashew; sesame; grass pollen; perennial ryegrass; olive tree pollen; *alternaria tenuis*; cat; house dust mite), asthma, food allergy, allergic rhinitis, eczema at 3 years of life	-
Best et al. [69]	as above	as above	skin prick test positivity (hens' egg; peanut; cashew; perennial ryegrass pollen; olive tree pollen; *alternaria tenuis*; cat; dog; 2 species of house dust mite), IgE-associated allergic disease symptoms (eczema, wheeze, or rhinitis) with sensitization at 6 years of life	less sensitisation to one species of house dust mite (13.4% vs. 20.3%; $p = 0.049$)
Bisgaard et al. [70]	pregnant women; $n = 736$	fish oil providing 2.4 g *n*-3 PUFAs daily including 1.32 g EPA and 0.89 g DHA; control group received olive oil; from 24 weeks of gestation until delivery	asthma, allergy, eczema; parental report of lung, skin, lower respiratory tract related symptoms; skin prick test positivity (hens' egg; cows' milk; cat; dog) at 6 and 18 months of life	less persistant wheeze/asthma from 3 to 5 years of life (hazard ratio 0.68; $p = 0.02$)

One study has looked at maternal fish oil supplementation during lactation and immune outcomes in the offspring [77]. Mononuclear cells from 2.5 years old children of mothers who received fish oil supplements during lactation produced higher amounts of interferon-γ. This observation was interpreted by the authors to reflect faster maturation of the immune system. Unfortunately, the study did not assess clinical outcomes.

One study has investigated the effect of fish oil given to infants from birth until 6 months of age on immune outcomes [78] and allergic disease [79]. The infants were at high-risk of developing allergy. Mononuclear cells from infants who had received fish oil produced less of the Th2 cytokine IL-13 when stimulated ex vivo with housedust mite [78]. They also produced more of the Th1 cytokines interferon-γ and tumour necrosis factor when stimulated with phytohaemagglutinin. These observations would suggest a favourable shift in the Th1 vs. Th2 balance with fish oil supplementation. The study found that low plasma DHA and low red blood cell EPA were both predictive of eczema by age 12 months [78]. At 12 months of age, clinical outcomes (any allergic disease, total or any specific sensitization, eczema, food allergy, wheeze) were not different between infants who had received fish oil or placebo [79]. However, infants who were most complaint to the intervention had a lower risk of eczema at age 12 months. Furthermore, infants with a higher red blood cell EPA, red blood cell ratio of EPA to ARA or plasma DHA at 6 months of age were less likely to develop eczema by 12 months of age [79]. Infants with higher plasma DHA or EPA + docosapentaenoic acid + DHA at 6 months were less likely to develop recurrent wheeze by 12 months of age [79].

Table 2. Summary of the findings of the meta-analysis of Best et al. [76] of randomized controlled trials of *n*-3 PUFAs in pregnancy reporting on allergic outcomes in the offspring.

Outcome	Finding (Risk Ratio; 95% Confidence Interval; *p*)	Studies Included
atopic eczema (eczema with positive skin prick test) in the first 12 months of life	0.53; 0.35–0.81; 0.004	[65,67]
any eczema (eczema with or without a positive skin prick test) in the first 12 months of life	0.85; 0.67–1.07; 0.16	[65,67]
cumulative incidence of IgE-mediated rhino-conjunctivitis (rhino-conjuctivitis with a postive skin prick test) in the first 3 years of life	0.81; 0.44–1.47; 0.49	[66,68]
positive skin prick test to any allergen in the first 12 months of life	0.68; 0.52–0.89; 0.006	[62,65,67]
positive skin prick test to hens' egg in the first 12 months of life	0.54; 0.39–0.75; 0.0003	[62,65,67]
positive skin prick test to any food extract in the first 12 months of life	0.58; 0.45–0.75; <0.0001	[62,65,67]

One study has examined the long-term effect on allergic diseases of fish oil supplementation of infants [80–84]. There was decreased prevalence of wheeze in the fish oil group at 18 months of age and higher plasma *n*-3 PUFA levels were associated with less bronchodilator use [80,81]. At 3 years of age the fish oil group had reduced cough, but not wheeze and there was no effect of fish oil on other outcomes such as eczema, serum IgE concentration, or doctor diagnosis of asthma [82]. At 5 years of age there was no significant effect of fish oil on any of the clinical outcomes relating to lung function [32], allergy [83], or asthma [84]. Reasons for the lack of beneficial effects of long chain *n*-3 PUFAs at 5 years of age may be suboptimal adherence to the intervention (50% and 56% compliance in the intervention and control group, respectively), the low dose of fish oil used, loss to follow-up, and lack of power.

Taken together, these studies provide evidence that early exposure to the *n*-3 PUFAs EPA and DHA induces immune effects that may be associated with reduced allergic sensitization and with a reduction in allergic manifestations. However, the data available are not fully consistent and so it is not possible to draw a certain conclusion at this stage. More studies in this area are needed and, where these are interventions, it is important that they be sufficiently powered, that they measure both immune and clinical outcomes where possible, and that dose of *n*-3 PUFAs and duration are carefully considered.

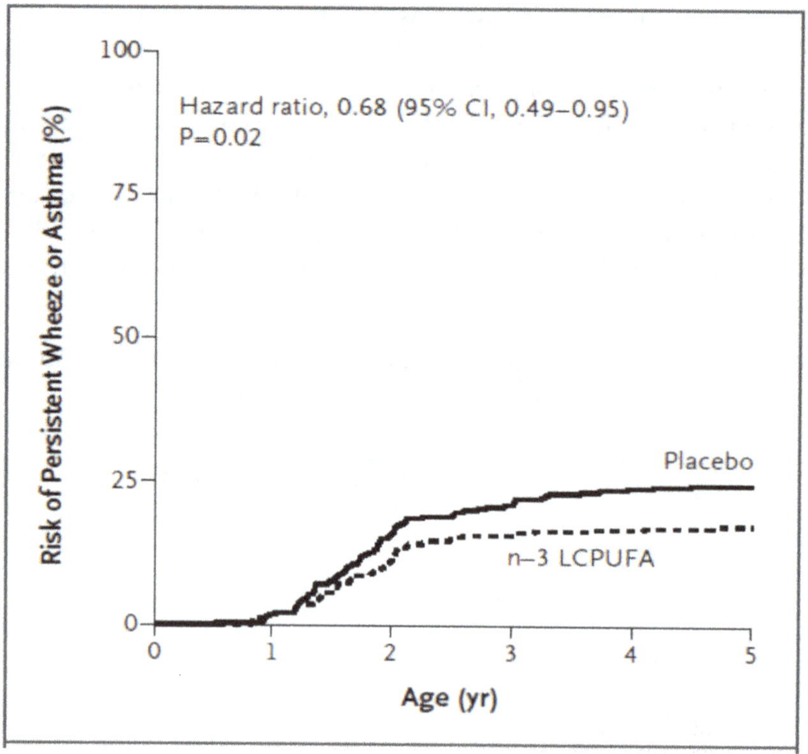

Figure 5. Risk of persistent wheeze or asthma in children according to maternal use of fish oil or placebo during pregnanacy. From New England Journal of Medicine, H. Bisgaard, J. Stokholm, B.L. Chawes, N.H. Vissing, E. Bjarnadóttir, A.M. Schoos, H.M. Wolsk, T.M. Pedersen, R.K. Vinding, S. Thorsteinsdóttir, N.V. Følsgaard, N.R. Fink, J. Thorsen, A.G. Pedersen, J. Waage, M.A. Rasmussen, K.D. Stark, S.F. Olsen, K. Bønnelykke, Fish Oil-Derived Fatty Acids in Pregnancy and Wheeze and Asthma in Offspring, Volume 375, Page 2530–2539. Copyright © 2016 Massachusetts Medical Society. Reprinted with permission from Massachusetts Medical Society.

6. The Salmon in Pregnancy Study

A systematic review published in 2011 identified that intake of fish, fatty fish, and omega-3 fatty acids in pregnancy is associated with reduced risk of allergic disease in the offspring infants [57]. As with its advice to other adults, the UK Government advises that pregnant women should consume two portions of fish per week, at least one of which should be fatty [85]. The Salmon in Pregnancy Study was a randomised, controlled dietary intervention testing this advice in the context of offspring allergic disease. Pregnant women who were low consumers of fatty fish and who were at risk of giving birth to an infant who would become allergic were recruited [86]. The women were randomized to two groups: one group maintained their habitual diet while the other included salmon twice per week in their diet from week 19 of pregnancy until delivery. Women in the salmon group had a higher dietary intake of EPA and DHA: intake of EPA + DHA from the diet was equivalent to 0.03 g/day in the control group and was 0.4 g/day in the salmon group [86]. Women in the control group showed a decline in the percentage of both EPA and DHA in plasma phosphatidylcholine from week 19 to week 38 pregnancy [86], consistent with other reports [87,88]. However, in the salmon group this decline did not occur and EPA and DHA were seen to increase in plasma phosphatidylcholine over the course of pregnancy [86]. Furthermore, both EPA and DHA were significantly higher in the umbilical cord plasma phosphatidylcholine in the salmon group compared with the control group [86]. Thus, by consuming salmon twice per week mothers were providing more EPA and DHA to their growing fetus. There were also some differences in umbilical cord blood immune cell responses between the two groups, including a lower production of pro-allergic PGE_2 by cord blood mononuclear cells in response to inflammatory stimuli in the salmon group [89]. Breast milk DHA was higher from women in salmon group at days 1, 5, 14, and 28 after birth, even though women ceased consuming salmon at birth [90]. Thus, women in the salmon group were most likely able to provide a greater amount of DHA to their newborn infant during the early weeks of lactation. Despite, these important findings, at 6 months of age there was no significant difference between the two groups in the number of infants with atopic eczema or in the severity of atopic eczema, in the number of infants showing positive skin prick test responses to common allergens, or in various allergic manifestations [89]. However, the number of infants affected was low in both groups. It is possible that the amount of EPA and DHA provided through two servings of salmon per week (equivalent to 0.4 g/day) was too low to influence the clinical outcomes despite the higher n-3 PUFA status in cord blood and the altered cord blood immune cell responses.

7. Summary and Conclusions

There are two main families of PUFAs, the n-6 and the n-3 families. Intake of the major plant n-6 PUFA LA increased over the second half of the 20th century. This increase in LA intake coincided with increased incidence and prevalence of allergic diseases. A causal link between n-6 PUFA intake and allergic disease has been suggested and this is supported by biologically plausible mechanisms, largely related to the roles of eicosanoid mediators produced from the n-6 PUFA AA. There is some evidence that high LA intake is associated with increased risk of allergic sensitization and allergic manifestations. Fish and fish oils are sources of the long chain n-3 PUFAs EPA and DHA. These fatty acids act to oppose the actions of n-6 PUFAs particularly with regard to eicosanoid synthesis. Thus, n-3 PUFAs may protect against allergic sensitisation and allergic manifestations. Epidemiological studies investigating the association between maternal fish intake during pregnancy and allergic outcomes in infants/children of those pregnancies suggest protective associations, but findings from these studies are not consistent. Fish oil provision to pregnant women is associated with immunologic changes in cord blood and such changes may persist. Studies performed to date indicate that provision of fish oil during pregnancy may reduce sensitisation to common food allergens and reduce prevalence and severity of atopic dermatitis in the first year of life, with a possible persistence until adolescence. A recent study reported that fish oil consumption in pregnancy reduces persistent wheeze and asthma in the offspring at ages 3 to 5 years. Eating oily fish or fish oil supplementation in pregnancy may be a strategy to prevent infant and childhood allergic disease. Further studies of increased long chain n-3 PUFA provision during pregnancy, lactation, and infancy are needed to more clearly identify the immunologic and clinical effects in infants and children and to identify protective effects and their persistence.

Author Contributions: Both authors contributed to the writing of the manuscript and are responsible fo its content.

Abbreviations

The following abbreviations are used in this manuscript:

AA	Arachidonic acid
ALA	α-Linolenic acid
COX	Cyclooxygenase
DHA	Docosahexaenoic acid
EPA	Eicosapentaenoic acid
Ig	Immunoglobulin
IL	Interleukin
LA	Linoleic acid
LOX	Lipoxygenase
LT	Leukotriene

PG	Prostaglandin
PUFA	Polyunsaturated fatty acid
TX	Thromboxane

References

1. Barker, D.J. The developmental origins of adult disease. *J. Am. Coll. Nutr.* **2004**, *23*, 588S–595S. [CrossRef] [PubMed]
2. Gluckman, P.D.; Hanson, M.A.; Cooper, C.; Thornburg, K.L. Effect of in utero and early-life conditions on adult health and disease. *N. Engl. J. Med.* **2008**, *359*, 61–73. [CrossRef] [PubMed]
3. Jackson, A.A. Nutrients, growth, and the development of programmed metabolic function. *Adv. Exp. Med. Biol.* **2000**, *478*, 41–55. [PubMed]
4. Langley-Evans, S.C. Nutrition in early life and the programming of adult disease: A review. *J. Hum. Nutr. Diet.* **2015**, *28* (Suppl. 1), 1–14. [CrossRef] [PubMed]
5. Zusman, I.; Gurevich, P.; Ben-Hur, H. Two secretory immune systems (mucosal and barrier) in human intrauterine development, normal and pathological. *Int. J. Mol. Med.* **2005**, *16*, 127–133. [CrossRef] [PubMed]
6. Levy, O. Innate immunity of the newborn: Basic mechanisms and clinical correlates. *Nat. Rev. Immunol.* **2007**, *7*, 379–390. [CrossRef] [PubMed]
7. Simon, A.K.; Hollander, G.A.; McMichael, A. Evolution of the immune system in humans from infancy to old age. *Proc. R. Soc. B* **2015**, *282*, 2014–3085. [CrossRef] [PubMed]
8. Calder, P.C.; Krauss-Etschmann, S.; de Jong, E.C.; Dupont, C.; Frick, J.-S.; Frokiaer, H.; Garn, H.; Koletzko, S.; Lack, G.; Mattelio, G.; et al. Workshop report: Early nutrition and immunity—Progress and perspectives. *Br. J. Nutr.* **2006**, *96*, 774–790. [PubMed]
9. Hodge, L.; Peat, J.; Salome, C. Increased consumption of polyunsaturated oils may be a cause of increased prevalence of childhood asthma. *Aust. N. Z. J. Med.* **1994**, *24*, 727. [CrossRef] [PubMed]
10. Black, P.N.; Sharp, S. Dietary fat and asthma: Is there a connection? *Eur. Resp. J.* **1997**, *10*, 6–12. [CrossRef]
11. Calder, P.C.; Kremmyda, L.S.; Vlachava, M.; Noakes, P.S.; Miles, E.A. Is there a role for fatty acids in early life programming of the immune system? *Proc. Nutr. Soc.* **2010**, *69*, 373–380. [CrossRef] [PubMed]
12. Blasbalg, T.L.; Hibbeln, J.R.; Ramsden, C.E.; Majchrzak, S.F.; Rawlings, R.R. Changes in consumption of omega-3 and omega-6 fatty acids in the United States during the 20th century. *Am. J. Clin. Nutr.* **2011**, *93*, 950–962. [CrossRef] [PubMed]
13. British Nutrition Foundation. *Briefing Paper: N-3 Fatty Acids and Health*; British Nutrition Foundation: London, UK, 1999.
14. Yaqoob, P.; Calder, P.C. Fatty acids and immune function: New insights into mechanisms. *Br. J. Nutr.* **2007**, *98*, S41–S45. [CrossRef] [PubMed]
15. Calder, P.C. Immunomodulation by omega-3 fatty acids. *Prostagland Leukotr. Essent. Fatty Acids* **2007**, *77*, 327–335. [CrossRef] [PubMed]
16. Calder, P.C. The relationship between the fatty acid composition of immune cells and their function. *Prostagland Leukotr. Essent. Fatty Acids* **2008**, *79*, 101–108. [CrossRef] [PubMed]
17. Calder, P.C. Marine omega-3 fatty acids and inflammatory processes: Effects, mechanisms and clinical relevance. *Biochim. Biophys. Acta Mol. Cell. Biol. Lipids* **2015**, *1851*, 469–484. [CrossRef] [PubMed]
18. Calder, P.C.; Miles, E.A. Fatty acids and atopic disease. *Pediat. Allergy Immunol.* **2000**, *11* (Suppl. 13), 29–36. [CrossRef]
19. Calder, P.C. Abnormal fatty acid profiles occur in atopic dermatitis but what do they mean? *Clin. Exp. Allergy* **2006**, *36*, 138–141. [CrossRef] [PubMed]
20. Nicolaou, A. Prostanoids. In *Bioactive Lipids*; Nicolaou, A., Kafatos, G., Eds.; The Oily Press: Bridgewater, UK, 2004; pp. 197–222.
21. Fiore, S. Leukotrienes and lipoxins. In *Bioactive Lipids*; Nicolaou, A., Kafatos, G., Eds.; The Oily Press: Bridgewater, UK, 2004; pp. 223–243.
22. Lewis, R.A.; Austen, K.F.; Soberman, R.J. Leukotrienes and other products of the 5-lipoxygenase pathway: Biochemistry and relation to pathobiology in human diseases. *N. Engl. J. Med.* **1990**, *323*, 645–655. [PubMed]
23. Tilley, S.L.; Coffman, T.M.; Koller, B.H. Mixed messages: Modulation of inflammation and immune responses by prostaglandins and thromboxanes. *J. Clin. Investig.* **2001**, *108*, 15–23. [CrossRef] [PubMed]

24. Kalinski, P. Regulation of immune responses by prostaglandin E2. *J. Immunol.* **2012**, *188*, 21–28. [CrossRef] [PubMed]
25. Moore, M.L.; Peebles, R.S. Update on the role of prostaglandins in allergic lung inflammation: Separating friends from foes, harder than you might think. *J. Allegy Clin. Immunol.* **2006**, *117*, 1036–1039. [CrossRef] [PubMed]
26. Park, G.Y.; Christman, J.W. Involvement of cyclooxygenase-2 and prostaglandins in the molecular pathogenesis of inflammatory lung diseases. *Am. J. Physiol. Lung Cell. Mol. Physiol.* **2006**, *290*, L797–L805. [CrossRef] [PubMed]
27. Fajt, M.L.; Gelhaus, S.L.; Freeman, B.; Uvalle, C.E.; Trudeau, J.B.; Holgun, F.; Wenzel, S.E. Prostaglandn D2 pathway upregulation: Relation to asthma severity, control, and TH2 inflammation. *J. Allergy Clin. Immunol.* **2013**, *131*, 1504–1512. [CrossRef] [PubMed]
28. Levy, B.D.; Clish, C.B.; Schmidt, B.; Gronert, K.; Serhan, C.N. Lipid mediator class switching during acute inflammation: Signals in resolution. *Nat. Immunol.* **2001**, *2*, 612–619. [CrossRef] [PubMed]
29. Vachier, I.; Chanez, P.; Bonnans, C.; Godard, P.; Bousquet, J.; Chavis, C. Endogenous anti-inflammatory mediators from arachidonate in human neutrophils. *Biochem. Biophys. Res. Commun.* **2002**, *290*, 219–224. [CrossRef] [PubMed]
30. Serhan, C.N.; Jain, A.; Marleau, S.; Clish, C.; Kantarci, A.; Behbehani, B.; Colgan, S.P.; Stahl, G.L.; Merched, A.; Petasis, N.A.; et al. Reduced inflammation and tissue damage in transgenic rabbits overexpressing 15-lipoxygenase and endogenous anti-inflammatory lipid mediators. *J. Immunol.* **2003**, *171*, 6856–6865. [CrossRef] [PubMed]
31. Gewirtz, A.T.; Collier-Hyams, L.S.; Young, A.N.; Kucharzik, T.; Guilford, W.J.; Parkinson, J.F.; Williams, I.R.; Neish, A.S.; Madara, J.L. Lipoxin A4 analogs attenuate induction of intestinal epithelial proinflammatory gene expression and reduce the severity of dextran sodium sulfate induced colitis. *J. Immunol.* **2002**, *168*, 5260–5267. [CrossRef] [PubMed]
32. Von Mutius, E.; Martinez, F.D.; Fritzsch, C.; Nicolai, T.; Roell, G.; Thiemann, H.H. Prevalence of asthma and atopy in two areas of West and East Germany. *Am. J. Resp. Crit. Care Med.* **1994**, *149*, 358–364. [CrossRef] [PubMed]
33. Poysa, L.; Korppi, M.; Pietikainen, M.; Remes, K.; Juntunen-Backman, K. Asthma, allergic rhinitis and atopic eczema in finnish children and adolescents. *Allergy* **1991**, *46*, 161–165. [CrossRef] [PubMed]
34. Von Mutius, E.; Weiland, S.K.; Fritzsch, C.; Duhme, H.; Keil, U. Increasing prevalence of hay fever and atopy among children in Leipzig, East Germany. *Lancet* **1998**, *351*, 862–866. [CrossRef]
35. Dunder, T.; Kuikka, L.; Turtinen, J.; Rasanen, L.; Uhari, M. Diet, serum fatty acids, and atopic diseases in childhood. *Allergy* **2001**, *56*, 425–428. [CrossRef] [PubMed]
36. Haby, M.M.; Peat, J.K.; Marks, G.B.; Woolcock, A.J.; Leeder, S.R. Asthma in preschool children: Prevalence and risk factors. *Thorax* **2001**, *56*, 589–595. [CrossRef] [PubMed]
37. Bolte, G.; Frye, C.; Hoelscher, B.; Meyer, I.; Wjst, M.; Heinrich, J. Margarine consumption and allergy in children. *Am. J. Respir. Crit. Care Med.* **2001**, *163*, 277–279. [CrossRef] [PubMed]
38. Kim, J.L.; Elfman, L.; Mi, Y.; Johansson, M.; Smedje, G.; Norback, D. Current asthma and respiratory symptoms among pupils in relation to dietary factors and allergens in the school environment. *Indoor Air* **2005**, *15*, 170–182. [CrossRef] [PubMed]
39. Oddy, W.H.; de Klerk, N.H.; Kendall, G.E.; Mihrshahi, S.; Peat, J.K. Ratio of omega-6 to omega-3 fatty acids and childhood asthma. *J. Asthma* **2004**, *41*, 319–326. [CrossRef] [PubMed]
40. Sala-Vila, A.; Miles, E.A.; Calder, P.C. Fatty acid composition abnormalities in atopic disease: Evidence explored and role in the disease process examined. *Clin. Exp. Allergy* **2008**, *38*, 1432–1450. [CrossRef] [PubMed]
41. Nwaru, B.I.; Erkkola, M.; Lumia, M.; Kronberg-Kippilä, C.; Ahonen, S.; Kaila, M.; Ilonen, J.; Simell, O.; Knip, M.; Veijola, R.; et al. Maternal intake of fatty acids during pregnancy and allergies in the offspring. *Br. J. Nutr.* **2012**, *108*, 720–732. [CrossRef] [PubMed]
42. Yaqoob, P.; Pala, H.S.; Cortina-Borja, M.; Newsholme, E.A.; Calder, P.C. Encapsulated fish oil enriched in α-tocopherol alters plasma phospholipid and mononuclear cell fatty acid compositions but not mononuclear cell functions. *Eur. J. Clin. Investig.* **2000**, *30*, 260–274. [CrossRef] [PubMed]
43. Healy, D.A.; Wallace, F.A.; Miles, E.A.; Calder, P.C.; Newsholme, P. The effect of low to moderate amounts of dietary fish oil on neutrophil lipid composition and function. *Lipids* **2000**, *35*, 763–768. [CrossRef] [PubMed]

44. Rees, D.; Miles, E.A.; Banerjee, T.; Wells, S.J.; Roynette, C.E.; Wahle, K.W.J.W.; Calder, P.C. Dose-related effects of eicosapentaenoic acid on innate immune function in healthy humans: A comparison of young and older men. *Am. J. Clin. Nutr.* **2006**, *83*, 331–342. [PubMed]
45. Browning, L.M.; Walker, C.G.; Mander, A.P.; West, A.L.; Madden, J.; Gambell, J.M.; Young, S.; Wang, L.; Jebb, S.A.; Calder, P.C. Incorporation of eicosapentaenoic and docosahexaenoic acids into lipid pools when given as supplements providing doses equivalent to typical intakes of oily fish. *Am. J. Clin. Nutr.* **2012**, *96*, 748–758. [CrossRef] [PubMed]
46. Walker, C.G.; West, A.L.; Browning, L.M.; Madden, J.; Gambell, J.M.; Jebb, S.A.; Calder, P.C. The pattern of fatty acids displaced by EPA and DHA following 12 Months supplementation varies between blood cell and plasma fractions. *Nutrients* **2015**, *7*, 6281–6293. [CrossRef] [PubMed]
47. Calder, P.C. *N*-3 polyunsaturated fatty acids, inflammation, and inflammatory diseases. *Am. J. Clin. Nutr.* **2006**, *83*, 1505S–1519S. [PubMed]
48. Wada, M.; DeLong, C.J.; Hong, Y.H.; Rieke, C.J.; Song, I.; Sidhu, R.S.; Yuan, C.; Warnock, M.; Schmaier, A.H.; Yokoyama, C.; et al. Enzymes and receptors of prostaglandin pathways with arachidonic acid-derived versus eicosapentaenoic acid-derived substrates and products. *J. Biol. Chem.* **2007**, *282*, 22254–22266. [CrossRef] [PubMed]
49. Bannenberg, G.; Serhan, C.N. Specialized pro-resolving lipid mediators in the inflammatory response: An update. *Biochim. Biophys. Acta Mol. Cell. Biol. Lipids* **2010**, *1801*, 1260–1273. [CrossRef] [PubMed]
50. Serhan, C.N.; Chiang, N.; van Dyke, T.E. Resolving inflammation: Dual anti-inflammatory and pro-resolution lipid mediators. *Nat. Rev. Immunol.* **2008**, *8*, 349–361. [CrossRef] [PubMed]
51. Serhan, C.N.; Chiang, N. Resolution phase lipid mediators of inflammation: Agonists of resolution. *Curr. Opin. Pharmacol.* **2013**, *13*, 632–640. [CrossRef] [PubMed]
52. Kang, Z.B.; Ge, Y.; Chen, Z.; Cluette-Brown, J.; Laposata, M.; Leaf, A.; Kang, J.X. Adenoviral gene transfer of *Caenorhabditis elegans n*-3 fatty acid desaturase optimizes fatty acid composition in mammalian cells. *Proc. Natl. Acad. Sci. USA* **2001**, *98*, 4050–4054. [CrossRef] [PubMed]
53. Bilal, S.; Haworth, O.; Wu, L.; Weylandt, K.H.; Levy, B.D.; Kang, J.X. Fat-1 transgenic mice with elevated omega-3 fatty acids are protected from allergic airway responses. *Biochim. Biophys. Acta Mol. Cell. Biol. Lipids* **2011**, *1812*, 1164–1169. [CrossRef] [PubMed]
54. Aoki, H.; Hisada, T.; Ishizuka, T.; Utsugi, M.; Kawata, T.; Shimizu, Y.; Okajima, F.; Dobashi, K.; Mori, M. Resolvin E1 dampens airway inflammation and hyperresponsiveness in a murine model of asthma. *Biochem. Biophys. Res. Commun.* **2008**, *367*, 509–515. [CrossRef] [PubMed]
55. Haworth, O.; Cernadas, M.; Yang, R.; Serhan, C.N.; Levy, B.D. Resolvin E1 regulates interleukin 23, interferon-gamma and lipoxin A4 to promote the resolution of allergic airway inflammation. *Nat. Immunol.* **2008**, *9*, 873–879. [CrossRef] [PubMed]
56. Rogerio, A.P.; Haworth, O.; Croze, R.; Oh, S.F.; Uddin, M.; Carlo, T.; Pfeffer, M.A.; Priluck, R.; Serhan, C.N.; Levy, B.D. Resolvin D1 and aspirin triggered resolvin D1 promote resolution of allergic airways responses. *J. Immunol.* **2012**, *189*, 1983–1991. [CrossRef] [PubMed]
57. Kremmyda, L.-S.; Vlachava, M.; Noakes, P.S.; Diaper, N.D.; Miles, E.A.; Calder, P.C. Atopy risk in infants and children in relation to early exposure to fish, oily fish, or long-chain omega-3 fatty acids: A systematic review. *Clin. Rev. Allergy Immunol.* **2011**, *41*, 36–66. [CrossRef] [PubMed]
58. Zhang, G.-Q.; Liu, B.; Li, J.; Luo, C.-Q.; Zhang, Q.; Chen, J.-L.; Sinha, A.; Li, Z.-Y. Fish intake during pregnancy or infancy and allergic outcomes in children: Asystematic review and meta-analysis. *Pediatr. Allergy Immunol.* **2017**, *28*, 152–161.
59. Lumia, M.; Luukkainen, P.; Tapanainen, H.; Kaila, M.; Erkkola, M.; Uusitalo, L.; Niinistö, S.; Kenward, M.G.; Ilonen, J.; Simell, O.; et al. Dietary fatty acid composition during pregnancy and the risk of asthma in the offspring. *Pediatr. Allergy Immunol.* **2011**, *22*, 827–835. [CrossRef] [PubMed]
60. Miyake, Y.; Sasaki, S.; Tanaka, K.; Ohfuji, S.; Hirota, Y. Maternal fat consumption during pregnancy and risk of wheeze and eczema in Japanese infants aged 16–24 months: The Osaka Maternal and Child Health Study. *Thorax* **2009**, *64*, 815–821. [CrossRef] [PubMed]
61. Pike, K.C.; Calder, P.C.; Inskip, H.M.; Robinson, S.M.; Roberts, G.C.; Cooper, C.; Godfrey, K.M.; Lucas, J.S.A. Maternal plasma phosphatidylcholine fatty acids and atopy and wheeze in the offspring at age of 6 years. *Clin. Dev. Immunol.* **2012**, 474–613. [CrossRef] [PubMed]

62. Dunstan, J.A.; Mori, T.A.; Barden, A.; Beilin, L.J.; Taylor, A.L.; Holt, P.G.; Prescott, S.L. Fish oil supplementation in pregnancy modifies neonatal allergen-specific immune responses and clinical outcomes in infants at high risk of atopy: A randomized, controlled trial. *J. Allergy Clin. Immunol.* **2003**, *112*, 1178–1184. [CrossRef] [PubMed]
63. Olsen, S.F.; Osterdal, M.L.; Salvig, J.D.; Mortensen, L.M.; Rytter, D.; Secher, N.J.; Henriksen, T.B. Fish oil intake compared with olive oil intake in late pregnancy and asthma in the offspring: 16 y of registry-based follow-up from a randomized controlled trial. *Am. J. Clin. Nutr.* **2008**, *88*, 167–175. [PubMed]
64. Hansen, S.; Strøm, M.; Maslova, E.; Dahl, R.; Hoffmann, H.J.; Rytter, D.; Bech, B.H.; Henriksen, T.B.; Granström, C.; Halldorsson, T.I.; et al. Fish oil supplementation during pregnancy and allergic respiratory disease in the adult offspring. *J. Allergy Clin. Immunol.* **2017**, *139*, 104–111. [CrossRef] [PubMed]
65. Furuhjelm, C.; Warstedt, K.; Larsson, J.; Fredriksson, M.; Böttcher, M.F.; Fälth-Magnusson, K.; Duchén, K. Fish oil supplementation in pregnancy and lactation may decrease the risk of infant allergy. *Acta Paediatr.* **2009**, *98*, 1461–1467. [CrossRef] [PubMed]
66. Furuhjelm, C.; Warstedt, K.; Fagerås, M.; Fälth-Magnusson, K.; Larsson, J.; Fredriksson, M.; Duchén, K. Allergic disease in infants up to 2 years of age in relation to plasma omega-3 fatty acids and maternal fish oil supplementation in pregnancy and lactation. *Pediatr. Allergy Immunol.* **2011**, *22*, 505–514. [CrossRef] [PubMed]
67. Palmer, D.J.; Sullivan, T.; Gold, M.S.; Prescott, S.L.; Heddle, R.; Gibson, R.A.; Makrides, M. Effect of *n*-3 long chain polyunsaturated fatty acid supplementation in pregnancy on infants' allergies in first year of life: Randomised controlled trial. *Br. Med. J.* **2012**, *344*, e184. [CrossRef] [PubMed]
68. Palmer, D.J.; Sullivan, T.; Gold, M.S.; Prescott, S.L.; Heddle, R.; Gibson, R.A.; Makrides, M. Randomized controlled trial of fish oil supplementation in pregnancy on childhood allergies. *Allergy* **2013**, *68*, 1370–1376. [CrossRef] [PubMed]
69. Best, K.P.; Sullivan, T.; Palmer, D.; Gold, M.; Kennedy, D.J.; Martin, J.; Makrides, M. Prenatal fish oil supplementation and allergy: 6-year follow-up of a randomized controlled trial. *Pediatrics* **2016**, *137*, e20154443. [CrossRef] [PubMed]
70. Bisgaard, H.; Stokholm, J.; Chawes, B.L.; Vissing, N.H.; Bjarnadóttir, E.; Schoos, A.M.; Wolsk, H.M.; Pedersen, T.M.; Vinding, R.K.; Thorsteinsdóttir, S.; et al. Fish oil-derived fatty acids in pregnancy and wheeze and asthma in offspring. *N. Engl. J. Med.* **2016**, *375*, 2530–2539. [CrossRef] [PubMed]
71. Krauss-Etschmann, S.; Hartl, D.; Rzehak, P.; Heinrich, J.; Shadid, R.; del Carmen Ramírez-Tortosa, M.; Campoy, C.; Pardillo, S.; Schendel, D.J.; Decsi, T.; et al. Nutraceuticals for Healthier Life Study Group. Decreased cord blood IL-4, IL-13, and CCR4 and increased TGF-beta levels after fish oil supplementation of pregnant women. *J. Allergy Clin. Immunol.* **2008**, *121*, 464–470. [CrossRef] [PubMed]
72. Dunstan, J.A.; Mori, T.A.; Barden, A.; Beilin, L.J.; Taylor, A.L.; Holt, P.G.; Prescott, S.L. Maternal fish oil supplementation in pregnancy reduces interleukin-13 levels in cord blood of infants at high risk of atopy. *Clin. Exp. Allergy* **2003**, *33*, 442–448. [CrossRef] [PubMed]
73. Prescott, S.L.; Barden, A.E.; Mori, T.A.; Dunstan, J.A. Maternal fish oil supplementation in pregnancy modifies neonatal leukotriene production by cord-blood-derived neutrophils. *Clin. Sci.* **2006**, *113*, 409–416. [CrossRef] [PubMed]
74. Denburg, J.A.; Hatfield, H.M.; Cyr, M.M.; Hayes, L.; Holt, P.G.; Sehmi, R.; Dunstan, J.A.; Prescott, S.L. Fish oil supplementation in pregnancy modifies neonatal progenitors at birth in infants at risk of atopy. *Pediatr. Res.* **2005**, *57*, 276–281. [CrossRef] [PubMed]
75. Warstedt, K.; Furuhjelm, C.; Duchen, K.; Falth-Magnusson, K.; Fageras, M. The effects of omega-3 fatty acid supplementation in pregnancy on maternal eicosanoid, cytokine, and chemokine secretion. *Pediatr. Res.* **2009**, *66*, 212–217. [CrossRef] [PubMed]
76. Best, K.P.; Gold, M.; Kennedy, D.; Martin, J.; Makrides, M. Omega-3 long-chain PUFA intake during pregnanacy and allergic disease outcomes in the offspring: A systematic review and meta-analysis of observational studies and randomized controlled trials. *Am. J. Clin. Nutr.* **2016**, *103*, 128–143. [CrossRef] [PubMed]
77. Lauritzen, L.; Kjaer, T.M.R.; Fruekilde, M.B.; Michaelsen, K.F.; Frokiaer, H. Fish oil supplementation of lactating mothers affects cytokine production in 2 1/2-year-old children. *Lipids* **2005**, *40*, 669–676. [CrossRef] [PubMed]

78. D'Vaz, N.; Meldrum, S.J.; Dunstan, J.A.; Lee-Pullen, T.F.; Metcalfe, J.; Holt, B.J.; Serralha, M.; Tulic, M.K.; Mori, T.A.; Prescott, S.L. Fish oil supplementation in early infancy modulates developing infant immune responses. *Clin. Exp. Allergy* **2012**, *42*, 1206–1216. [CrossRef] [PubMed]
79. D'Vaz, N.; Meldrum, S.J.; Dunstan, J.A.; Martino, D.; McCarthy, S.; Metcalfe, J.; Tulic, M.K.; Mori, T.A.; Prescott, S.A. Postnatal fish oil supplementation in high-risk infants to prevent allergy: Randomized controlled trial. *Pediatrics* **2012**, *130*, 674–682. [CrossRef] [PubMed]
80. Mihrshahi, S.; Peat, J.K.; Marks, G.B.; Mellis, C.M.; Tovey, E.R.; Webb, K.; Britton, W.J.; Leeder, S.R. Childhood Asthma Prevention Study. Eighteen-month outcomes of house dust mite avoidance and dietary fatty acid modification in the Childhood Asthma Prevention Study (CAPS). *J. Allergy Clin. Immunol.* **2003**, *111*, 162–168. [CrossRef] [PubMed]
81. Mihrshahi, S.; Peat, J.K.; Webb, K.; Oddy, W.; Marks, G.B.; Mellis, C.M. Effect of omega-3 fatty acid concentrations in plasma on symptoms of asthma at 18 months of age. *Pediatr. Allergy. Immunol.* **2004**, *15*, 517–522. [CrossRef] [PubMed]
82. Peat, J.K.; Mihrshahi, S.; Kemp, A.S.; Marks, G.B.; Tovey, E.R.; Webb, K.; Mellis, C.M.; Leeder, S.R. Three-year outcomes of dietary fatty acid modification and house dust mite reduction in the Childhood Asthma Prevention Study. *J. Allergy Clin. Immunol.* **2004**, *114*, 807–813. [CrossRef] [PubMed]
83. Marks, G.B.; Mihrshahi, S.; Kemp, A.S.; Tovey, E.R.; Webb, K.; Almqvist, C.; Ampon, R.D.; Crisafulli, D.; Belousova, E.G.; Mellis, C.M.; et al. Prevention of asthma during the first 5 years of life: A randomized controlled trial. *J. Allergy Clin. Immunol.* **2006**, *118*, 53–61. [CrossRef] [PubMed]
84. Almqvist, C.; Garden, F.; Xuan, W.; Mihrshahi, S.; Leeder, S.R.; Oddy, W.; Webb, K.; Marks, G.B.; CAPS team. Omega-3 and omega-6 fatty acid exposure from early life does not affect atopy and asthma at age 5 years. *J. Allergy Clin. Immunol.* **2007**, *119*, 1438–1444. [CrossRef] [PubMed]
85. SACN/COT (Scientific Advisory Committee on Nutrition/Committee on Toxicity). *Advice on Fish Consumption: Benefits and Risks*; TSO: London, UK, 2004.
86. Miles, E.A.; Noakes, P.S.; Kremmyda, L.S.; Vlachava, M.; Diaper, N.D.; Rosenlund, G.; Urwin, H.; Yaqoob, P.; Rossary, A.; Farges, M.C.; et al. The Salmon in Pregnancy Study: Study design, subject characteristics, maternal fish and marine *n*-3 fatty acid intake, and marine *n*-3 fatty acid status in maternal and umbilical cord blood. *Am. J. Clin. Nutr.* **2011**, *94*, 1986S–1992S. [CrossRef] [PubMed]
87. Al, M.D.; van Houwelingen, A.C.; Kester, A.D.; Hasaart, T.H.; de Jong, A.E.; Hornstra, G. Maternal essential fatty acid patterns during normal pregnancy and their relationship to the neonatal essential fatty acid status. *Br. J. Nutr.* **1995**, *74*, 55–68. [CrossRef] [PubMed]
88. Otto, S.J.; Houwelingen, A.C.; Antal, M.; Manninen, A.; Godfrey, K.; López-Jaramillo, P.; Hornstra, G. Maternal and neonatal essential fatty acid status in phospholipids: An international comparative study. *Eur. J. Clin. Nutr.* **1997**, *51*, 232–242. [CrossRef] [PubMed]
89. Noakes, P.S.; Vlachava, M.; Kremmyda, L-S.; Diaper, N.D.; Miles, E.A.; Erlewyn-Lajeunesse, M.; Williams, A.P.; Godfrey, K.M.; Calder, P.C. Increased intake of oily fish in pregnancy: Effects on neonatal immune responses and on clinical outcomes in infants at 6 months. *Am. J. Clin. Nutr.* **2012**, *95*, 395–404. [CrossRef] [PubMed]
90. Urwin, H.J.; Miles, E.A.; Noakes, P.S.; Kremmyda, L.S.; Vlachava, M.; Diaper, N.D.; Pérez-Cano, F.J.; Godfrey, K.M.; Calder, P.C.; Yaqoob, P. Salmon consumption during pregnancy alters fatty acid composition and secretory IgA concentration in human breast milk. *J. Nutr.* **2012**, *142*, 1603–1610. [CrossRef] [PubMed]

13

Maternal Folic Acid Supplementation during Pregnancy and Childhood Allergic Disease Outcomes: A Question of Timing?

Catrina L. McStay [1], Susan L. Prescott [2,3,4], Carol Bower [3] and Debra J. Palmer [2,3,4,*]

1 Department of Health Western Australia, Perth 6004, Western Australia, Australia; Catrina.Mcstay@health.wa.gov.au
2 School of Paediatrics and Child Health, The University of Western Australia, Subiaco 6008, Western Australia, Australia; Susan.Prescott@telethonkids.org.au
3 Telethon Kids Institute, The University of Western Australia, Subiaco 6008, Western Australia, Australia; Carol.Bower@telethonkids.org.au
4 Members of the in-FLAME International Inflammation Network, Perth 6000, Western Australia, Australia
* Correspondence: debbie.palmer@uwa.edu.au

Abstract: Since the early 1990s, maternal folic acid supplementation has been recommended prior to and during the first trimester of pregnancy, to reduce the risk of infant neural tube defects. In addition, many countries have also implemented the folic acid fortification of staple foods, in order to promote sufficient intakes amongst women of a childbearing age, based on concerns surrounding variable dietary and supplementation practices. As many women continue to take folic acid supplements beyond the recommended first trimester, there has been an overall increase in folate intakes, particularly in countries with mandatory fortification. This has raised questions on the consequences for the developing fetus, given that folic acid, a methyl donor, has the potential to epigenetically modify gene expression. In animal studies, folic acid has been shown to promote an allergic phenotype in the offspring, through changes in DNA methylation. Human population studies have also described associations between folate status in pregnancy and the risk of subsequent childhood allergic disease. In this review, we address the question of whether ongoing maternal folic acid supplementation after neural tube closure, could be contributing to the rise in early life allergic diseases.

Keywords: allergic disease; epigenetics; folate; folic acid; maternal diet; pregnancy

---

1. Introduction

The dramatic increase in childhood allergic disease is now a serious public health issue in high-income countries [1–4]. Current evidence points to a multifactorial aetiology with a complex genetic predisposition, interacting with key environmental factors, including dietary changes. Both epidemiologic and mechanistic studies have linked specific and general consequences of recent dietary intake patterns, to biological effects in early life, including early immune dysregulation, an enhanced predisposition to inflammation, and inappropriate responses to normally harmless ubiquitous antigens, such as allergens, in very early life. The impact of diet is complex and is influenced through changing food sources and changes in specific nutrient intakes, with secondary immune and metabolic effects. These nutritional factors (including folate) have the potential to induce persistent developmental changes in gene expression through epigenetic modifications, and thereby, alter developing immune pathways, organ systems, and subsequent disease predisposition [5–7].

The developing fetus is highly responsive to environmental cues. One of the best described examples is the ability to modulate metabolic activity in response to the maternal nutrient supply—activating gene modules that conserve energy when maternal nutrition is restricted [8]. While these short term adaptations may provide short term advantages, they may also increase the risk of long term disease [8]. Some epigenetic modifications may also prompt early onset disease, such as allergic disease [9], although the evolutionary drivers of these adaptations are not well understood. In this context, there has been a focused interest on specific nutrients that are known to have direct effects on the epigenetic pathways that control gene expression during early development, such as folate.

Epigenetic mechanisms are finely coordinated processes that regulate the expression of genes, without alterations in the underlying gene sequence [10]. This includes DNA methylation, histone modifications, and non-coding RNAs, which coordinate gene expression to allow a responsive interface between the genes and the environment. Variations in the nutrient status can alter the epigenome, for example folate, which in addition to a myriad of biological actions, plays an essential role in the methylation of the universal methyl donor S-adenosylmethionine (SAM), and critically influences methionine metabolism pathways, protein synthesis and metabolism, cell multiplication, and tissue growth [11]. Changes in methyl donor activity of DNA methyl transferase enzymes, and an increased methylation of CpG sites of specific regions of DNA and associated changes in the chromatin structure, can silence gene transcription, thereby altering cellular activities [12].

Maternal nutrition is a critical factor, not only in providing the nutrient building blocks for fetal development, but also in steering the patterns of fetal gene expression that dictate the phenotype, patterns of metabolic and physiological responses, and future disease risk [13], even though subtle shifts in the profile of the nutrient supply. In this way, the epigenetic effects of maternal nutrition on fetal immune development are likely to be an important factor in the risk of allergic disease, particularly as differences in immune function can already be detected at birth, in those who go on to develop the disease [14]. This demonstrates lasting effects of in utero exposures on immune development, but also provides a window of opportunity for preventing immune-related diseases, and reversing the rising disease burden [7,15,16].

The hormonal milieu of pregnancy promotes tolerance at the materno-fetal interface, including immune regulatory responses and Type 2 T helper cell (TH2) responses, to protect the fetus from Type 1 T helper cell (TH1) alloantigen responses [17]. Fetal responses to allergens and other environmental exposures develop during this period, and are similarly TH2-skewed [17]. Specific regulatory responses in utero [18] have also been shown to be modified by the maternal environment [19]. Thus, variations in maternal environmental conditions may strongly set the scene for how the newborn responds to the postnatal environment, including the capacity to dampen inflammatory responses and to down-regulate TH2 responses in the postnatal period [20]. Disruption of these aspects of early immune regulation may interfere with normal TH1 maturation in the postnatal period, and lead to an allergic phenotype [21].

Of immediate relevance here are the antenatal effects of folate, shown to promote allergic predisposition in animal studies. Specifically, a landmark murine asthma model demonstrated that maternal folic acid supplementation promoted allergic airway disease in the offspring, by modifying DNA methylation and the expression of fetal genes associated with the development of an allergic phenotype [22]. Moreover, these epigenetic changes and the disease predisposition were inherited by the second generation. These biological actions of folic acid, together with epidemiological associations between infant allergic disease and maternal folate consumption in humans (below), raise questions on the unintended consequences of ongoing folic acid supplementation during pregnancy, potentially at higher than recommended requirements, after the window of risk for neural tube defects has passed.

Here, we examine world-wide changes in public health strategies, aimed at improving folic acid status over the past 25 years, and summarise the current evidence for a link between maternal folic acid supplementation during pregnancy and the development of childhood allergic diseases. This is based on a literature search for studies investigating the relationship between maternal folic acid supplement use in pregnancy, folate status, and childhood allergic disease outcomes; together with changes in folate- and folic acid-related public health strategies. The electronic databases of PubMed, Medline, Cochrane Library, and Google Scholar were searched, to identify articles published before the end of August 2016, using multiple combinations of the following search terms: allergic disease, atopy, epigenetics, DNA methylation, folate, folic acid, maternal diet, and pregnancy. Reference lists of recent review articles and key studies were also examined, to identify any other relevant studies not found during the initial database search. Multiple publications from some of the cohorts were examined, for potential overlapping participants and results. All relevant studies were included in this review.

2. Folate Requirements in Pregnancy

Folate requirements increase in pregnancy, in order to meet the maternal and fetal metabolic needs, and greater DNA synthesis and rapid cell division, during fetal development. An inadequate periconceptional maternal folate status has been associated with neural tube defects, such as spina bifida and anencephaly, highlighting the importance of entering pregnancy with adequate folate stores [23]. The international reference range for folate levels during pregnancy have been derived from 10 studies; seven studies relating to serum folate levels and three studies relating to red cell folate for the use of clinicians interpreting laboratory results [24]. These have been set using 5th to 95th percentile laboratory analyte values for red cell folate, for the first, second, and third trimesters of pregnancy, and are 137–589 ng/mL, 94–828 ng/mL, and 109–663 ng/mL, respectively; and 2.6–15.0 ng/mL, 0.8–24.0 ng/mL, and 1.4–20.7 ng/mL, respectively, for serum folate. The target for women of reproductive age is a level of red cell folate >906 nmol/L, to maximally reduce the risk of neural tube defects [23,25]. There is no target reference value for serum folate in women of reproductive age, due to a lack of epidemiological evidence for deriving these levels. Dietary reference values for folic acid intake during pregnancy vary internationally, with estimated daily average requirement values of 250 μg in the United Kingdom (UK); 370 μg in Japan; 400 μg in Europe; and 520 μg in Australia, United States (US), Canada and New Zealand.

3. History of Folic Acid Supplementation

Investigations into the therapeutic benefit of folic acid commenced in the 1930s, when Wills and colleagues investigated the treatment of tropical megaloblastic anaemia with yeast and marmite, and identified the presence of an unidentified bioactive factor [26]. The consumption of yeast extract, which contains folic acid, to nourish pregnant women, was also promoted from the 1930s [27]. In the 1950s and 1960s, researchers found that treatment with folic acid supplementation prevented megaloblastic anaemia in pregnancy [28,29]. Recommendations for utilising prophylactic folic acid treatment of pregnant women to prevent folate deficiency-related anaemia followed, and were implemented at a hospital located in Staffordshire (England) in around 1958, and in some ante-natal clinics in Britain by the late 1960s [29–31]. It was also recommended in the US, by the Manual of Standards in Obstetric-Gynaecologic Practice, from 1965.

Early research into folate deficiency in pregnancy and adverse pregnancy outcomes of fetal abnormalities, suggested a beneficial effect of folic acid supplementation in pregnancy and the risk of neural tube defect outcomes, only emerged in the 1960s [32,33]. Evidence of "periconceptional" folate status, emerged during the late 1980s and early 1990s [34–39]. A meta-analysis examining the protective effect of daily folic acid supplementation (alone or in combination with other vitamins and minerals) in preventing neural tube defects, when compared with no interventions/placebo or vitamins and minerals without folic acid in randomized trials, found a risk ratio of 0.28, and a 95% confidence interval of 0.15 to 0.52 [40].

During the past two decades, folate recommendations to prevent neural tube defects have been implemented in many regions of the world for women who are pregnant, planning a pregnancy, and of childbearing age. Early recommendations were made by the US in 1991, the UK in 1992, Canada in 1993, and Australia in 1994. Daily 400 μg folic acid supplementation recommendations for women of a reproductive age, and those planning a pregnancy, have now been adopted world-wide, and were endorsed by the World Health Organisation (WHO) in 2006.

4. Time Trends in Folic Acid Supplementation Practices

Folic acid supplementation rates have been found to vary over the last few decades. Public health education has been shown to increase the use of folic acid in planned pregnancy [41], although, research indicates that folic acid supplementation rates are increased amongst higher socioeconomic status (SES) groups, and that primary prevention strategies specifically targeting folic acid supplementation, even when supported with public health promotional activities, do not reach some socially disadvantaged groups, who are potentially at the greatest risk [42–45]. In particular, this includes younger women, those who are less educated, on low incomes, minority ethnic populations, and/or those with an unplanned pregnancy. A recent study from China supports this point. It found that pregnant women taking folic acid supplements after the first trimester, were more likely to be older, from urban areas, and have had a higher level of education, than those women who were not taking supplements in late pregnancy [46].

5. Dietary Intake of Folate from Food Sources

A recent systematic review and meta-analysis of dietary micronutrient intakes from food sources alone during pregnancy in developed countries [47], reported that the median dietary folate intakes (interquartile ranges) were 190 (190–232) μg/day for Australia/New Zealand, 334 (292–367) μg/day for the USA/Canada; 280 (260–315) μg/day for Europe, 217 (184–265) μg/day for the UK, and 276 (271–284) μg/day for Japan. Dietary intakes were consistent across the whole of the gestation for each geographical region. Importantly, estimated folate intakes were 13% to 63% less than each respective country's dietary folate intake recommendations; reinforcing the need for pregnant women to take folic acid supplements.

6. Folic Acid Food Fortification

The limitations of relying on consumer-driven supplementation as the primary public health approach, led to the consideration of other folic acid-related policies, in order to achieve more equitable folate status in women of reproductive age. To address this, in addition to the existing folate recommendations and preventive health campaigns, some countries introduced voluntary and/or mandatory food fortification [48,49]; including developed economies such as Australia, Canada, Finland, Ireland, New Zealand, Norway, South Africa, the UK, and the US; and developing economies such as Brazil, Chile, China, and Costa Rica. Voluntary fortification of bread and breakfast cereal commenced in the UK from the mid to late 1980s. Both Canada and the US introduced similar mandatory fortification of all cereal flour food products into regulations in 1996, with the enactment of fortification by 1998. The US mandatory fortification requires all cereal grain to be fortified with folic acid, at 140 μg/100 g of grain food. Following these mandatory fortification initiatives, the effectiveness on the reductions in neural tube defect rates in the US and Canada, were around 50% and 54%, respectively [50]. Mandatory folic acid fortification of food has now been introduced in around 79 countries world-wide.

The governments of Australia and New Zealand implemented voluntary folate fortification of some foods in the mid-1990s, with manufacturers primarily fortifying breakfast cereals and bread products [49,51]. Following this, a 30% reduction in neural tube defects was reported in Western Australia; likely reflecting the combined influence of a folate promotion project and voluntary fortification measures [52]. Similar reductions in neural tube defects were reported in other countries, following mandatory folic acid fortification of staple foods, including Chile (43% reduction after 2000) [53], Brazil (35% reduction after 2004) [54], and South Africa (30% reduction) [55].

Evidence that the prevalence of neural tube defects was higher in Australia and New Zealand than the US, the UK, and Canada, led to the Australian and New Zealand Food Regulation Ministerial

Council determination that neural tube defects posed a public health issue of sufficient severity, warranting a mandatory fortification approach. This led to the mandatory fortification of bread-making wheat flour with folic acid that came into effect in Australia in September 2009, with a two year phase-in period from 2007. A recent evaluation of this measure found significant reductions in the rates of neural tube defects of 14% in the states for which data were available, and 74% amongst the offspring of Australian Indigenous women in the same states. At this time, New Zealand delayed implementation of this food standard, mainly due to both industry and political issues [48]. Some countries, for example Sweden, have not introduced any fortification of foods, opting instead for a precautionary approach to minimise the risk of unintentional consequences [48].

7. Dietary Intake and Folate Status Post Folic Acid Food Fortification

In Australia, the aim of the mandatory folic acid fortification was to increase folic acid intake by 100 μg/day [56]. After the commencement of mandatory fortification, folic acid intake in the target population group of women of reproductive age, was estimated to have increased by 159 μg/day, when calculated using dietary modelling based on measured folic acid levels in bread samples in 2010 [56]. There was an expectation that folic acid supplementation would still be required to meet the required folate status for preventing neural tube defects [57]. The most recent Australian national dietary folate intake data, recorded by the Australian Health Survey in 2011/12, captured dietary intake of folate post fortification in Australia, including natural folate in food, and folic acid intake from fortified foods and supplements [58]. The mean daily intake for females aged 14–18 years, 19–30 years, and 31–50 years was 559.6 μg/day, 536.3 μg/day, and 529.4 μg/day, respectively. Dietary intakes were influenced by consumption of the fortified foods, which is dependent on the variations in dietary patterns of subgroups in the population. Current popular low carbohydrate diets, and low grain-based diets, may impact on some consumers' fortified bread consumption [59], and hence lower their overall dietary folate intake.

The Australian Health Survey, conducted in 2011/12 [58], was the first national collection of biomedical results of folate status collected post implementation of mandatory folic acid fortification. Nutrient biomarker results reported median serum folate levels of 33.6 (interquartile range 26.5, 40.7) nmol/L, and mean red cell folate levels of 1601.0 (1366.0, 1848.4) nmol/L, for women of reproductive age (16–44 years of age). Nearly half of the female population surveyed (48.1%) had a serum folate level greater than 35.0 nmol/L; and 16.5% had a level greater than 45.0 nmol/L. These levels are in the upper range of the international reference range of 3–47 nmol/L [24]. Notably, a recent Canadian study found that folate levels post mandatory food fortification, were above the normal reference ranges for early and late pregnancy, and over twice the folate target range for women of reproductive age, with geometric mean (95% CI) red cell folate levels in early pregnancy (12–16 weeks) of 2417 nmol/L (2362, 2472), and late pregnancy (at delivery, 38–42 weeks) of 2793 nmol/L (2721, 2867) [60].

8. Timelines of Changing Folate Status and Increasing Prevalence of Allergic Diseases

The increased prevalence of childhood allergic diseases, including allergic rhinoconjuctivitis, eczema, and asthma, has been well-documented since the 1990s; although, for some countries that previously reported a high prevalence of asthma symptoms, the rates may now have plateaued or decreased [4,61]. This decrease in asthma prevalence is not consistent with the suggested role that folate supplementation may play in the development of asthma from animal studies. In a recent global survey of both developed and developing countries, the food allergy prevalence rates for children aged <5 years from nine countries with oral food, varied from 1% in Thailand, through to 10% in Australia, challenging proven food allergy data [4]. The rates of hospital emergency food-related anaphylaxis admissions have also increased in the UK, the US, and Australia, since 1990 [1]. The increase in food-related anaphylaxis admissions rates for 0–4 years old in Australia has occurred in parallel with the timeframes of implemented Australian folic acid related initiatives, although it should be highlighted that this does not imply any evidence of association (Figure 1).

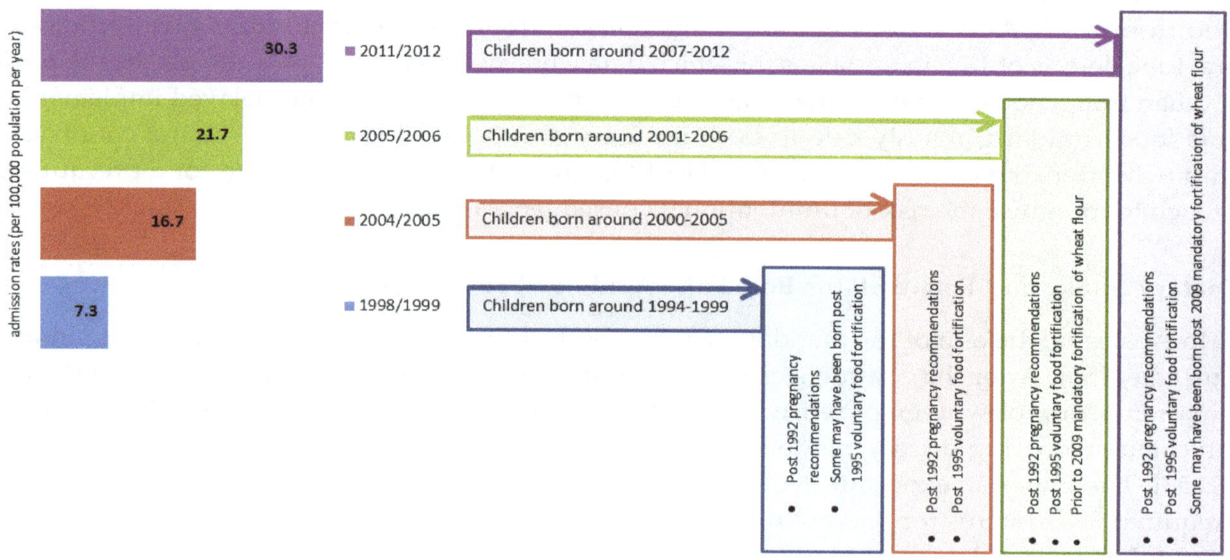

Figure 1. Food-related anaphylaxis hospital admissions rates (per 100,000 population per year) of children aged 0–4 years in Australia between 1998/99 and 2011/12, and the timing of Australian folic acid public health measures. Source: Adapted from Mullins, R.J. et al. [1].

9. Observational Studies Investigating the Relationship between Maternal Folic Acid Supplementation and/or Folate Status during Pregnancy and Childhood Allergic Disease

Ten publications [62–71] reporting the findings of the relationships between folic acid supplementation and/or folate status in pregnancy, and allergic disease outcomes in children, were identified. These studies encompassed folic acid supplementation use at differing time periods during pregnancy. To date, there have been no randomised, controlled trials investigating the effect of folic acid supplementation during pregnancy on childhood allergic disease outcomes. The observational studies differed in the investigated allergic disease outcomes; the methods used to determine the disease outcomes, such as clinical history (parental reported symptoms, parental reported diagnosis by medical practitioner, medical practitioner diagnosis); sensitization using skin prick tests and allergen specific IgE; and the "at risk" status of the children, due to the family history of allergic disease. The study time periods also cross decades; with differing levels of folic acid supplementation use, dietary folate intakes, and different folic acid food fortification policies. None of the studies were conducted in countries where there is a mandatory folic acid fortification in place.

9.1. Periconceptional and First Trimester Folic Acid Supplementation

The relationship between preconception and first trimester folic acid supplementation, or folate status in early pregnancy and allergic disease in children, has been investigated in two prospective mother and child birth cohort studies. In the Netherlands, the maternal plasma folate status at 13.5 $\pm$ 2.0 weeks' gestation, of >16.2 nmol/L, was associated with and increased prevalence of atopic dermatitis outcomes in children up to 4 years of age [67]. This study recruited pregnant women residing in the Netherlands from the year 2000 onwards, at a time when dietary folate intakes may have been influenced by voluntary food fortification. A Norwegian study found that maternal-reported first trimester folic acid supplementation use, was associated with an increased risk of maternal-reported wheeze in children at 18 months of age [66]. Folate rich diets and folic acid supplementation in pregnancy recommendations, were the initiatives implemented in Norway during the study recruitment period.

9.2. *Folate Status and/or Folic Acid Supplementation at Some Time during Pregnancy*

In a recent Finnish study, folate intake and folic acid supplement use during pregnancy, were associated with an increased risk of a cow's milk allergy in the offspring [70]. Finland had no voluntary folic acid fortification in place at the time of this study. In the Netherlands, folic acid use during pregnancy was associated with an increased risk of respiratory wheeze at the age of one year, but not at two-eight years; however, there was no association with other allergic diseases, such as asthma and eczema [62]. In a separate birth cohort study in the Netherlands, researchers found no association with asthma, wheeze, eczema, atopic dermatitis, and specific IgE sensitization, at multiple follow ups, between three months and six-seven years [69]; although, there was an association between higher maternal folate levels measured at around 35 weeks gestation, and a reduced asthma risk in offspring aged six-seven years. Dietary folate exposure may have been influenced by voluntary food fortification in The Netherlands at this time.

A South Korean cohort study of pregnant women at 12 to 28 weeks gestation, found that serum folate at a level of ≥9.5 ng/mL, was associated with a reduced risk of maternal-reported atopic dermatitis in offspring at 24 months; although, no relationship was found for late pregnancy (29–42 weeks gestation) [68]. This finding is contrary to the other studies described here, adding to the uncertainty of the potential role of folic acid supplementation on allergy development. This may reflect differences between countries. Also of interest in this study [68], is that higher serum folate levels were associated with increased levels of the immunoregulatory cytokine IL-10 in cord blood.

9.3. *Second and Third Trimester Pregnancy Folic Acid Supplementation*

Publications from those studies examining later pregnancy folate supplementation and allergic disease in the offspring outcomes, have also reported variable results (Table 1). These longitudinal studies provide evidence from cohorts of mother-child pairs across England, Norway, and Australia.

An English study found no association between maternal folic acid supplementation at 18 weeks and childhood atopy; although, there was some evidence of an association between maternal folic acid supplementation at 32 weeks and a child's genotype (T allelle), and childhood atopy [64]. This is the earliest of the studies described here, where the cohort study time period occurred after voluntary permission to fortify bread and breakfast cereal in the mid/late 1980s, and prior to the 1992–1993 folic acid supplementation recommendations in the UK.

In a Norwegian cohort study, no association between late pregnancy folic acid supplementation use (after 12 weeks), and childhood allergic disease outcomes, was found; whereas, in a case control study nested in the same cohort, the risk of asthma was found to be increased in children at three years of age, with increasing quintiles of maternal plasma folate levels at 18 weeks [65,66]. Norway had dietary folate recommendations for pregnancy, but there was no fortification of food in place at the time of these studies.

Intriguingly, two Australian cohort studies found positive associations between folic acid supplementation in late pregnancy and the risk of asthma at 3.5 years [71]; and between higher doses of folic acid (>500 μg/day) from supplements in the third trimester and eczema at 12 months, along with a reduced risk of sensitization for fetal serum folate levels between 50 to 75 nmol/L after adjusting for confounders, including maternal allergy [63]. Only voluntary fortification of some food was implemented in Australia at the time of these studies.

Table 1. Studies investigating the relationship between later pregnancy maternal folic acid supplementation and childhood allergic disease.

Reference	Study Design	Study Characterisitics	Key Allergic Disease Outcomes	Main Findings
Granell et al. 2008 [64] United Kingdom	Prospective cohort, pregnant women due date 1991–1992 with live births (n = 14,062); children aged 7–8 years (n = 5364).	Reported early and late pregnancy folic acid supplementation use; dietary folate intake at 32 weeks gestation, maternal and offspring methylenetetrahydrofolate reductase (*MTHFR*) C677T allele.	Skin prick test where positive SPT $\geq$ 2 mm weal; maternal reported child wheeze, and/or asthma diagnosed by physician.	No association between *MTHFR* C677T variant and atopy in children and maternal folic acid supplementation at 18 weeks and 32 weeks, or maternal folate intake at 32 weeks gestation.
Håberg et al. 2009 [66] Norway	Prospective cohort, pregnant women with children aged 18 months (n = 32,077) born 2000–2005.	Pregnant women reported maternal folic acid supplementation use in 1st trimester and after 1st trimester.	Maternal reported episodes of wheeze in children aged 18 months.	No association with folic acid supplement use after 12 weeks gestation and allergic disease outcomes.
Whitrow et al. 2009 [71] Australia	Prospective cohort, pregnant women (n = 557); mothers and their children aged 3.5 years (n = 490), 5.5 years (n = 423) recruited 1998–2000.	Pregnant women recruited in first 16 weeks of gestation. Reported food folate intake, inventory of supplement use at <16 weeks (early gestation) and at 30–34 weeks (late gestation).	Parental report of physician-diagnosed asthma of their child aged 3.5 and 5.5 years.	Late pregnancy folic acid supplementation use (weeks 30–34) was positively associated with risk of physician-diagnosed asthma at 3.5 years.
Håberg et al. 2011 [65] Norway	Case control, children aged 3 years (n = 1455 controls; 507 cases) born 2002–2004	Pregnant women reported maternal folic acid supplementation use after week 13 gestation; plasma folate at median gestation 18 weeks.	Maternal reported asthma diagnosis in children.	Asthma risk at 3 years increased in offspring with increasing quintile of maternal folate intake. Supplementation use associated with 2nd trimester folate status (Spearman correlation = 0.46).
Dunstan et al. 2012 [63] Australia	Prospective cohort, pregnant women (n = 628) with a history of allergic disease (n = 592); skin prick test positive (n = 615), children aged 12 months (n = 484), born 2002–2009	Maternal: food folate intake, folic acid supplement use in 3rd trimester. Calcuated dietary folate equivalants, serum folate; Cord blood: serum folate.	Medically diagnosed allergic diseases in infants aged 12 months of eczema and IgE mediated food allergy (symptoms on contact and sensitization by skin prick test).	Doses of folic acid > 500 µg/day from supplements in 3rd trimester associated with diagnosed eczema at 12 months. Reduced risk of sensitization for fetal serum levels between 50–75 nmol/L

The limitations of observational epidemiological studies should be highlighted here, given that the statistical significance of associations does not infer causality. Many of the observational studies were reliant on maternal-reported folic acid supplementation use and parental-reported allergic disease outcomes, which are subject to reporting bias. There is a lack of randomised clinical trials investigating the effect of the single dietary exposure of folic acid supplementation use during the second and third trimester of pregnancy. Randomisation of exposures is critical for accounting for the multiple confounding modifiable environmental factors that have been identified as potentially influencing the in-utero environment and related allergic disease outcomes in children, including other nutritional factors, such as vitamin D, gut microbiota, smoking, rural environments, pet keeping, and high SES-related health seeking behaviours [5,7,13,16].

10. Epigenetic Effect of Folate on Immune Gene Regulation

Following the hallmark study by Hollingsworth et al., in 2008, [22] demonstrating the transgenerational effects of folic acid on epigenetic regulation, and the predisposition to allergic disease, there has been intense interest in the effects of folate on immune development. In a randomised, controlled trial of healthy subjects (n = 20), where participants were allocated a daily folic acid supplement of 1.2 mg over a 12 week period (n = 10, 70% female), or a placebo (n = 10, 80% female), the folate status was found to influence the proteome, including the proteins involved in immune function [72]. Maternal use of folic acid supplements around the time of conception, has been found to be associated with increased methylation of genes in their children, such as insulin-like growth factor 2 (IGF2) in early childhood [73].

Recently, DNA methylation signatures from mononuclear blood cells, were found to predict clinical food allergy in infants aged 11–15 months [74]. Another study identified the longitudinal stable methylation differences in CD4+ T cells, from 12 month old infants with a diagnosed food allergy, highlighting the potential for epigenetic changes in these cells to influence the allergy phenotype via changes during T-cell development [75]. Interestingly, there is also evidence linking whole blood-isolated DNA methylation profiles and an active cow's milk allergy; therefore indicating the potential of a link between the epigenetic changes in DNA methylation and the findings of the Finnish association study described above. In an epigenome-wide association study in US children, using DNA from whole blood samples, the methylation of gene loci was identified as being associated with a cow's milk allergy [76]. A study of children in the Netherlands also found general hypermethylation in DNA regions, identified as being involved in immunological pathways of children, which challenge the proven cow's milk allergy evidence, when compared to controls [77]. Mononuclear cells from children with a cow's milk allergy have also been found to have distinct differences in the DNA methylation profiles for TH2- (IL-4, IL-5) and TH1(IL-10, IFN-γ)-associated cytokine genes, when compared to controls (healthy children) and tolerant children who had outgrown their previous cow's milk allergy [78]. Collectively, these observations emphasise the need to better understand the impact of folic acid supplementation practices on aspects of fetal development, including the immune system. It is important to note the limitations of this review described above; and frame the current extent of the evidence base as being mainly derived from animal and observational epidemiological studies, with some emerging evidence from DNA methylation studies.

11. Conclusions

Folic acid acts as a methyl donor, with the capacity to alter the methylation of DNA. In animal studies, folic acid has been found to modify gene expression, linked to the development of allergic disease in offspring. These actions of folic acid, coupled with results from several human population studies, provide some foundation to bring into question the role of folic acid exposure in late pregnancy in the development of allergic disease in children, after the critical period of time for protection against neural tube defects. However, the epidemiological cohort study results are conflicting, and there is a significant lack of conclusive human trials, including in folate-replete populations. The likelihood of a multifactorial aetiology of allergic diseases in children, further highlights the need to examine this potential hypothesis using a randomised control trial study design, in order to better understand the clinical plausibility of this epigenetic role of folic acid supplementation in late pregnancy. Given the global trend of increasing allergic disease prevalence, this field of research is of interest to researchers, health practitioners, and food regulators alike; and has important research translation potential for informing food policy and health communication decision making.

Acknowledgments: The preparation of this review manuscript received no specific grant or funding from any agency, commercial, or not-for-profit sectors.

Author Contributions: C.L.M. conceived the manuscript idea, conducted the review, and led the manuscript writing. D.J.P. and S.L.P. conceived the manuscript idea, participated in manuscript writing, and reviewed the manuscript. C.B. reviewed and provided critical comments on the manuscript.

References

1. Mullins, R.J.; Dear, K.B.; Tang, M.L. Time trends in Australian hospital anaphylaxis admissions in 1998–1999 to 2011–2012. *J. Allergy Clin. Immunol.* **2015**, *136*, 367–375. [CrossRef] [PubMed]
2. Osborne, N.J.; Koplin, J.J.; Martin, P.E.; Gurrin, L.C.; Lowe, A.J.; Matheson, M.C.; Ponsonby, A.L.; Wake, M.; Tang, M.L.; Dharmage, S.C.; et al. Prevalence of challenge-proven ige-mediated food allergy using population-based sampling and predetermined challenge criteria in infants. *J. Allergy Clin. Immunol.* **2011**, *127*, 668–676. [CrossRef] [PubMed]
3. Pawankar, R.; Canonica, G.W.; Holgate, S.T.; Lockey, R.F. Allergic diseases and asthma: A major global health concern. *Curr. Opin. Allergy Clin. Immunol.* **2012**, *12*, 39–41. [CrossRef] [PubMed]
4. Prescott, S.L.; Pawankar, R.; Allen, K.J.; Campbell, D.E.; Sinn, J.; Fiocchi, A.; Ebisawa, M.; Sampson, H.A.; Beyer, K.; Lee, B.W. A global survey of changing patterns of food allergy burden in children. *World Allergy Organ. J.* **2013**, *6*, 21. [CrossRef] [PubMed]
5. Barua, S.; Junaid, M.A. Lifestyle, pregnancy and epigenetic effects. *Epigenomics* **2015**, *7*, 85–102. [CrossRef] [PubMed]
6. Brown, S.B.; Reeves, K.W.; Bertone-Johnson, E.R. Maternal folate exposure in pregnancy and childhood asthma and allergy: A systematic review. *Nutr. Rev.* **2014**, *72*, 55–64. [CrossRef] [PubMed]
7. Campbell, D.E.; Boyle, R.J.; Thornton, C.A.; Prescott, S.L. Mechanisms of allergic disease—Environmental and genetic determinants for the development of allergy. *Clin. Exp. Allergy* **2015**, *45*, 844–858. [CrossRef] [PubMed]
8. Barker, D.J. In utero programming of chronic disease. *Clin. Sci.* **1998**, *95*, 115–128. [CrossRef] [PubMed]
9. Palmer, D.J.; Huang, R.C.; Craig, J.M.; Prescott, S.L. Nutritional influences on epigenetic programming: Asthma, allergy, and obesity. *Immunol. Allergy Clin. N. Am.* **2014**, *34*, 825–837. [CrossRef] [PubMed]
10. Waterland, R.A.; Michels, K.B. Epigenetic epidemiology of the developmental origins hypothesis. *Ann. Rev. Nutr.* **2007**, *27*, 363–388. [CrossRef] [PubMed]
11. Tsang, B.L.; Devine, O.J.; Cordero, A.M.; Marchetta, C.M.; Mulinare, J.; Mersereau, P.; Guo, J.; Qi, Y.P.; Berry, R.J.; Rosenthal, J.; et al. Assessing the association between the methylenetetrahydrofolate reductase (MTHFR) 677C>T polymorphism and blood folate concentrations: A systematic review and meta-analysis of trials and observational studies. *Am. J. Clin. Nutr.* **2015**, *101*, 1286–1294. [CrossRef] [PubMed]
12. Miles, E.A.; Calder, P.C. Maternal diet and its influence on the development of allergic disease. *Clin. Exp. Allergy* **2015**, *45*, 63–74. [CrossRef] [PubMed]
13. Prescott, S.L. Early-life environmental determinants of allergic diseases and the wider pandemic of inflammatory noncommunicable diseases. *J. Allergy Clin. Immunol.* **2013**, *131*, 23–30. [CrossRef] [PubMed]
14. Martino, D.; Prescott, S. Epigenetics and prenatal influences on asthma and allergic airways disease. *Chest* **2011**, *139*, 640–647. [CrossRef] [PubMed]
15. Amarasekera, M.; Prescott, S.L.; Palmer, D.J. Nutrition in early life, immune-programming and allergies: The role of epigenetics. *Asian Pac. J. Allergy Immunol.* **2013**, *31*, 175–182. [PubMed]

16. Ashley, S.; Dang, T.; Koplin, J.; Martino, D.; Prescott, S. Food for thought: Progress in understanding the causes and mechanisms of food allergy. *Curr. Opin. Allergy Clin. Immunol.* **2015**, *15*, 237–242. [CrossRef] [PubMed]
17. Prescott, S.L.; Macaubas, C.; Holt, B.J.; Smallacombe, T.B.; Loh, R.; Sly, P.D.; Holt, P.G. Transplacental priming of the human immune system to environmental allergens: Universal skewing of initial T cell responses toward the Th2 cytokine profile. *J. Immunol.* **1998**, *160*, 4730–4737. [PubMed]
18. Mold, J.E.; Michaelsson, J.; Burt, T.D.; Muench, M.O.; Beckerman, K.P.; Busch, M.P.; Lee, T.H.; Nixon, D.F.; McCune, J.M. Maternal alloantigens promote the development of tolerogenic fetal regulatory T cells in utero. *Science* **2008**, *322*, 1562–1565. [CrossRef] [PubMed]
19. Schaub, B.; Liu, J.; Hoppler, S.; Schleich, I.; Huehn, J.; Olek, S.; Wieczorek, G.; Illi, S.; von Mutius, E. Maternal farm exposure modulates neonatal immune mechanisms through regulatory T cells. *J. Allergy Clin. Immunol.* **2009**, *123*, 774–782. [CrossRef] [PubMed]
20. Tulic, M.K.; Hodder, M.; Forsberg, A.; McCarthy, S.; Richman, T.; D'Vaz, N.; van den Biggelaar, A.H.; Thornton, C.A.; Prescott, S.L. Differences in innate immune function between allergic and nonallergic children: New insights into immune ontogeny. *J. Allergy Clin. Immunol.* **2011**, *127*, 470–478. [CrossRef] [PubMed]
21. Prescott, S.L.; Macaubas, C.; Smallacombe, T.; Holt, B.J.; Sly, P.D.; Holt, P.G. Development of allergen-specific T-cell memory in atopic and normal children. *Lancet* **1999**, *353*, 196–200. [CrossRef]
22. Hollingsworth, J.W.; Maruoka, S.; Boon, K.; Garantziotis, S.; Li, Z.; Tomfohr, J.; Bailey, N.; Potts, E.N.; Whitehead, G.; Brass, D.M.; et al. In utero supplementation with methyl donors enhances allergic airway disease in mice. *J. Clin. Investig.* **2008**, *118*, 3462–3469. [CrossRef] [PubMed]
23. Daly, L.E.; Kirke, P.N.; Molloy, A.; Weir, D.G.; Scott, J.M. Folate levels and neural tube defects. Implications for prevention. *JAMA* **1995**, *274*, 1698–1702. [CrossRef] [PubMed]
24. Abbassi-Ghanavati, M.; Greer, L.G.; Cunningham, F.G. Pregnancy and laboratory studies: A reference table for clinicians. *Obstet. Gynecol.* **2009**, *114*, 1326–1331. [CrossRef] [PubMed]
25. Hursthouse, N.A.; Gray, A.R.; Miller, J.C.; Rose, M.C.; Houghton, L.A. Folate status of reproductive age women and neural tube defect risk: The effect of long-term folic acid supplementation at doses of 140 microg and 400 microg per day. *Nutrients* **2011**, *3*, 49–62. [CrossRef] [PubMed]
26. Wills, L. Treatment of "pernicious anaemia of pregnancy" and "tropical anaemia". *Br. Med. J.* **1931**, *1*, 1059–1064. [CrossRef] [PubMed]
27. Al-Gailani, S. Making birth defects 'preventable': Pre-conceptional vitamin supplements and the politics of risk reduction. *Stud. Hist. Philos. Biol. Biomed. Sci.* **2014**, *47 Pt B*, 278–289. [CrossRef] [PubMed]
28. Chanarin, I.; Macgibbon, B.M.; O'Sullivan, W.J.; Mollin, D.L. Folic-acid deficiency in pregnancy. The pathogenesis of megaloblastic anaemia of pregnancy. *Lancet* **1959**, *2*, 634–639. [CrossRef]
29. Giles, C. An account of 335 cases of megaloblastic anaemia of pregnancy and the puerperium. *J. Clin. Pathol.* **1966**, *19*, 1–11. [CrossRef] [PubMed]
30. Hansen, H.A. The incidence of pernicious anaemia and the etiology of folic acid deficiency in pregnancy. *Acta Obstet. Gynecol. Scand.* **1967**, *46* (Suppl. 7), 113–115. [CrossRef]
31. Willoughby, M.L.; Jewell, F.J. Investigation of folic acid requirements in pregnancy. *Br. Med. J.* **1966**, *2*, 1568–1571. [CrossRef] [PubMed]
32. Hibbard, B.M.; Hibbard, E.D. Folate deficiency in pregnancy. *Br. Med. J.* **1968**, *4*, 452–453. [CrossRef] [PubMed]
33. Hibbard, B.M.; Hibbard, E.D.; Jeffcoate, T.N. Folic acid and reproduction. *Acta Obstet. Gynecol. Scand.* **1965**, *44*, 375–400. [CrossRef] [PubMed]
34. Bower, C.; Stanley, F.J. Dietary folate as a risk factor for neural-tube defects: Evidence from a case-control study in Western Australia. *MJA* **1989**, *150*, 613–619. [PubMed]
35. Czeizel, A.E.; Dudas, I. Prevention of the first occurrence of neural-tube defects by periconceptional vitamin supplementation. *NEJM* **1992**, *327*, 1832–1835. [CrossRef] [PubMed]
36. Milunsky, A.; Jick, H.; Jick, S.S.; Bruell, C.L.; MacLaughlin, D.S.; Rothman, K.J.; Willett, W. Multivitamin/folic acid supplementation in early pregnancy reduces the prevalence of neural tube defects. *JAMA* **1989**, *262*, 2847–2852. [CrossRef] [PubMed]
37. Mulinare, J.; Cordero, J.F.; Erickson, J.D.; Berry, R.J. Periconceptional use of multivitamins and the occurrence of neural tube defects. *JAMA* **1988**, *260*, 3141–3145. [CrossRef] [PubMed]

38. Smithells, R.W.; Sheppard, S.; Schorah, C.J.; Seller, M.J.; Nevin, N.C.; Harris, R.; Read, A.P.; Fielding, D.W. Possible prevention of neural-tube defects by periconceptional vitamin supplementation. *Lancet* **1980**, *1*, 339–340. [CrossRef]
39. Smithells, R.W.; Sheppard, S.; Schorah, C.J.; Seller, M.J.; Nevin, N.C.; Harris, R.; Read, A.P.; Fielding, D.W. Apparent prevention of neural tube defects by periconceptional vitamin supplementation. *Arch. Dis. Child.* **1981**, *56*, 911–918. [CrossRef] [PubMed]
40. De-Regil, L.M.; Fernandez-Gaxiola, A.C.; Dowswell, T.; Pena-Rosas, J.P. Effects and safety of periconceptional folate supplementation for preventing birth defects. *Cochrane Database Syst. Rev.* **2010**, CD007950. [CrossRef]
41. Bower, C.; Blum, L.; O'Daly, K.; Higgins, C.; Loutsky, F.; Kosky, C. Promotion of folate for the prevention of neural tube defects: Knowledge and use of periconceptional folic acid supplements in Western Australia, 1992 to 1995. *Aust. N. Z. J. Public Health* **1997**, *21*, 716–721. [CrossRef] [PubMed]
42. Bower, C.; Miller, M.; Payne, J.; Serna, P. Promotion of folate for the prevention of neural tube defects: Who benefits? *Paediatr. Perinat. Epidemiol.* **2005**, *19*, 435–444. [CrossRef] [PubMed]
43. Mallard, S.R.; Houghton, L.A. Folate knowledge and consumer behaviour among pregnant New Zealand women prior to the potential introduction of mandatory fortification. *Asia Pac. J. Clin. Nutr.* **2012**, *21*, 440–449. [PubMed]
44. Stockley, L.; Lund, V. Use of folic acid supplements, particularly by low-income and young women: A series of systematic reviews to inform public health policy in the UK. *Public Health Nutr.* **2008**, *11*, 807–821. [CrossRef] [PubMed]
45. Watson, L.F.; Brown, S.J.; Davey, M.A. Use of periconceptional folic acid supplements in Victoria and New South Wales, Australia. *Aust. N. Z. J. Public Health* **2006**, *30*, 42–49. [CrossRef] [PubMed]
46. Wang, S.; Ge, X.; Zhu, B.; Xuan, Y.; Huang, K.; Rutayisire, E.; Mao, L.; Huang, S.; Yan, S.; Tao, F. Maternal continuing folic acid supplementation after the first trimester of pregnancy increased the risk of large-for-gestational-age birth: A population-based birth cohort study. *Nutrients* **2016**, *8*. [CrossRef] [PubMed]
47. Blumfield, M.L.; Hure, A.J.; Macdonald-Wicks, L.; Smith, R.; Collins, C.E. A systematic review and meta-analysis of micronutrient intakes during pregnancy in developed countries. *Nutr. Rev.* **2013**, *71*, 118–132. [CrossRef] [PubMed]
48. Crider, K.S.; Bailey, L.B.; Berry, R.J. Folic acid food fortification-its history, effect, concerns, and future directions. *Nutrients* **2011**, *3*, 370–384. [CrossRef] [PubMed]
49. Lawrence, M.A.; Chai, W.; Kara, R.; Rosenberg, I.H.; Scott, J.; Tedstone, A. Examination of selected national policies towards mandatory folic acid fortification. *Nutr. Rev.* **2009**, *67* (Suppl. 1), S73–S78. [CrossRef] [PubMed]
50. Mills, J.L.; Signore, C. Neural tube defect rates before and after food fortification with folic acid. *Birth Defects Res. A Clin. Mol. Teratol.* **2004**, *70*, 844–845. [CrossRef] [PubMed]
51. Mallard, S.R.; Gray, A.R.; Houghton, L.A. Periconceptional bread intakes indicate New Zealand's proposed mandatory folic acid fortification program may be outdated: Results from a postpartum survey. *BMC Pregnancy Childbirth* **2012**, *12*, 8. [CrossRef] [PubMed]
52. Bower, C.; Ryan, A.; Rudy, E.; Miller, M. Trends in neural tube defects in Western Australia. *Aust. N. Z. J. Public Health* **2002**, *26*, 150–151. [CrossRef] [PubMed]
53. Hertrampf, E.; Cortes, F. National food-fortification program with folic acid in Chile. *Food Nutr. Bull.* **2008**, *29*, S231–S237. [CrossRef] [PubMed]
54. Chakraborty, H.; Nyarko, K.A.; Goco, N.; Moore, J.; Moretti-Ferreira, D.; Murray, J.C.; Wehby, G.L. Folic acid fortification and women's folate levels in selected communities in Brazil—A first look. *Int. J. Vitam. Nutr. Res.* **2014**, *84*, 286–294. [CrossRef] [PubMed]
55. Sayed, A.R.; Bourne, D.; Pattinson, R.; Nixon, J.; Henderson, B. Decline in the prevalence of neural tube defects following folic acid fortification and its cost-benefit in South Africa. *Birth Defects Res. A Clin. Mol. Teratol.* **2008**, *82*, 211–216. [CrossRef] [PubMed]
56. Dugbaza, J.; Cunningham, J. Estimates of total dietary folic acid intake in the Australian population following mandatory folic acid fortification of bread. *J. Nutr. Metab.* **2012**, *2012*, 492353. [CrossRef] [PubMed]
57. Emmett, J.K.; Lawrence, M.; Riley, M. Estimating the impact of mandatory folic acid fortification on the folic acid intake of Australian women of childbearing age. *Aust. N. Z. J. Public Health* **2011**, *35*, 442–450. [CrossRef] [PubMed]

58. Australian Bureau of Statistics. Australian Health Survey. Nutrition First Results: Foods and Nutrients, 2011–12. Mean Daily Energy and Nutrient Intake. Available online: http://www.abs.gov.au/ausstats/abs@.nsf/detailspage/4364.0.55.0072011-12 (accessed on 1 November 2016).
59. Frigolet, M.E.; Ramos Barragan, V.E.; Tamez Gonzalez, M. Low-carbohydrate diets: A matter of love or hate. *Ann. Nutr. Metab.* **2011**, *58*, 320–334. [CrossRef] [PubMed]
60. Plumptre, L.; Masih, S.P.; Ly, A.; Aufreiter, S.; Sohn, K.J.; Croxford, R.; Lausman, A.Y.; Berger, H.; O'Connor, D.L.; Kim, Y.I. High concentrations of folate and unmetabolized folic acid in a cohort of pregnant canadian women and umbilical cord blood. *Am. J. Clin. Nutr.* **2015**, *102*, 848–857. [CrossRef] [PubMed]
61. Asher, M.I.; Montefort, S.; Bjorksten, B.; Lai, C.K.; Strachan, D.P.; Weiland, S.K.; Williams, H.; Group, I.P.T.S. Worldwide time trends in the prevalence of symptoms of asthma, allergic rhinoconjunctivitis, and eczema in childhood: Isaac phases one and three repeat multicountry cross-sectional surveys. *Lancet* **2006**, *368*, 733–743. [CrossRef]
62. Bekkers, M.B.; Elstgeest, L.E.; Scholtens, S.; Haveman-Nies, A.; de Jongste, J.C.; Kerkhof, M.; Koppelman, G.H.; Gehring, U.; Smit, H.A.; Wijga, A.H. Maternal use of folic acid supplements during pregnancy, and childhood respiratory health and atopy. *Eur. Respir. J.* **2012**, *39*, 1468–1474. [CrossRef] [PubMed]
63. Dunstan, J.A.; West, C.; McCarthy, S.; Metcalfe, J.; Meldrum, S.; Oddy, W.H.; Tulic, M.K.; D'Vaz, N.; Prescott, S.L. The relationship between maternal folate status in pregnancy, cord blood folate levels, and allergic outcomes in early childhood. *Allergy* **2012**, *67*, 50–57. [CrossRef] [PubMed]
64. Granell, R.; Heron, J.; Lewis, S.; Davey Smith, G.; Sterne, J.A.; Henderson, J. The association between mother and child MTHFR C677T polymorphisms, dietary folate intake and childhood atopy in a population-based, longitudinal birth cohort. *Clin. Exp. Allergy* **2008**, *38*, 320–328. [CrossRef] [PubMed]
65. Haberg, S.E.; London, S.J.; Nafstad, P.; Nilsen, R.M.; Ueland, P.M.; Vollset, S.E.; Nystad, W. Maternal folate levels in pregnancy and asthma in children at age 3 years. *J. Allergy Clin. Immunol.* **2011**, *127*, 262–264. [CrossRef] [PubMed]
66. Haberg, S.E.; London, S.J.; Stigum, H.; Nafstad, P.; Nystad, W. Folic acid supplements in pregnancy and early childhood respiratory health. *Arch. Dis. Child.* **2009**, *94*, 180–184. [CrossRef] [PubMed]
67. Kiefte-de Jong, J.C.; Timmermans, S.; Jaddoe, V.W.; Hofman, A.; Tiemeier, H.; Steegers, E.A.; de Jongste, J.C.; Moll, H.A. High circulating folate and vitamin b-12 concentrations in women during pregnancy are associated with increased prevalence of atopic dermatitis in their offspring. *J. Nutr.* **2012**, *142*, 731–738. [CrossRef] [PubMed]
68. Kim, J.H.; Jeong, K.S.; Ha, E.H.; Park, H.; Ha, M.; Hong, Y.C.; Bhang, S.Y.; Lee, S.J.; Lee, K.Y.; Lee, S.H.; et al. Relationship between prenatal and postnatal exposures to folate and risks of allergic and respiratory diseases in early childhood. *Pediatr. Pulmonol.* **2015**, *50*, 155–163. [CrossRef] [PubMed]
69. Magdelijns, F.J.; Mommers, M.; Penders, J.; Smits, L.; Thijs, C. Folic acid use in pregnancy and the development of atopy, asthma, and lung function in childhood. *Pediatrics* **2011**, *128*, e135–e144. [CrossRef] [PubMed]
70. Tuokkola, J.; Luukkainen, P.; Kaila, M.; Takkinen, H.M.; Niinisto, S.; Veijola, R.; Virta, L.J.; Knip, M.; Simell, O.; Ilonen, J.; et al. Maternal dietary folate, folic acid and vitamin d intakes during pregnancy and lactation and the risk of cows' milk allergy in the offspring. *Br. J. Nutr.* **2016**, *116*, 710–718. [CrossRef] [PubMed]
71. Whitrow, M.J.; Moore, V.M.; Rumbold, A.R.; Davies, M.J. Effect of supplemental folic acid in pregnancy on childhood asthma: A prospective birth cohort study. *Am. J. Epidemiol.* **2009**, *170*, 1486–1493. [CrossRef] [PubMed]
72. Duthie, S.J.; Horgan, G.; de Roos, B.; Rucklidge, G.; Reid, M.; Duncan, G.; Pirie, L.; Basten, G.P.; Powers, H.J. Blood folate status and expression of proteins involved in immune function, inflammation, and coagulation: Biochemical and proteomic changes in the plasma of humans in response to long-term synthetic folic acid supplementation. *J. Proteome Res.* **2010**, *9*, 1941–1950. [CrossRef] [PubMed]
73. Steegers-Theunissen, R.P.; Obermann-Borst, S.A.; Kremer, D.; Lindemans, J.; Siebel, C.; Steegers, E.A.; Slagboom, P.E.; Heijmans, B.T. Periconceptional maternal folic acid use of 400 microg per day is related to increased methylation of the IGF2 gene in the very young child. *PLoS ONE* **2009**, *4*, e7845. [CrossRef] [PubMed]
74. Martino, D.; Dang, T.; Sexton-Oates, A.; Prescott, S.; Tang, M.L.; Dharmage, S.; Gurrin, L.; Koplin, J.; Ponsonby, A.L.; Allen, K.J.; et al. Blood DNA methylation biomarkers predict clinical reactivity in

food-sensitized infants. *J. Allergy Clin. Immunol.* **2015**, *135*, 1319–1328. [CrossRef] [PubMed]

75. Martino, D.; Joo, J.E.; Sexton-Oates, A.; Dang, T.; Allen, K.; Saffery, R.; Prescott, S. Epigenome-wide association study reveals longitudinally stable DNA methylation differences in CD4+ T cells from children with IgE-mediated food allergy. *Epigenetics* **2014**, *9*, 998–1006. [CrossRef] [PubMed]
76. Hong, X.; Ladd-Acosta, C.; Hao, K.; Sherwood, B.; Ji, H.; Keet, C.A.; Kumar, R.; Caruso, D.; Liu, X.; Wang, G.; et al. Epigenome-wide association study links site-specific DNA methylation changes with cow's milk allergy. *J. Allergy Clin. Immunol.* **2016**, *138*, 908–911. [CrossRef] [PubMed]
77. Petrus, N.C.; Henneman, P.; Venema, A.; Mul, A.; van Sinderen, F.; Haagmans, M.; Mook, O.; Hennekam, R.C.; Sprikkelman, A.B.; Mannens, M. Cow's milk allergy in Dutch children: An epigenetic pilot survey. *Clin. Transl. Allergy* **2016**, *6*, 16. [CrossRef] [PubMed]
78. Berni Canani, R.; Paparo, L.; Nocerino, R.; Cosenza, L.; Pezzella, V.; Di Costanzo, M.; Capasso, M.; Del Monaco, V.; D'Argenio, V.; Greco, L.; et al. Differences in DNA methylation profile of Th1 and Th2 cytokine genes are associated with tolerance acquisition in children with IgE-mediated cow's milk allergy. *Clin. Epigenet.* **2015**, *7*, 38. [CrossRef] [PubMed]

14

Gut Microbiota as a Target for Preventive and Therapeutic Intervention against Food Allergy

Rosita Aitoro [1], Lorella Paparo [1], Antonio Amoroso [1], Margherita Di Costanzo [1], Linda Cosenza [1], Viviana Granata [1], Carmen Di Scala [1], Rita Nocerino [1], Giovanna Trinchese [1], Mariangela Montella [1], Danilo Ercolini [2,3] and Roberto Berni Canani [1,3,4,5,*]

1 Department of Translational Medical Science-Pediatric Section, University of Naples "Federico II", 80131 Naples, Italy; aitoro.rosita@gmail.com (R.A.); paparolorella@gmail.com (L.P.); antonioamoroso87@gmail.com (A.A.); mara.dicostanzo@live.it (M.D.C.); lindacosenza@libero.it (L.C.); vivianagranata@gmail.com (V.G.); carmendiscala@gmail.com (C.D.S.); ritanocerino@alice.it (R.N.); giovanna.trinchese@unina.it (G.T.); mariangelamontella@libero.it (M.M.)

2 Department of Agricultural Sciences, Division of Microbiology, University of Naples "Federico II", 80055 Portici, Italy; ercolini@unina.it

3 Task Force on Microbiome Studies, University of Naples "Federico II", 80131 Naples, Italy

4 European Laboratory for the Investigation of Food Induced Diseases, University of Naples "Federico II", 80131 Naples, Italy

5 CEINGE Advanced Biotechnologies, University of Naples "Federico II", 80131 Naples, Italy

* Correspondence: berni@unina.it

Abstract: The gut microbiota plays a pivotal role in immune system development and function. Modification in the gut microbiota composition (dysbiosis) early in life is a critical factor affecting the development of food allergy. Many environmental factors including caesarean delivery, lack of breast milk, drugs, antiseptic agents, and a low-fiber/high-fat diet can induce gut microbiota dysbiosis, and have been associated with the occurrence of food allergy. New technologies and experimental tools have provided information regarding the importance of select bacteria on immune tolerance mechanisms. Short-chain fatty acids are crucial metabolic products of gut microbiota responsible for many protective effects against food allergy. These compounds are involved in epigenetic regulation of the immune system. These evidences provide a foundation for developing innovative strategies to prevent and treat food allergy. Here, we present an overview on the potential role of gut microbiota as the target of intervention against food allergy.

Keywords: cow's milk allergy; diet; immune tolerance; dysbiosis; probiotics; short chain fatty acids; butyrate

1. Introduction

During the last several decades, a changing patterns in the epidemiology of food allergy [FA] have been observed, with an increased prevalence, severity of clinical manifestations, and risk of persistence until later ages [1]. Atopic family history, ethnicity, atopic dermatitis (AD), and related genetic polymorphisms have been associated with FA development [2]. Although genetic factors may predispose individuals to the development of FA among selected individuals, they cannot explain the changes in epidemiology over this short time frame, suggesting that environmental factors promote FA [3]. FA develops following loss of immune tolerance, which results in allergic sensitization and subsequent disease manifestation and progression.

The initial exposure to food allergens occurs predominantly via the gastrointestinal tract or skin. An impaired skin barrier could lead to increased transcutaneous passage of antigens and subsequent sensitization. An association between the early onset of AD and development of FA has been shown [4]. In the gastrointestinal tract, the two main factors influencing immune tolerance are dietary factors and microbiota composition and function [5]. Kim et al. demonstrated that under normal physiological conditions, macromolecules from the diet induce the bulk of regulatory T cells (Tregs) development, which is essential for suppressing a default immune response to dietary antigens [5]. Observational studies have suggested that the early introduction of peanut [6], egg [7], or cow's milk [8] may prevent the development of allergy to these foods. A randomized controlled trial (Learning Early about Peanut Allergy, LEAP) showed that the early consumption of peanut in high-risk infants with severe eczema, egg allergy, or both reduced the development of peanut allergy by 80% by 5 years of age [9]. The Persistence of Oral Tolerance to Peanut (LEAP-On) study showed that the absence of reactivity is maintained in these subjects [10].

The gut microbiota could be defined as the trillions of microbes that collectively inhabit the gut lumen [4,11], and increasing evidence shows that altered patterns of microbial exposure [dysbiosis] early in life can lead to FA development by negatively influencing immune system development [12]. Thus, the gut microbiota could be considered a potential target for preventive and therapeutic intervention against FA. Recent studies have reported the efficacy of intervention in the gut microbiota against FA.Here, we review the current understanding of the potential role of gut microbiota as potential target against FA.

2. Importance of Microbial Exposure for the Development of Immune Tolerance

Immune tolerance is the state of unresponsiveness of the immune system to substances or tissues that have the potential to induce an immune response. Tolerance is achieved through both central tolerance and peripheral tolerance mechanisms [13]. The exact mechanisms involved in the development of immune tolerance have not been not fully defined [14]. Current evidence suggests that the gut microbiota and its metabolites (mainly short chain fatty acids), together with to exposure to dietary factors in early life, critically influence the establishment of immune tolerance to food antigens [5] (Figure 1). Germ-free mice are unable to achieve immune tolerance to food antigens [15]. During the early stage of post-natal life, development of the gut microbiota parallels maturation of the immune system [16]. During vaginal delivery, infants receive their first bacterial inoculum from the maternal vaginal tract, skin tissue, and often fecal matter, exposing the immature immune system of newborns to a significant bacterial load [17]. Maturation of a healthy gut microbiota in early life allows for a change in the Th2/Th1 balance, favoring a Th1 cell response [18], while dysbiosis alters host-microbiota homeostasis, favoring a shift in the Th1/Th2 cytokine balance toward a Th2 response [19]. Gut microbes induce the activation of Tregs which are depleted in germ-free mice [20]. Microbiota-induced Tregs express the nuclear hormone receptor RORγt and differentiate along a pathway that also leads to Th17 cells; while in the absence of RORγt in Tregs, there is an expansion of GATA-3-expressing Tregs, as well as conventional Th2 cells, and Th2-associated pathology is exacerbated [21]. Moreover, it has been demonstrated that under normal physiological conditions, macromolecules obtained via the diet induce Treg cell development in the small intestinal lamina propria, which is essential for suppressing the default strong immune response to dietary antigens [5]. The presence of both diet- and microbe-induced populations of Treg cells may be required to induce complete tolerance to food antigens [5].

It has been speculated that microbiota can activate MyD88 signaling in the lamina propria and follicular dendritic cells (DCs) [22]. Mucosal plasma cells, upon induction by DCs, produce secretory IgA (sIgA). The sIgA system is considered important in the pathogenesis of FA. Delayed development of IgA-producing cells or insufficient sIgA-dependent function at the intestinal surface barrier appears to contribute substantially to FA [21]. This agrees with previous study of minor dysregulations of both innate and adaptive immunity (particularly low levels of IgA) in children with multiple FAs [23]. Furthermore, the gut microbiota stimulates DCs in the Peyer's patches to secrete transforming growth factor (TGF)-β, C-X-C motif chemokine ligand 13, and B-cell activating protein, which leads to IgA production and class switching [24].

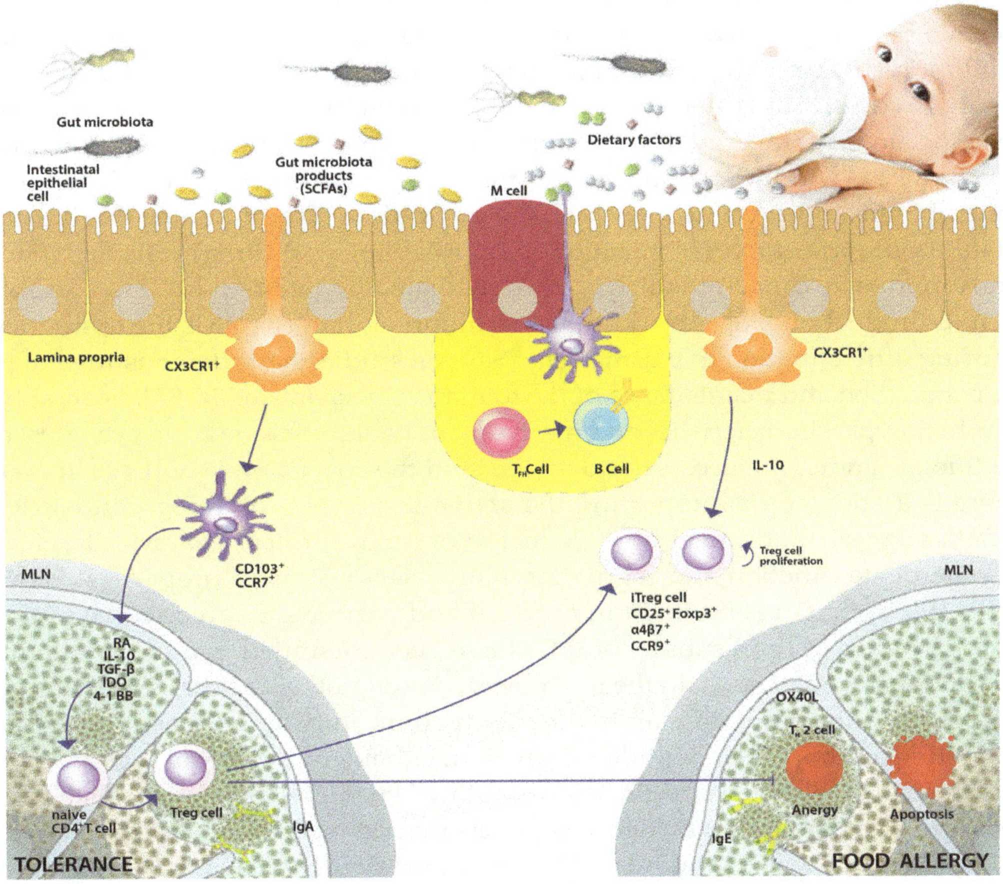

Figure 1. Immune tolerance network in the intestinal lumen: interaction between microbiome and the gut immune system in early-life. The immune tolerance network is mainly composed by the well-modulated activity of different components: gut microbiota (without gut microbiota, it is not possible to achieve oral tolerance); dietary factors (mainly dietary peptides, as amino acids are unable to drive immune tolerance); epithelial cells; dendritic cells; and regulatory T cells. Food antigens and intestinal microbiota constitute the majority of the antigen load in the intestine. CX3CR1$^+$ cells (likely macrophages) extend dendrites between intestinal epithelial cells, sample antigens in the gut lumen, and transfer captured antigens via gap junctions to CD103$^+$CCR7$^+$ dendritic cells (DCs). This subset of DCs migrates from the lamina propria to the draining lymph nodes, where the DCs express transforming growth factor-β (TGFβ), retinoic acid (RA), interleukin-10 (IL-10) and also express the enzyme indoleamine 2,3-dioxygenase (IDO), thereby inducing naïve CD4$^+$ T cells to differentiate into regulatory T (Treg) cells. Macrophages also appear to secrete IL-10, leading to Treg cell proliferation. Treg cell express integrin α4β7, which results in homing to the gut where Treg cells may dampen the immune response. CD103$^+$ DCs also sample antigens that pass through the epithelial barrier via M cell-mediated transcytosis or by extending a process through a transcellular pore in an M cell. Recent evidence suggests a role for regulatory B cells in activating Tregs after stimulation with microbial factors recognized by Toll-like receptors. B cell clones expressing antibodies specific for food allergen may undergo isotype switching in secondary lymphoid organs with the aid of follicular T helper (TFH) cells. Food tolerance is associated with IgA. For a broader prospective, the complex interaction between intestinal contents and immune and non-immune cells creates an environment that favors tolerance by the inducting IgA antibodies and Tregs, which produce IL-10, a molecule crucial for the induction of tolerance to food antigens.

Accordingly, it has been recently demonstrated that dietary elements, including fibers and vitamin A, are essential for the tolerogenic function of CD103^{+} DCs and maintenance of mucosal homeostasis, including IgA production and epithelial barrier function [25].Moreover, in experimental studies, some mice are protected from the development of FA (non-responders) compared with animals showing marked systemic FA symptoms after immunizations [26,27]. This differential immune response is associated with a distinct microbiota composition in mice with a non-responding phenotype [28]. Recent findings have also suggested that neonatal gut microbiome dysbiosis promotes CD4^{+} T cell dysfunction associated with allergy [29] and supports age-sensitive interactions with microbiota [30]. Early-life may be a key "window of opportunity" for intervention given the age-dependent association of the gut microbiome and FA outcomes [31].The microbiota also promotes B cell receptor editing within the lamina propria upon colonization [32]. Regulatory B (Breg) cells are characterized by their immunosuppressive capacity, which is often mediated by interleukin (IL)-10 secretion, but also IL-35 and TGF-β production [33]. An additional immunoregulatory role is the up-regulation of IgG4 antibodies during differentiation to plasma cells. Several studies have demonstrated a potential role for Breg in the induction and maintenance of the tolerance mechanism [34–36]. Several types of Bregs with distinct phenotypic characteristics and mechanisms of suppression have been described [34–36]; therefore, additional studies are necessary to understand the effective role of Bregs in oral tolerance.In addition, there is a body of data reporting the activation of non-immune pathways in food oral tolerance. Data suggest that a healthy gut microbiota may protect against allergic sensitization by affecting enterocyte function and regulating its barrier-protective properties. Similarly, innate lymphoid cells (ILCs) that are abundant in mucosal and barrier sites are involved in these defence mechanisms [37]. While several subsets of ILCs have been identified, particular attention has been given to ILC3 and its interactions with the microbiota. Among other factors, these cells produce IL-22, a cytokine of central importance in maintaining tissue immunity and physiology via its pleiotropic action in promoting antimicrobial peptide production, enhancing epithelial regeneration, increasing mucus production, and regulating intestinal permeability [38]. How the microbiota affects the turnover of ILC3 remains unclear, but recent evidence supports that defined commensals preferentially impact this subset. Particularly, Clostridia-induced IL-22 has been demonstrated to be an innate mechanism by which the microbiota can regulate the permeability of the epithelial barrier and contribute to protection against food allergen sensitization [15]. In contrast, gut microbiota dysbiosis induces alterations in intestinal epithelial function resulting in aberrant Th2 responses toward allergic, rather than tolerogenic, responses [39].

3. Gut Microbiota in FA

Epidemiological studies have established a correlation between factors that disrupt the microbiota during childhood and immune and metabolic conditions later in life. Several factors responsible for dysbiosis have been associated with the occurrence of FA, such as caesarean delivery [40], lack of breast milk [41], drug use (mainly antibiotics and gastric acidity inhibitors) [42], antiseptic agent use, and low fiber/high fat diet [43] (Figure 2). Emerging data from human studies link the use of antimicrobial agents to the increasing prevalence of FA. Neonatal antibiotic treatment reduced microbial diversity and bacterial load in both fecal and ileal samples and enhanced food allergen sensitization [15]. Even low-dose early-life antibiotic exposure can lead to long-lasting effects on metabolic and immune responsiveness [44]. Maternal use of antibiotics before and during pregnancy, as well as antibiotic courses during the first months of life, are associated with an increased risk of cow's milk allergy (CMA) in infants [45].

Data characterizing the microbiota of patients with FA are still preliminary because of multiple environmental stimuli that profoundly influence the composition of the gut microbiota [46]. Some studies have failed to identify differences in infant microbiota according to later allergic status, or have found different changes in gut microbiota depending on the cases and groups of subjects. Although compelling evidence for the association of gut microbiota dysbiosis with FA is emerging, heterogeneities in study design, including sampling time points, methods used to characterize the microbiota, and different allergic phenotypes under study, make it difficult to establish a clear correlation between specific bacterial taxa and allergy development. To better identify microbiota changes associated with the emergence of FA, well-phenotyped birth cohorts are needed with long-term follow up.

First studies using bacterial cultures showed that infants allergic to cow's milk had higher total bacteria and anaerobic counts [47]. There was no association between culturable bacteria and food sensitization by 18 months of age in three cohorts of European infants [48]. Kendler et al. found no association between culturable gut bacteria and sensitization to food including milk, egg, peanut, and hazelnut [49].Pyrosequencing technology can identify approximately 80% more bacteria in the gut than those identified by conventional culture-based methods, revealing the high complexity and diversity of the gut microbiota.Recent evidence suggests that gut dysbiosis precedes FA and influences during early life affected the subsequent development of allergic disease [50]. Nakayama et al. profiled the fecal bacteria compositions of allergic and non-allergic infants and correlated changes in gut microbiota composition with allergy development in later years [51]. They found that in the allergic group, the genus *Bacteroides* at 1 month and genera *Propionibacterium* and *Klebsiella* at 2 months were more abundant, while the genera *Acinetobacter* and *Clostridium* at 1 month were less abundant than in the non-allergic group [51]. Additionally, the relative abundance of total *Proteobacteria*, excluding genus *Klebsiella*, was significantly lower in the allergic than in the non-allergic group at the age of 1 month. Allergic infants with high colonization of *Bacteroides* and/or *Klebsiella* showed less colonization of *Clostridium* within the major phylotypes, suggesting antagonism between these bacterial groups in the gut. *Bacteroides* are sensitive to short-chain fatty acids (SCFAs), particularly under low pH conditions [52], suggesting that the observed antagonism is attributable to an SCFA produced by *Clostridium* [52]. Azad et al. found that an increased *Enterobacteriaceae/Bacteroidaceae* ratio and low *Ruminococcaceae* (*Clostridia* class) abundance, in the context of low gut microbiota richness in early infancy, are associated with subsequent food sensitization, suggesting that early gut dysbiosis contributes to subsequent development of FA [53]. A low level of microbial diversity with reduced *Clostridiales*, and increased *Bacteroidales* have been also observed in the gut microbiota of allergic patients [54].

Cross-sectional studies comparing the intestinal microbial composition of food allergies in healthy subjects have also been performed. Fecal microbial composition was assessed using 16 S rRNA sequencing to determine the differences between children with FA (n = 17 with IgE-mediated FA, n = 17 with non-IgE-mediated FA) and healthy controls (n = 45) [55]. There was no difference in microbial diversity between groups. Subjects with IgE-mediated FA showed increased levels of *Clostridium sensu stricto* and *Anaerobacter* (*Clostridia* class) and decreased levels of *Bacteroides* and *Clostridium* XVIII. Levels of *C. sensu stricto* were also correlated with the levels of IgE [56]. Chen et al. recently showed that children with food sensitization in early life have an altered fecal microbiota and lower microbiota diversity compared to healthy controls. Children with food sensitization showed significantly decreased numbers of *Bacteroidetes* and a significantly increased number of *Firmicutes* compared to healthy children. The most differentially abundant taxa in children with food sensitization were characterized by increased abundances of *Clostridium* IV and *Subdoligranulum* (*Clostridia* class) and decreased abundances of *Bacteroides* and *Veillonella* (*Clostridia* class) [56]. Recently, enriched taxa from the *Clostridia* class and *Firmicutes* phylum were observed in children with a more favourable CMA disease course [57]. Accordingly, a low abundance of some sub-taxa belonging to *Clostridia* may be associated with the development of FA. The *Clostridia* class has become one of the largest genera of bacteria, and presently contains more than 100 species. Some *Clostridia* groups possess pathogenic species; however, most *Clostridia* have a commensal relationship with the host [58].In agreement with this view, a pivotal study by Atarashi et al. showed that the spore-forming component of gut microbiota, particularly clusters IV and XIVa of the genus *Clostridium*, promoted Tregs accumulation in the colonic mucosa. Colonization of mice by a defined mix of *Clostridium* strains provided an environment rich in TGF-β and affected the number and function of colonic Tregs expressing the Foxp3 transcription factor (Foxp3$^+$ Tregs) [59]. Foxp3$^+$ Tregs play a critical role in oral tolerance [60]. In a subsequent study, Atarashi et al. isolated 17 strains within *Clostridia* clusters XIVa, IV and XVIII from a human fecal sample and demonstrated that these strains affect Tregs differentiation, accumulation and function in mouse colon [61].

Many bacterial metabolites are an important communication tools between the host immune system and commensal microbiota, establishing a broad basis for mutualism [62]. Among these, SCFAs are among the most abundant, and play a critical role in mucosal integrity, and local and systemic metabolic function, and stimulate regulatory immune responses [63–65]. *Clostridia* species belonging to cluster IV and XIVa are prominent source of SCFAs in the colon. SCFAs have been implicated in the regulation of both the proportions and functional capabilities of colonic Tregs [62], which, in some studies, has been specifically attributed to butyrate production by spore-forming *Clostridiales* [63]. Moreover, SCFAs can increase epithelial barrier functions, as measured by fluorescein isothiocyanate-dextran permeability assay, in a GPR43-dependent manner [25] or through the stabilization of hypoxia-inducible factor-alpha, particularly by butyrate [66]. Therefore, SCFAs can promote the barrier functions of the intestine, suggesting another protective role of butyrate against FA. In FA children compared to healthy subjects, different levels of fecal SCFAs, particularly butyrate, have been described [67–69]. As recently demonstrated, dysbiosis in *Faecalibacterium prausnitzii* is associated with AD, but it was shown that the presence of subspecies is more associated with AD than with the species overall [70]. Dysbiosis results in the suppression of high-butyrate-producer subspecies, leading to a reduction in overall butyrate production. Thus, different types of dysbiosis may share the same metabolic features leading to similar effects in term of SCFAs or of other metabolites levels that could facilitate the occurrence of FA. Interestingly, substantial correlations exist between the 16S rRNA profile, predicted metagenome, and metabolome of neonatal fecal samples, indicating a deterministic relationship between the bacterial community composition and metabolic microenvironment of the neonatal gut [29].It is also crucial that studies move beyond cataloguing of bacteria and toward functional characterization and mechanistic understanding. Metatranscriptomic studies will provide information regarding not only which bacteria and bacterial genes are present in a sample, but also the transcriptional activity of the community [71]. Metabolomics can reveal how bacterial metabolites facilitate interactions with the host and how they may influence the health state of the host [72,73]. Fine-level characterization of bacterial species can help reveal the function of the microbiome, which is affected by interactions among closely related bacteria that may compete for the same niche but have distinct activities. Together, these studies will provide a high-resolution picture of bacteria-host interactions that can lead to disease.Moreover, studies on germ-free mice may enable more precise determination of how microbial imbalances result in disease.

4. Modulation of the Gut Microbiota in FA

Primary prevention via microbiota-directed therapy is particularly appealing for potentially decreasing the incidence of FA. Children exposed to farm environments show a decreased risk for the development of allergic disease [74,75]. Although it has not been proven, a plausible explanation for the protective effect of early-life farm exposure is the role of microbiota, as individuals exposed to a farm environment exhibit a different microbial composition than those with other lifestyles [76]. Other epidemiologic factors protective against FA include having older siblings and pet exposure in early life [77]. Pet ownership is associated with a high microbial diversity in the home environment [78]. A recent study examining the influence of dietary patterns on the development of FA at the age of two years suggests that dietary habits influence FA development by changing the composition of the gut microbiota [43]. During infancy, breast milk provides various benefits to the new-born. Oligosaccharides, which are enriched in breast milk, favour the colonization of the SCFA-producing bacteria *Bifidobacterium* spp. [79]. Breast milk plays a critical role in the maturation of the gut microbiota by providing an initial source of commensal bacteria to the infant [80]. It has been recently demonstrated that higher levels of TGF-β2 in breast milk are associated with an increased relative abundance of several bacteria, including members of *Streptococcaceae* and *Ruminococcaceae*, and lower relative abundance of distinct *Staphylococcaceae* taxa [81]. One intervention that can modify the gut microbiota most significantly is diet, either by introducing new species or bacterial genes or by modulating the abundance of existing microbes in the community [82]. It has been demonstrated that an infant diet consisting of high levels of fruits, vegetables, and home-prepared foods was associated with fewer FA [43] (Figure 2). A high-fiber diet favours the outgrowth of bacteria capable of fermenting dietary fibers, such as *Bifidobacterium* and *Lactobacillus*, followed by an increase in serum SCFA levels. Neonatal prebiotic supplementation studies have failed to demonstrate any effect of prebiotics on the development of FA, but showed positive results for other allergic manifestations such as eczema [83].

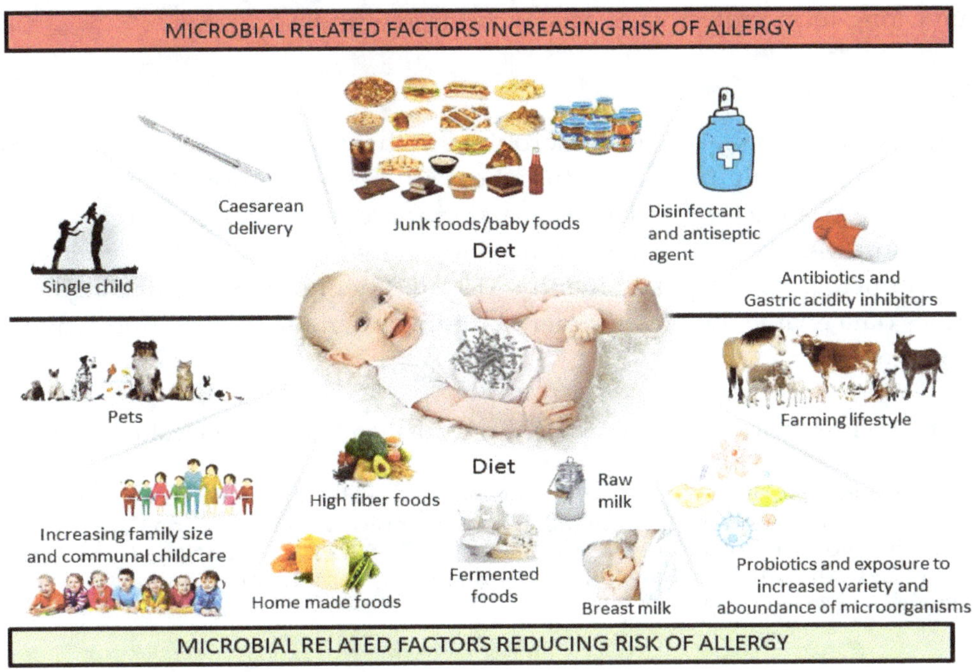

Figure 2. Environmental and lifestyle factors related to microbial exposure and their putative effect on the risk of developing food allergy.

Probiotics, defined as ingested microbes that provide health benefits to the host [84], may be beneficial by changing the microbiota. Recently published guidelines for atopic disease prevention from the World Allergy Organization concluded that there is a likely benefit to using probiotics in preventing eczema in children with a family history of allergic disease, but the evidence is very low in quality [85]. The most important factor in using probiotics against allergy is that this effect on the immune system is strain-specific. Thus, the results of studies for a selected bacterial strain cannot be adopted to other probiotic strains [84].Selected probiotics, such as *Lactobacillus rhamnosus* GG (LGG), were found to lower the risk of eczema when used by women during the last trimester of pregnancy, by breastfeeding mothers, or when given to infants [86].Studies examining the efficacy of currently available probiotics in treating FA have yielded conflicting results. It was recently demonstrated that oral immunotherapy supplemented with the probiotic *L. rhamnosus* CGMCC 1.3724 led to peanut unresponsiveness in 82% of allergic children [87]. In one randomized, double-blind, placebo-controlled study of infants with challenge-proven CMA, administration of *Lactobacillus casei* CRL431 and *Bifidobacterium lactis* Bb12 for 12 months did not affect the acquisition of tolerance to cow's milk [88]. In contrast, we demonstrated in different studies that an extensively hydrolyzed casein formula (EHCF) containing LGG accelerated the development of tolerance acquisition in infants with CMA and reduced the incidence of other allergic manifestations [89–91]. When we compared the fecal microbiota of infants receiving this tolerance-inducing probiotic-supplemented formula to that obtained from infants receiving EHCF alone, we found significant positive correlations between the abundance of butyrate-producing genera, and an increase concentration of fecal butyrate [68]. The mechanisms of action of butyrate are multiple, but many of these involve epigenetic regulation of gene expression by inhibiting histone deacetylase (HDAC). Inhibition of HDAC 9 and 6 increased FoxP3 gene expression, and the production and suppressive function of Tregs [92]. We demonstrated that the use of EHCF+LGG induces stronger epigenetic regulation of Th1 and Th2 cytokines genes as revealed by the significantly different levels of promoter region methylation [93]. Similar results were obtained by examining the FoxP3 Treg-specific demethylated region (TSDR) methylation profile. FoxP3 TSDR demethylation and expression were significantly higher in children treated with EHCF+LGG compared to in children treated with other dietary strategies [94]. These results strongly suggest that acting on gut microbiota composition and function can have long-term protective effects in children with FA.

5. Conclusions

Our understanding of the role of gut microbiota in the development of FA continues to evolve. Larger studies, preferably longitudinal birth cohort studies with more homogenous designs, are needed to clarify the presence or absence of a defined dysbiotic signature associated with FA. In addition, larger interventional trials are required to evaluate the roles of different probiotic strains in modulating gut microbiota composition and function. Integrating these findings with epigenetics and metabolomics data enable the development targeted microbiota with innovative approaches to prevent and manage FA.

Acknowledgments: This paper was supported in part by the Italian Ministry of Health Grant PE-2011-02348447.

Author Contributions: Rosita Aitoro, Margherita Di Costanzo and Roberto Berni Canani conceptualized the review and drafted the initial manuscript. Lorella Paparo, Antonio Amoroso, Linda Cosenza, Viviana Granata, Carmen Di Scala, Rita Nocerino, Mariangela Montella and Danilo Ercolini revised and approved the final manuscript as submitted. All authors approved the final manuscript as submitted and agree to be accountable for all aspects of the work.

References

1. Sicherer, S.H.; Sampson, H.A. Food allergy: Epidemiology, pathogenesis, diagnosis, and treatment. *J. Allergy Clin. Immunol.* **2014**, *133*, 291–307. [CrossRef] [PubMed]
2. Du Toit, G.; Tsakok, T. Prevention of food allergy. *J. Allergy Clin. Immunol.* **2016**, *137*, 998–1010. [CrossRef] [PubMed]
3. Gilbert, J.A.; Quinn, R.A. Microbiome-wide association studies link dynamic microbial consortia to disease. *Nature* **2016**, *535*, 94–103. [CrossRef] [PubMed]
4. Tsakok, T.; Marrs, T. Does atopic dermatitis cause food allergy? A systematic review. *J. Allergy Clin. Immunol.* **2016**, *137*, 1071–1078. [CrossRef] [PubMed]
5. Kim, K.S.; Hong, S.W. Dietary antigens limit mucosal immunity by inducing regulatory T cells in the small intestine. *Science* **2016**, *351*, 858–863. [CrossRef] [PubMed]
6. Du Toit, G.; Katz, Y. Early consumption of peanuts in infancy is associated with a low prevalence of peanut allergy. *J. Allergy Clin. Immunol.* **2008**, *122*, 984–991. [CrossRef] [PubMed]
7. Koplin, J.J.; Osborne, N.J. Can early introduction of egg prevent egg allergy in infants? A population-based study. *J. Allergy Clin. Immunol.* **2010**, *126*, 807–813. [CrossRef] [PubMed]
8. Katz, Y.; Rajuan, N. Early exposure to cow's milk protein is protective against IgE-mediated cow's milk protein allergy. *J. Allergy Clin. Immunol.* **2010**, *126*, 77–82. [CrossRef] [PubMed]
9. Du Toit, G.; Roberts, G. Randomized trial of peanut consumption in infants at risk for peanut allergy. *N. Engl. J. Med.* **2015**, *372*, 803–813. [CrossRef] [PubMed]
10. Du Toit, G.; Sayre, P.H.N. Effect of Avoidance on Peanut Allergy after Early Peanut Consumption. *N. Engl. J. Med.* **2016**, *374*, 1435–1443. [CrossRef] [PubMed]

11. Sekirov, I.; Russell, S.L. Gut microbiota in health and disease. *Physiol. Rev.* **2010**, *90*, 859–904. [CrossRef] [PubMed]
12. Tamburini, S.; Shen, N. The microbiome in early life: Implications for health outcomes. *Nat. Med.* **2016**, *22*, 713–722. [CrossRef] [PubMed]
13. Eberl, G. Immunity by equilibrium. *Nat. Rev. Immunol.* **2016**, *16*, 524–532. [CrossRef] [PubMed]
14. Pabst, O.; Mowat, A.M. Oral tolerance to food protein. *Mucosal Immunol.* **2012**, *5*, 232–239. [CrossRef] [PubMed]
15. Stefka, A.T.; Feehley, T. Commensal bacteria protect against food allergen sensitization. *Proc. Natl. Acad. Sci. USA* **2014**, *111*, 13145–13150. [CrossRef] [PubMed]
16. Maynard, C.L.; Elson, C.O. Reciprocal interactions of the intestinal microbiota and immune system. *Nature* **2012**, *489*, 231–241. [CrossRef] [PubMed]
17. Yatsunenko, T.; Rey, F.E. Human gut microbiome viewed across age and geography. *Nature* **2012**, *486*, 222–227. [CrossRef] [PubMed]
18. Tulic, M.K.; Hodder, M. Differences in innate immune function between allergic and non-allergic children: New insights into immune ontogeny. *J. Allergy Clin. Immunol.* **2011**, *127*, 470–478. [CrossRef] [PubMed]
19. Mazmanian, S.K.; Liu, C.H. An immunomodulatory molecule of symbiotic bacteria directs maturation of the host immune system. *Cell* **2005**, *122*, 107–118. [CrossRef] [PubMed]
20. Berni Canani, R.; Gilbert, J.A. The role of the commensal microbiota in the regulation of tolerance to dietary antigens. *Curr. Opin. Allergy Clin. Immunol.* **2015**, *15*, 243–249. [CrossRef] [PubMed]
21. Ohnmacht, C.; Park, J.-H. The microbiota regulates type 2 immunity through RORgt1 T cells. *Science* **2015**, *349*, 989–993. [CrossRef] [PubMed]
22. Wang, S.; Villablanca, E.J. MyD88-dependent TLR1/2 signals educate dendritic cells with gut-specific imprinting properties. *J. Immunol.* **2011**, *187*, 141–150. [CrossRef] [PubMed]
23. Latcham, F. A consistent pattern of minor immunodeficiency and subtle enteropathy in children with multiple food allergy. *J. Pediatr.* **2003**, *143*, 39–47. [CrossRef]
24. Suzuki, K.; Maruya, M. The sensing of environmental stimuli by follicular dendritic cells promotes immunoglobulin A generation in the gut. *Immunity* **2010**, *33*, 71–83. [CrossRef] [PubMed]
25. Tan, J.; McKenzie, C. Dietary Fiber and Bacterial SCFA Enhance Oral Tolerance and Protect against Food Allergy through Diverse Cellular Pathways. *Cell Rep.* **2016**, *15*, 2809–2824. [CrossRef] [PubMed]
26. Diesner, S.C.; Knittelfelder, R. Dose-dependent food allergy induction against ovalbumin under acid-suppression: A murine food allergy model. *Immunol. Lett.* **2008**, *121*, 45–51. [CrossRef] [PubMed]
27. Untersmayr, E.; Diesner, S.C. Nitration of the egg-allergen ovalbumin enhances protein allergenicity but reduces the risk for oral sensitization in a murine model of food allergy. *PLoS ONE* **2010**, *5*, e14210. [CrossRef] [PubMed]
28. Diesner, S.C.; Bergmayr, C. A distinct microbiota composition is associated with protection from food allergy in an oral mouse immunization model. *Clin. Immunol.* **2016**, *173*, 10–18. [CrossRef] [PubMed]
29. Fujimura, K.E.; Sitarik, A.R. Neonatal gut microbiota associates with childhood multisensitized atopy and T cell differentiation. *Nat. Med.* **2016**, *22*, 1187–1191. [CrossRef] [PubMed]
30. Olszak, T.; An, D. Microbial exposure during early life has persistent effects on natural killer T cell function. *Science* **2012**, *336*, 489–493. [CrossRef] [PubMed]
31. Huang, Y.J.; Marsland, B.J. The Microbiome in Allergic Disease: Current Understanding and Future Opportunities—2017 PRACTALL Document of the American Academy of Allergy, Asthma & Immunology and the European Academy of Allergy and Clinical Immunology. *J. Allergy Clin. Immunol.* **2017**, *139*, 1099–1110. [PubMed]
32. Wesemann, D.R.; Portuguese, A.J. Microbial colonization influences early B-lineage development in the gut lamina propria. *Nature* **2013**, *501*, 112–115. [CrossRef] [PubMed]
33. Rosser, E.C.; Mauri, C. Regulatory B cells: Origin, phenotype, and function. *Immunity* **2015**, *42*, 607–612. [CrossRef] [PubMed]
34. Van de Veen, W.; Stanic, B. IgG4 production is confined to human IL-10-producing regulatory B cells that suppress antigen-specific immune responses. *J. Allergy Clin. Immunol.* **2013**, *131*, 1204–1212. [CrossRef] [PubMed]
35. Liu, Z.Q.; Wu, Y.; Song, J.P. Tolerogenic CX3CR1+ B cells suppress food allergy-induced intestinal inflammation in mice. *Allergy* **2013**, *68*, 1241–1248. [CrossRef] [PubMed]

36. Amu, S.; Saunders, S.P. Regulatory B cells prevent and reverse allergic airway inflammation via FoxP3-positive T regulatory cells in a murine model. *J. Allergy Clin. Immunol.* **2010**, *125*, 1114–1124. [CrossRef] [PubMed]
37. Tait Wojno, E.D.; Artis, D. Emerging concepts and future challenges in innate lymphoid cell biology. *J. Exp. Med.* **2016**, *213*, 2229–2248. [CrossRef] [PubMed]
38. Eyerich, K.; Dimartino, V. IL-17 and IL-22 in immunity: Driving protection and pathology. *Eur. J. Immunol.* **2017**, *47*, 607–614. [CrossRef] [PubMed]
39. Plunkett, C.H.; Nagler, C.R. The Influence of the Microbiome on Allergic Sensitization to Food. *J. Immunol.* **2017**, *198*, 581–589. [CrossRef] [PubMed]
40. Papathoma, E.; Triga, M. Cesarean section delivery and development of food allergy and atopic dermatitis in early childhood. *Pediatr. Allergy Immunol.* **2016**, *27*, 419–424. [CrossRef] [PubMed]
41. Muraro, A.; Halken, S. EAACI food allergy and anaphylaxis guidelines. Primary prevention of food allergy. *Allergy* **2014**, *69*, 590–601. [CrossRef] [PubMed]
42. Anita Trikha, M.D.; Jacques, G. Baillargeon Development of food allergies in patients with Gastroesophageal Reflux Disease treated with gastric acid suppressive medications. *Pediatr Allergy Immunol.* **2013**, *24*, 582–588. [CrossRef] [PubMed]
43. Grimshaw, K.E.; Maskell, J. Diet and food allergy development during infancy: Birth cohort study findings using prospective food diary data. *J. Allergy Clin. Immunol.* **2014**, *133*, 511–519. [CrossRef] [PubMed]
44. Cox, L.M.; Yamanishi, S. Altering the intestinal microbiota during a critical developmental window has lasting metabolic consequences. *Cell* **2014**, *158*, 705–721. [CrossRef] [PubMed]
45. Metsälä, J.; Lundqvist, A. Mother's and offspring's use of antibiotics and infant allergy to cow's milk. *Epidemiology* **2013**, *24*, 303–309. [CrossRef] [PubMed]
46. Marrs, T.; Bruce, K.D. Is there an association between microbial exposure and food allergy? A systematic review. *Pediatr. Allergy Immunol.* **2013**, *24*, 311–320. [CrossRef] [PubMed]
47. Thompson-Chagoyan, O.C.; Vieites, J.M. Changes in faecal microbiota of infants with cow's milk protein allergy—a Spanish prospective case-control 6-month follow-up study. *Pediatr. Allergy Immunol.* **2010**, *21 Pt 2*, e394–e400. [CrossRef] [PubMed]
48. Adlerberth, I.; Strachan, D.P. Gut microbiota and development of atopic eczema in 3 European birth cohorts. *J. Allergy Clin. Immunol.* **2007**, *120*, 343–350. [CrossRef] [PubMed]
49. Kendler, M.; Uter, W. Comparison of fecal microflora in children with atopic eczema/dermatitis syndrome according to IgE sensitization to food. *Pediatr. Allergy Immunol.* **2006**, *17*, 141–147. [CrossRef] [PubMed]
50. Arrieta, M.C.; Stiemsma, L.T. Early infancy microbial and metabolic alterations affect risk of childhood asthma. *Sci. Transl. Med.* **2015**, *7*, 307ra152. [CrossRef] [PubMed]
51. Nakayama, J.; Kobayashi, T. Aberrant structures of fecal bacterial community in allergic infants profiled by 16S rRNA gene pyrosequencing. *FEMS Immunol. Med. Microbiol.* **2011**, *63*, 397–406. [CrossRef] [PubMed]
52. Duncan, S.H.; Louis, P. The role of pH in determining the species composition of the human colonic microbiota. *Environ. Microbiol.* **2009**, *11*, 2112–2122.
53. Azad, M.B.; Konya, T. Infant gut microbiota and food sensitization: Associations in the first year of life. *Clin. Exp. Allergy* **2015**, *45*, 623–643. [CrossRef] [PubMed]
54. Hua, X.; Goedert, J.J. Allergy associations with the adult fecal microbiota: Analysis of the American Gut Project. *EBioMedicine* **2015**, *3*, 172–179. [CrossRef] [PubMed]
55. Ling, Z.; Li, Z. Altered fecal microbiota composition associated with food allergy in infants. *Appl. Environ. Microbiol.* **2014**, *80*, 2546–2554. [CrossRef] [PubMed]
56. Chen, C.C.; Chen, K.J. Alterations in the gut microbiotas of children with food sensitization in early life. *Pediatr. Allergy Immunol.* **2016**, *27*, 254–262. [CrossRef] [PubMed]
57. Bunyavanich, S.; Shen, N. Early-life gut microbiome composition and milk allergy resolution. *J. Allergy Clin. Immunol.* **2016**, *138*, 1122–1130. [CrossRef] [PubMed]
58. Collins, M.D.; Lawson, P.A. The phylogeny of the genus Clostridium: Proposal of five new genera and eleven new species combinations. *Int. J. Syst. Bacteriol.* **1994**, *44*, 812–826. [CrossRef] [PubMed]
59. Atarashi, K.; Tanoue, T. Induction of colonic regulatory T cells by indigenous Clostridium species. *Science* **2011**, *331*, 337–341. [CrossRef] [PubMed]
60. Xie, X.; Stubbington, M.J. The Regulatory T Cell Lineage Factor Foxp3 Regulates Gene Expression through Several Distinct Mechanisms Mostly Independent of Direct DNA Binding. *PLoS Genet.* **2015**, *11*, e1005251. [CrossRef] [PubMed]

61. Atarashi, K.; Tanoue, T. Treg induction by a rationally selected mixture of Clostridia strains from the human microbiota. *Nature* **2013**, *500*, 232–236. [CrossRef] [PubMed]
62. Arpaia, N.; Campbell, C. Metabolites produced by commensal bacteria promote peripheral regulatory T cell generation. *Nature* **2013**, *504*, 451–455. [CrossRef] [PubMed]
63. Furusawa, Y.; Obata, Y. Commensal microbe-derived butyrate induces differentiation of colonic regulatory T cells. *Nature* **2013**, *504*, 446–450. [CrossRef] [PubMed]
64. Smith, P.M.; Howitt, M.R. The microbial metabolites, short-chain fatty acids, regulate colonic Treg cell homeostasis. *Science* **2013**, *341*, 569–573. [CrossRef] [PubMed]
65. Maslowski, K.M.; Mackay, C.R. Diet, gut microbiota and immune responses. *Nat. Immunol.* **2011**, *12*, 5–9. [CrossRef] [PubMed]
66. Kelly, C.J.; Zheng, L. Crosstalk between Microbiota-Derived Short-Chain Fatty Acids and Intestinal Epithelial HIF Augments Tissue Barrier Function. *Cell Host Microbe* **2015**, *17*, 662–671. [CrossRef] [PubMed]
67. Sandin, A.; Bråbäck, L. Faecal short chain fatty acid pattern and allergy in early childhood. *Acta Paediatr.* **2009**, *98*, 823–827. [CrossRef] [PubMed]
68. Berni Canani, R.; Sangwan, N. Lactobacillus rhamnosus GG supplemented formula expands butyrate producing bacterial strains in food allergic infants. *ISME J.* **2016**, *10*, 742–750. [CrossRef] [PubMed]
69. Geuking, M.B.; McCoy, K.D. Metabolites from intestinal microbes shape Treg. *Cell Res* **2013**, *23*, 1339–1340. [CrossRef] [PubMed]
70. Song, H.; Yoo, Y. Faecalibacterium prausnitzii subspecies-level dysbiosis in the human gut microbiome underlying atopic dermatitis. *J. Allergy Clin. Immunol.* **2015**, *137*, 852–860. [CrossRef] [PubMed]
71. Franzosa, E.A. Relating the metatranscriptome and metagenome of the human gut. *Proc. Natl. Acad. Sci. USA* **2014**, *111*, e2329–e2338. [CrossRef] [PubMed]
72. Sellitto, M. Proof of concept of microbiome–metabolome analysis and delayed gluten exposure on celiac disease autoimmunity in genetically at-risk infants. *PLoS ONE* **2012**, *7*, e33387. [CrossRef] [PubMed]
73. Stewart, C.J. Preterm gut microbiota and metabolome following discharge from intensive care. *Sci. Rep.* **2015**, *5*, 17141. [CrossRef] [PubMed]
74. Riedler, J.; Braun-Fahrländer, C. Exposure to farming in early life and development of asthma and allergy: A cross-sectional survey. *Lancet* **2001**, *358*, 1129–1133. [CrossRef]
75. Schuijs, M.J.; Willart, M.A. Farm dust and endotoxin protect against allergy through A20 induction in lung epithelial cells. *Science* **2015**, *349*, 1106–1110. [CrossRef] [PubMed]
76. Dicksved, J.; Flöistrup, H. Molecular fingerprinting of the fecal microbiota of children raised according to different lifestyles. *Appl. Environ. Microbiol.* **2007**, *73*, 2284–2289. [CrossRef] [PubMed]
77. Peters, R.L.; Allen, K.J. Differential factors associated with challenge-proven food allergy phenotypes in a population cohort of infants: A latent class analysis. *Clin. Exp. Allergy* **2015**, *45*, 953–963. [CrossRef] [PubMed]
78. Fujimura, K.E.; Johnson, C.C. Man's best friend? The effect of pet ownership on house dust microbial communities. *J. Allergy Clin. Immunol.* **2010**, *126*, 410–412. [CrossRef] [PubMed]
79. Turroni, F.; Peano, C. Diversity of bifidobacteria within the infant gut microbiota. *PLoS ONE* **2012**, *7*, e36957. [CrossRef] [PubMed]
80. Harmsen, H.J.; Wildeboer-Veloo, A.C. Analysis of intestinal flora development in breast-fed and formula-fed infants by using molecular identification and detection methods. *J. Pediatr. Gastroenterol. Nutr.* **2000**, *30*, 61–67. [CrossRef] [PubMed]
81. Sitarik, A.R.; Bobbitt, K.R. Breast Milk TGF [beta] is Associated with Neonatal Gut Microbial Composition. *J. Pediatr. Gastroenterol. Nutr.* **2017**. [CrossRef] [PubMed]
82. Wu, G.D.; Chen, J. Linking long-term dietary patterns with gut microbial enterotypes. *Science* **2011**, *334*, 105–108. [CrossRef] [PubMed]
83. Osborn, D.A.; Sinn, J.K. Probiotics in infants for prevention of allergic disease and food hypersensitivity. *Cochrane Database Syst. Rev.* **2007**, CD006475.
84. Hill, C.; Guarner, F. Expert consensus document. The International Scientific Association for Probiotics and Prebiotics consensus statement on the scope and appropriate use of the term probiotic. *Nat. Rev. Gastroenterol. Hepatol.* **2014**, *11*, 506–514. [CrossRef] [PubMed]
85. Fiocchi, A.; Pawankar, R. World Allergy Organization-McMaster University Guidelines for Allergic Disease Prevention [GLAD-P]: Probiotics. *WAO J.* **2015** *8*, 4. [CrossRef] [PubMed]

86. Elazab, N.; Mendy, A. Probiotic administration in early life, atopy, and asthma: A meta-analysis of clinical trials. *Pediatrics* **2013**, *132*, e666–e676. [CrossRef] [PubMed]
87. Tang, M.L.; Ponsonby, A.L. Administration of a probiotic with peanut oral immunotherapy: A randomized trial. *J. Allergy Clin. Immunol.* **2015**, *135*, 737–744. [CrossRef] [PubMed]
88. Hol, J.; van Leer, E.H. The acquisition of tolerance toward cow's milk through probiotic supplementation: A randomized, controlled trial. *J. Allergy Clin. Immunol.* **2008**, *121*, 1448–1454. [CrossRef] [PubMed]
89. Berni Canani, R.; Nocerino, R. Effect of Lactobacillus GG on tolerance acquisition in infants with cow's milk allergy: A randomized trial. *J. Allergy Clin. Immunol.* **2012**, *129*, 580–582. [CrossRef] [PubMed]
90. Berni Canani, R.; Nocerino, R. Formula selection for management of children with cow's milk allergy influences the rate of acquisition of tolerance: A prospective multicenter study. *J. Pediatr.* **2013**, *163*, 771–777. [CrossRef] [PubMed]
91. Berni Canani, R.; Di Costanzo, M. Extensively hydrolyzed casein formula containing Lactobacillus rhamnosus GG reduces the occurrence of other allergic manifestations in children with cow's milk allergy: 3-year randomized controlled trial. *J. Allergy Clin. Immunol.* **2017**, *139*, 1906–1913. [CrossRef] [PubMed]
92. Tao, R.; de Zoeten, E.F. Deacetylase inhibition promotes the generation and function of regulatory T cells. *Nat. Med.* **2007**, *13*, 1299–1307. [CrossRef] [PubMed]
93. Berni Canani, R.; Paparo, L. Differences in DNA methylation profile of Th1 and Th2 cytokine genes are associated with tolerance acquisition in children with IgE-mediated cow's milk allergy. *Clin. Epigenetics* **2015**, *31*, 7–38. [CrossRef] [PubMed]
94. Paparo, L.; Nocerino, R. Epigenetic features of FoxP3 in children with cow's milk allergy. *Clin. Epigenetics* **2016**, *12*, 8–86. [CrossRef] [PubMed]

Permissions

All chapters in this book were first published by MDPI; hereby published with permission under the Creative Commons Attribution License or equivalent. Every chapter published in this book has been scrutinized by our experts. Their significance has been extensively debated. The topics covered herein carry significant findings which will fuel the growth of the discipline. They may even be implemented as practical applications or may be referred to as a beginning point for another development.

The contributors of this book come from diverse backgrounds, making this book a truly international effort. This book will bring forth new frontiers with its revolutionizing research information and detailed analysis of the nascent developments around the world.

We would like to thank all the contributing authors for lending their expertise to make the book truly unique. They have played a crucial role in the development of this book. Without their invaluable contributions this book wouldn't have been possible. They have made vital efforts to compile up to date information on the varied aspects of this subject to make this book a valuable addition to the collection of many professionals and students.

This book was conceptualized with the vision of imparting up-to-date information and advanced data in this field. To ensure the same, a matchless editorial board was set up. Every individual on the board went through rigorous rounds of assessment to prove their worth. After which they invested a large part of their time researching and compiling the most relevant data for our readers.

The editorial board has been involved in producing this book since its inception. They have spent rigorous hours researching and exploring the diverse topics which have resulted in the successful publishing of this book. They have passed on their knowledge of decades through this book. To expedite this challenging task, the publisher supported the team at every step. A small team of assistant editors was also appointed to further simplify the editing procedure and attain best results for the readers.

Apart from the editorial board, the designing team has also invested a significant amount of their time in understanding the subject and creating the most relevant covers. They scrutinized every image to scout for the most suitable representation of the subject and create an appropriate cover for the book.

The publishing team has been an ardent support to the editorial, designing and production team. Their endless efforts to recruit the best for this project, has resulted in the accomplishment of this book. They are a veteran in the field of academics and their pool of knowledge is as vast as their experience in printing. Their expertise and guidance has proved useful at every step. Their uncompromising quality standards have made this book an exceptional effort. Their encouragement from time to time has been an inspiration for everyone.

The publisher and the editorial board hope that this book will prove to be a valuable piece of knowledge for researchers, students, practitioners and scholars across the globe.

List of Contributors

Lieve van Brakel, Ronald P. Mensink and Jogchum Plat
Department of Nutrition and Movement Sciences, NUTRIM (School of Translational Research in Metabolism), Maastricht University Medical Center, 6200 MD Maastricht, The Netherlands

Geertjan Wesseling
Department of Respiratory Medicine, Maastricht University Medical Center, 6200 MD Maastricht, The Netherlands

Eliza Wasilewska and Ewa Jassem
Department of Pulmonology and Allergology, Medical University of Gdansk, Debinki str 7, 90-211 Gdańsk, Poland

Sylwia Małgorzewicz and Marta Gruchała-Niedoszytko
Department of Clinical Nutrition, Medical University of Gdansk, Debinki str 7, 90-211 Gdańsk, Poland

Magdalena Skotnicka
Department of Food Commodity Science, Medical University of Gdansk, Debinki str 7, 90-211 Gdańsk, Poland

Naser A. Alsharairi
Heart, Mind & Body Research Group, Menzies Health Institute Queensland, Grith University, Gold Coast 4215, Australia

Daniel Munblit
Department of Paediatrics, Imperial College London, London W2 1NY, UK
Faculty of Pediatrics, Federal State Autonomous Educational Institution of Higher Education I.M. Sechenov First Moscow State Medical University of the Ministry of Health of the Russian Federation., Moscow 119991, Russia
International Inflammation (in-FLAME) network of the World Universities Network, Perth 6000, WA, Australia
The In-FLAME Global Network, an Affiliate of the World Universities Network (WUN), West New York, NJ 07093, USA

Diego G. Peroni
International Inflammation (in-FLAME) network of the World Universities Network, Perth 6000, WA, Australia
Department of Clinical and Experimental Medicine, Section of Paediatrics, University of Pisa, Pisa 56126, Italy
Department of Paediatrics, Imperial College London, London W2 1NY, UK

Alba Boix-Amorós and Maria Carmen Collado
Department of Paediatrics, Imperial College London, London W2 1NY, UK
Institute of Agrochemistry and Food Technology, National Research Council (IATA-CSIC), 46980 Valencia, Spain

Peter S. Hsu
Department of Paediatrics, Imperial College London, London W2 1NY, UK
Allergy and Immunology, The Kids Research Institute, The Children's Hospital at Westmead, Sydney, NSW 2145, Australia

Melvin C. L. Gay
Department of Paediatrics, Imperial College London, London W2 1NY, UK
School of Molecular Sciences, The University of Western Australia, Perth, WA 6009, Australia

Anastasia Kolotilina
Faculty of Pediatrics, I.M. Sechenov First Moscow State Medical University, 119991 Moscow, Russia

Chrysanthi Skevaki
Department of Paediatrics, Imperial College London, London W2 1NY, UK
Institute of Laboratory Medicine and Pathobiochemistry, Molecular Diagnostics, Philipps University Marburg, University Hospital Giessen and Marburg GmbH Baldingerstr, 35043 Marburg, Germany

Attilio L. Boner
Department of Life and Reproduction Sciences, Section of Paediatrics, University of Verona, Verona 37124 Italy

Robert J. Boyle
The In-FLAME Global Network, an Affiliate of the World Universities Network (WUN), West New York, NJ 07093, USA
Department of Paediatrics, Imperial College London, London W2 1NY, UK

Ralph Nanan
Charles Perkins Centre Nepean, University of Sydney, Sydney, NSW 2747, Australia

Carolyn Slupsky
Department of Nutrition, University of California, Davis, CA 95616-5270, USA

Belinda van't Land
Department of Paediatric Immunology, University Medical Center Utrecht/Wilhelmina Children's Hospital, 3584 EA Utrecht, The Netherlands
Nutricia Research, 3584 CT Utrecht, The Netherlands

Johan Garssen
Nutricia Research, 3584 CT Utrecht, The Netherlands
Utrecht Institute for Pharmaceutical Sciences, Faculty of Science, Utrecht University, 3584 CG Utrecht, The Netherlands

Donna T. Geddes
International Inflammation (in-FLAME) network of the World Universities Network, Perth 6000, WA, Australia School of Molecular Sciences, The University of Western Australia, Perth, WA 6009, Australia
Department of Paediatrics, Imperial College London, London W2 1NY, UK

Ganesa Wegienka
Department of Paediatrics, Imperial College London, London W2 1NY, UK
Department of Public Health Sciences, Henry Ford Health System, Detroit, MI 48202, USA
Center for Urban Responses to Environmental Stressors, Detroit, MI 48202, USA

Anita L. Kozyrskyj
Department of Pediatrics, University of Alberta, Edmonton, AB T6G 1C9, Canada

John O. Warner
Department of Paediatrics, Imperial College London, London W2 1NY, UK
International Inflammation (in-FLAME) network of the World Universities Network, Perth 6000, WA, Australia

Yvan Vandenplas
Kidz Health Castle, UZ Brussel, Vrije UniversiteitBrussel, Laarbeeklaan 101, 1090 Brussels, Belgium

Tomasz P. Wypych and Benjamin J. Marsland
Faculty of Biology and Medicine, University of Lausanne, Service de Pneumologie, CHUV, Epalinges 1066, Switzerland

Tabea Brick and Andreas Böck
Dr. von Hauner Children's Hospital, Ludwig Maximilians University Munich, Lindwurm Str. 4, 80337 Munich, Germany
Comprehensive Pneumology Centre Munich (CPC-M), Member of the German Center of Lung Research (DZL), 80337 Munich, Germany

Erika von Mutius
Dr. von Hauner Children's Hospital, Ludwig Maximilians University Munich, Lindwurm Str. 4, 80337 Munich, Germany
Comprehensive Pneumology Centre Munich (CPC-M), Member of the German Center of Lung Research (DZL), 80337 Munich, Germany
Helmholtz Zentrum München—German Research Center for Environmental Health, Institute for Asthma and Allergy Prevention, Ingolstädter Landstr. 1, 85764 Neuherberg, Germany

Markus Ege
Dr. von Hauner Children's Hospital, Ludwig Maximilians University Munich, Lindwurm Str. 4, 80337 Munich, Germany

Kasper Hettinga
Dairy Science and Technology, Food Quality and Design Group, Wageningen University, 6708 PB Wageningen, The Netherlands

Sjef Boeren and Jacques Vervoort
Laboratory of Biochemistry, Wageningen University, 6708 WE Wageningen, The Netherlands

Marina Treneva and Alexander Pampura
International Inflammation (in-FLAME) network of the World Universities Network, Perth 6000, WA, Australia
Allergy Department, Veltischev Clinical Pediatric Research Institute of Pirogov Russian National Research Medical University, Moscow 125412, Russia

Silvia Colicino
National Heart and Lung Institute, Imperial College London, London SW3 6NP, UK

Li Yan Chow
Department of Paediatrics, Imperial College London, London W2 1NY, UK

Shobana Dissanayeke
Royal Holloway University of London School of Biological Sciences, Biomedical Sciences, London TW20 0EX, UK

Attilio L. Boner
Department of Life and Reproduction Sciences, Section of Paediatrics, University of Verona, Verona 37124 Italy

Malgorzata Teodorowicz and Huub Savelkoul
Cell Biology and Immunology Group, Wageningen University & Research, 6708 WD Wageningen, The Netherlands
Allergy Consortium Wageningen, Wageningen University & Research, 6708 WD Wageningen, The Netherlands

Joost van Neerven
Cell Biology and Immunology Group, Wageningen University & Research, 6708 WD Wageningen, The Netherlands
Friesland Campina, 3818 LE Amersfoort, The Netherlands

Lies Hulshof
Department of Paediatric Respiratory Medicine and Allergy, Emma Children's Hospital Academic Medical Center, 1105 AZ Amsterdam, The Netherlands

Belinda van't Land
Department of Paediatric Immunology, University Medical Center Utrecht/Wilhelmina Children's Hospital, 3584 EA Utrecht, The Netherlands
Nutricia Research, 3584 CT Utrecht, The Netherlands

Aline B. Sprikkelman
Department of Paediatric Pulmonology and Paediatric Allergology, University Medical Center Groningen, 9713 GZ Groningen, The Netherlands

Johan Garssen
Nutricia Research, 3584 CT Utrecht, The Netherlands
Utrecht Institute for Pharmaceutical Sciences, Faculty of Science, Utrecht University, 3584 CG Utrecht, The Netherlands

Alessandra Mazzocchi and Carlo Agostoni
Pediatric Intermediate Care Unit, Fondazione IRCCS Ospedale Ca' Granda-Ospedale Maggiore Policlinico, Department of Clinical Sciences and Community Health, University of Milan, 20122 Milan, Italy

Carina Venter
Section of Allergy and Immunology, Children's Hospital Colorado, University of Colorado, Aurora, CO 80045, USA

Kate Maslin
MRC Lifecourse Epidemiology Unit, University of Southampton, Southampton SO16 6YD, UK

Elizabeth A. Miles
Human Development and Health Academic Unit, Faculty of Medicine, University of Southampton, Southampton SO16 6YD, UK

Philip C. Calder
Human Development and Health Academic Unit, Faculty of Medicine, University of Southampton, Southampton SO16 6YD, UK
NIHR Southampton Biomeducal Research Centre, University Hospital Southampton NHS Foundation Trust and University of Southampton, Southampton SO16 6YD, UK

Catrina L. McStay
Department of Health Western Australia, Perth 6004, Western Australia, Australia

Susan L. Prescott and Debra J. Palmer
School of Paediatrics and Child Health, The University of Western Australia, Subiaco 6008, Western Australia, Australia
Telethon Kids Institute, The University of Western Australia, Subiaco 6008, Western Australia, Australia
Members of the in-FLAME International Inflammation Network, Perth 6000, Western Australia, Australia

Carol Bower
Telethon Kids Institute, The University of Western Australia, Subiaco 6008, Western Australia, Australia

Rosita Aitoro, Lorella Paparo, Antonio Amoroso, Margherita Di Costanzo, Linda Cosenza, Viviana Granata, Carmen Di Scala, Rita Nocerino, Giovanna Trinchese and Mariangela Montella
Department of Translational Medical Science-Pediatric Section, University of Naples "Federico II", 80131 Naples, Italy

Danilo Ercolini
Department of Agricultural Sciences, Division of Microbiology, University of Naples "Federico II", 80055 Portici, Italy
Task Force on Microbiome Studies, University of Naples "Federico II", 80131 Naples, Italy

Roberto Berni Canani
Department of Translational Medical Science-Pediatric Section, University of Naples "Federico II", 80131 Naples, Italy

Index

www.ingramcontent.com/pod-product-compliance
Lightning Source LLC
LaVergne TN
LVHW060512210926
848485LV00005B/1069